OCCUPATIONAL MEDICINE SECRETS

OCCUPATIONAL MEDICINE SECRETS

ROSEMARIE M. BOWLER, PH.D., M.P.H.
Professor, Department of Psychology
San Francisco State University
San Francisco, California

JAMES E. CONE, M.D., M.P.H.
Chief, Occupational Health Branch
California Department of Health Services
Oakland, California
Assistant Clinical Professor
Department of Medicine
University of California
San Francisco, School of Medicine

HANLEY & BELFUS, INC./ Philadelphia

Publisher: HANLEY & BELFUS, INC.
                  Medical Publishers
                  210 South 13th Street
                  Philadelphia, PA 19107
                  (215) 546-7293; 800-962-1892
                  FAX (215) 790-9330
                  Web site: http://www.hanleyandbelfus.com

Note to the reader: Although the information in this book has been carefully reviewed for correctness of dosage and indications, neither the authors nor the editors nor the publisher can accept any legal responsibility for any errors or omissions that may be made. Neither the publisher nor the editors make any warranty, expressed or implied, with respect to the material contained herein. Before prescribing any drug, the reader must review the manufacturer's current product information (package inserts) for accepted indications, absolute dosage recommendations, and other information pertinent to the safe and effective use of the product described.

Library of Congress Cataloging-in-Publication Data

    Occupational medicine secrets / edited by Rosemarie M. Bowler, James E.
    Cone.
        p.   cm. — (The Secrets Series)
      Includes bibliographical references and index.
      ISBN 1-56053-161-4 (alk. paper)
      1. Medicine, Industrial— Miscellanea.   I. Bowler, Rosemarie M.,
    1942–   II. Cone, James.   III. Series.
      [DNLM: 1. Occupational Diseases—prevention & control Examination
    Questions.   2. Occupational Medicine—methods Examination Questions.
    3. Hazardous Substances—adverse effects Examination Questions.
    WA 18.2 O15 1999]
    RC 963.3.O25   1999
    616.9'803—dc21
    DNLM/DLC
    for Library of Congress   99-19893
                                                                       CIP

OCCUPATIONAL MEDICINE SECRETS   ISBN 1-56053-161-4

Last digit is the print number: 9   8   7   6   5   4   3   2   1

CONTENTS

III. SPECIAL GROUPS AT RISK

IV. DISEASES

CONTRIBUTORS

Wasif Muhammad Alam, M.D., M.S.P.H.
Resident, Environmental and Occupational Medicine, University of South Florida, Tampa, Florida

Carol M. Baldwin, R.N., Ph.D.
Research Assistant Professor, Department of Medicine; Research Professor, Department of Psychology; Research Scientist, Respiratory Sciences Center, University of Arizona, Tucson; Research Scientist, Department of Psychiatry, Tucson Veterans Affairs Medical Center, Tucson, Arizona

John R. Balmes, M.D.
Chief, Division of Occupational and Environmental Medicine, San Francisco General Hospital; Professor, Department of Medicine, University of California, San Francisco, School of Medicine, San Francisco, California

William S. Beckett, M.D., M.P.H.
Professor of Environmental Medicine and Medicine, Occupational Medicine Division, University of Rochester School of Medicine and Dentistry, Rochester, New York

Iris R. Bell, M.D., Ph.D.
Associate Professor of Psychiatry, Psychology, and Family & Community Medicine, Department of Psychiatry, University of Arizona, Tucson; Director, Geriatric Psychiatry Program, Tucson Veterans Affairs Medical Center, Tucson, Arizona

Neal L. Benowitz, M.D.
Professor, Department of Medicine, University of California, San Francisco, School of Medicine, and San Francisco General Hospital Medical Center, San Francisco, California

Richard B. Berry, M.D.
Associate Professor of Medicine, Department of Medicine, University of California, Irvine; Director of the Sleep Laboratory, Long Beach, California

Margit L. Bleecker, M.D., Ph.D.
Director, Center for Occupational and Environmental Neurology, Baltimore, Maryland

Rosemarie M. Bowler, Ph.D., M.P.H.
Professor, Department of Psychology, San Francisco State University, San Francisco; Private Practice, Neuropsychological Assessment and Research, San Francisco, California

Russell P. Bowler, M.D.
Fellow, Pulmonary and Critical Care Medicine, Department of Pulmonary and Critical Care, University of Colorado Health Sciences Center, Denver, Colorado

Stuart M. Brooks, M.D.
Professor and Chairman, Department of Environmental and Occupational Health, and Professor of Medicine, Department of Internal Medicine, Divisions of Pulmonary, Critical Care, Occupational Medicine, Allergy and Clinical Immunology, University of South Florida College of Medicine, Tampa, Florida

Thomas C. Bruff, M.D., M.P.H.
Clinical Fellow, Department of Environmental Health Sciences, School of Hygiene and Public Health, Johns Hopkins University, and Johns Hopkins Hospital, Baltimore, Maryland

Judith A. Calder, M.S., R.N.
Child Day Care Health Consultant, Berkeley, California

Thomas J. Callender, M.D.
Medical Director, Environmental and Occupational Toxicology, Internal Medicine, Our Lady of Lourdes Hospital, Lafayette, Louisiana

Martin Cherniack, M.D., M.P.H.
Medical Director, Ergonomics Technology of Connecticut, University of Connecticut Health Center, Farmington, Connecticut

James E. Cone, M.D., M.P.H.
Chief, Occupational Health Branch, California Department of Health Services, Oakland; Assistant Clinical Professor, Department of Medicine, University of California, San Francisco, School of Medicine, San Francisco, California

Feroza Daroowalla, M.D., M.P.H.
Medical Officer, Division of Respiratory Disease Studies, National Institute for Occupational Safety and Health, Centers for Disease Control and Prevention, Morgantown, West Virginia

Stephen L. Demeter, M.D., M.P.H.
Professor and Head, Pulmonary Medicine and Critical Care Medicine, Northeastern Ohio Universities College of Medicine, Rootstown; Head of Preventive Medicine, Akron General Medical Center, Akron, Ohio

Jonathan Dropkin, M.S., P.T.
Ergonomics Coordinator, Mount Sinai School of Medicine, Mount Sinai Medical Center, New York, New York

Bradley Evanoff, M.D., M.P.H.
Assistant Professor of Medicine, Department of Medicine, Washington University School of Medicine, St. Louis, Missouri

R. William Field, Ph.D.
Associate Research Scientist, Division of Epidemiology, and Adjunct Professor, Division of Occupational and Environmental Health, Department of Preventive Medicine, University of Iowa, Iowa City, Iowa

David R. Franz, D.V.M., Ph.D.
Vice President, Chemical and Biological Defense Division, Southern Research Institute, Frederick, Maryland

Sharmeen S. Gettner, M.S., Ph.D.
Epidemiologist, CMRI, San Francisco, California

Mark Goldberg, Ph.D., C.I.H.
Assistant Professor, Urban Public Health Program, Environmental and Occupational Health, Hunter College–City University of New York, New York, New York

E. Brigitte Gottschall, M.D.
Instructor Fellow, Division of Environmental and Occupational Health and Safety, National Jewish Medical and Research Center, Denver, Colorado

Rene Gratz, Ph.D.
Associate Professor of Health Sciences, Department of Health Sciences, University of Wisconsin–Milwaukee, Milwaukee, Wisconsin

Michael R. Grey, M.D., M.P.H.
Associate Professor of Clinical Medicine, Department of Medicine, University of Connecticut School of Medicine, Farmington, Connecticut

Robert Harrison, M.D., M.P.H.
Associate Clinical Professor, Division of Occupational and Environmental Medicine, University of California, San Francisco, San Francisco, California

Robin Herbert, M.D.
Assistant Professor, Department of Community and Preventive Medicine, Mount Sinai School of Medicine, New York, New York

Karen L. Hipkins, R.N., N.P.-C., M.P.H.
Nurse Practitioner, Occupational Lead Poisoning Prevention Program, Public Health Institute, Berkeley, California

Franklin T. Hoagland, M.D.
Professor Emeritus, Department of Orthopaedic Surgery, University of California, San Francisco, School of Medicine, San Francisco, California

Perrine Hoet, M.D., M.I.H., M.Sc.
Assistant Professor, Industrial Toxicology and Occupational Medicine Unit, Catholic University of Louvain, Faculty of Medicine, and Cliniques Universitaires Saint Luc, Brussels, Belgium

Ronald A. House, M.D., M.Sc., FRCPC
Assistant Professor, Department of Public Health Sciences, University of Toronto, Ontario, Canada

Hilton Kenneth Hudnell, Ph.D.
Neurotoxicologist, Neurotoxicology Division, National Health and Environmental Effects Research Laboratory, U.S. Environmental Protection Agency, Research Triangle Park, North Carolina

William G. Hughson, M.D., D.Phil.
Clinical Professor of Medicine, and Director, University of California, San Diego Center for Occupational and Environmental Medicine, University of California, San Diego, California

Eckardt Johanning, M.D., M.Sc.
Medical Director, Eastern New York Occupational and Environmental Health Center, Mount Sinai School of Medicine, Albany, New York

Elizabeth A. Katz, M.P.H., C.I.H.
Acting Chief, Hazard Evaluation System and Information Service. California Department of Health Services, Oakland, California

Robert L. Keith, M.D.
Senior Fellow, Division of Pulmonary Sciences and Critical Care Medicine, Department of Medicine, University of Colorado Health Sciences Center, Denver, Colorado

Gordon K. Klintworth, M.D., Ph.D.
Professor of Pathology and Joseph A.C. Wadsworth Research Professor of Ophthalmology, Department of Pathology and Ophthalmology, Duke University Medical Center, Durham, North Carolina

Ellen Kolber, M.S., M.A., O.T.C., C.H.T., C.I.E.
Principal, Diversified Ergonomics, New York, New York

Michael J. Kosnett, M.D., M.P.H.
Assistant Professor, Division of Clinical Pharmacology and Toxicology, Department of Medicine, University of Colorado Health Sciences Center, Denver, Colorado

Kathleen Kreiss, M.D.
Field Studies Branch Chief, Division of Respiratory Disease Studies, National Institute for Occupational Safety and Health, Morgantown, West Virginia

Ware G. Kuschner, M.D.
Assistant Professor of Medicine, Division of Pulmonary and Critical Care Medicine, Stanford University School of Medicine, Palo Alto, California

Marc Alan Lappé, Ph.D.
Director, Center for Ethics and Toxics (CETOS), Gualala, California

Elaine A. Lisko, J.D.
Research Professor, Health, Law, and Policy Institute, University of Houston Law Center, Houston, Texas

Gary M. Liss, M.D., M.S., FRCPC
Medical Consultant, Ontario Ministry of Labour, and Assistant Professor, Department of Public Health Sciences, University of Toronto, Ontario, Canada

Robert D. Madory, M.A.
Clinical Audiologist and Director of Professional Services, Department of Audiology, San Francisco Hearing and Speech Center, San Francisco, California

Donna Mergler, Ph.D.
Director, CINBOISE, and WHO-PAHO Collaborating Center in Occupational and Environmental Health, Université du Montréal Faculty of Medicine, Quebec, Canada

Gyl Midroni, M.D., FRCP(C)
Director, Department of Neurophysiology, and Assistant Professor, Department of Neurology, University of Toronto, Ontario, Canada

John E. Midtling, M.D., M.S.
Professor and Head, Department of Family and Community Medicine; Associate Dean, University of Illinois College of Medicine at Rockford, Rockford, Illinois

Deborah Nagin, M.P.H.
Director, Public Health Partnership and Environmental Health, New York State Department of Health (NYSDOH)–Metropolitan Region, New York, New York

Peter Orris, M.D., M.P.H.
Professor of Preventive and Internal Medicine, Rush Medical College, Chicago; Attending Physician, Cook County Hospital, Chicago, Illinois

Ana Maria Osorio, M.D., M.P.H.
Assistant Clinical Professor, Department of Occupational and Environmental Medicine, University of California, San Francisco, School of Medicine, San Francisco, California

Eric J. Poulsen, M.D.
Resident, Department of Ophthalmology, Duke University Medical Center, Durham, North Carolina

Cecile S. Rose, M.D., M.P.H.
Associate Professor of Medicine, Department of Occupational and Pulmonary Medicine, National Jewish Medical and Research Center, and University of Colorado Health Sciences Center, Denver, Colorado

Mary A. Ross, Ph.D.
Health Scientist, Office of Air Quality Planning and Standards, U.S. Environmental Protection Agency, Research Triangle Park, North Carolina

Jonathan S. Rutchik, M.D., M.P.H.
Medical Director, Division of Occupational and Environmental Neurology, Occupational Health and Rehabilitation, Inc., Boston, Massachusetts

Cornelius H. Scannell, M.D., M.P.H.
Assistant Professor, Department of Medicine, University of California, San Francisco, School of Medicine, San Francisco, California

Brian S. Schwartz, M.D., M.S.
Associate Professor and Director, Division of Occupational and Environmental Health, Johns Hopkins School of Hygiene and Public Health, Baltimore, Maryland

Neil W. Schluger, M.D.
Associate Professor of Medicine and Public Health, Division of Pulmonary, Allergy, and Critical Care Medicine, and Chief, Clinical Pulmonary Medicine, Columbia University, College of Physicians and Surgeons, New York, New York

Miriam Shipp, M.D., M.P.H.
Physician, University Health Services, University of California, Berkeley; Health Care Consultant, California Childcare Health Program, Oakland, California

Lynda Sisson, M.D., M.P.H.
Assistant Professor, Department of Medicine, University of California, San Francisco, School of Medicine, San Francisco, California

Robert Smither, Ph.D.
Director, The Organizational Behavior Program, Department of Psychology, Rollins College, Winter Park, Florida

Len Sperry, M.D., Ph.D.
Professor of Psychiatry and Preventive Medicine, Department of Psychiatry and Preventive Medicine, Medical College of Wisconsin, Milwaukee, Wisconsin

Jeanne Mager Stellman, Ph.D.
Associate Professor of Public Health, School of Public Health, Columbia University, New York, New York

Jaime Szeinuk, M.D.
Assistant Professor, Department of Community and Preventive Medicine, Mount Sinai School of Medicine, New York, New York

Marilyn Thatcher, Ph.D.
Private Practice, Kentfield, California

Gregory R. Wagner, M.D.
Director, Division of Respiratory Disease Studies, National Institute for Occupational Safety and Health, Centers for Disease Control and Prevention, Morgantown, West Virginia

PREFACE

Occupational Medicine Secrets is a selected overview of relevant principles, issues, diseases, and practices in the field of occupational medicine. The breadth of clinical and public health aspects of occupational medicine is so vast that not every subject could be covered; however, the perspectives of the medical, nursing, psychiatric, legal, multidisciplinary practitioners, and health professionals are well represented.

Each section stresses the importance of prevention, evaluation, and effective treatment in the practice of occupational health. The first section outlines the principles of occupational medicine, including a brief historical background, and defines toxicologic and epidemiologic concepts. The second section focuses on particular hazards, such as pesticides and metals. The third section examines two groups at particular risk for work-related injuries and illnesses: child care workers and women workers. The fourth section discusses specific work-related diseases, as well as psychological issues and organizational dynamics. Finally, the fifth section provides a solid background of the practice of occupational medicine, with chapters on Disability Evaluation, Workforce Violence, and Occupational Medicine and the Law.

In particular, we wish to thank Andrew Booty, editorial assistant, for working diligently with the editors and persevering with the many difficulties in locating, contacting, and communicating with the authors. We are grateful to Ms. Deborah Nagin and Dr. Robert Harrison for providing early input and guidance on the selection of topics and contributors. We also thank all of the authors for their contributions. Most of all, we appreciate the lessons we all have learned from our patients and colleagues, and hope that this book contributes to the prevention of work-related illness in the 21st century.

Rosemarie M. Bowler, Ph.D., M.P.H.
James E. Cone, M.D., M.P.H.

I. Principles

1. PRINCIPLES OF OCCUPATIONAL AND ENVIRONMENTAL EPIDEMIOLOGY

Ana Maria Osorio, M.D., M.P.H.

1. Define occupational and environmental epidemiology.
Epidemiology is the study of the distribution and determinants of disease in human populations. Occupational epidemiology involves exposures and diseases in the workplace, whereas environmental epidemiology concerns nonworkplace settings. Possible goals for an occupational or environmental epidemiologic study include:
- Data collection for setting occupational or environmental standards
- Description of mechanism of toxicity
- Determination of health consequences and exposure
- Estimation of individual risk and extent of problem in the general population
- Evaluation of dose-response relationship
- Recommendations for corrective action to eliminate or control exposure

2. List the rates and proportions used to measure disease.
1. **Incident rate:** number of newly occurring cases per person-time units.
2. **Mortality rate:** specialized form of incident rate. For example, 10 new lung cancers occur at midyear among 1000 workers followed for 1 year; lung cancer mortality rate = $10/(1000 - (0.5 \times 10)) = 0.01005$.
3. **Disease risk:** number of incident cases per number of persons at risk at beginning of the interval; indicates the probability of developing the disease during the study period. For example, 1-year risk of mortality from lung cancer = $10/1000 = 0.01$.
4. **Point prevalence:** number of cases that exist in a population at one point in time, usually expressed as percentage or proportion (period prevalence involves number of cases that exist during given period). For example, among 500 workers studied, 125 reported skin disease problems; skin disease prevalence = $(125/500) \times 100 = 25\%$.

3. What are the major types of studies or reports in the medical literature?
1. **Case studies or case series:** identification and reporting of a group of cases; not a true epidemiologic investigation.
2. **Cross-sectional study:** survey to determine the prevalence of disease and exposure at the same point in time.
3. **Proportional mortality study:** comparison of the proportion of total deaths from disease of interest among different subgroups; specialized form of cross-sectional study.
4. **Ecologic study:** study that involves investigations of the group rather than the individual as the unit of analysis; also called an aggregate or descriptive study.
5. **Cohort study:** an exposed group and a nonexposed group are followed over time to determine who develops the disease of interest; provides the most direct evaluation of health and disease patterns in a population; also called a longitudinal or follow-up study.
6. **Case-control study:** comparison of the exposure among individuals with disease (cases) and other individuals without disease (controls); involves a group of persons with disease and a

group similar in all respects except for disease. A retrospective evaluation is conducted to determine who was exposed and who was not exposed; also called case-referent or retrospective study.

7. **Surveillance program:** ongoing epidemiologic evaluation of a disease among populations of interest. Examples include child lead poisoning registries and pesticide poisoning reporting systems conducted by state health departments.

4. List the advantages and disadvantages of the three major epidemiologic study types.

Comparison of Cross-sectional, Cohort, and Case-control Studies

STUDY DESIGN	ADVANTAGES	DISADVANTAGES

Cross-sectional	Relatively inexpensive
	Needs short time period
	Relatively easier to conduct
	Good if population is difficult
	    to access or define
		Selection bias—may find survivor
		    population with ill individuals gone
		Measures only prevalence

Cohort	Measures risk	Quite expensive Long follow-up period Individuals may be lost to follow-up Large number of subjects

Case-control	Less expensive
	Shorter time period needed
	Good for rare diseases
		Recall bias—persons with disease may
		    tend to remember exposure better
		    than controls

5. What major methodologic issues need to be considered in an epidemiologic study?
   • **Precision:** reduction of random error, indicated by the variance of a measurement and associated confidence interval.
   • **Validity:** reduction of systematic error (or systematic bias), indicated by comparing what the study estimated and what it is intended to estimate.
   • **Selection bias:** any bias due to the manner in which participants are selected.
   • **Information bias:** bias related to instruments and techniques used to collect information about exposure, health outcomes, or other factors.
   • **Confounding bias:** due to failure to account for the effects of other factors related to the exposure and health outcome. A confounder must be a risk factor for the disease, must be associated with the exposure, and must not be an intermediate step in the causal pathway between exposure and disease outcome.

6. What are the common sources of epidemiologic data for exposure and health outcome information?
   For exposure information:
   • Work records provide years of employment, often by job title and department.
   • Vital records, such as death certificates, do not often have accurate data about occupation and residence at time of exposure.
   • Monitoring records at the workplace or in the environment allows calculation of a duration of exposure index.
   • Actual environmental measures are good indicators, when available (either area sampling or personal measures).
   • The best indicators are biologic monitoring to estimate body burden (e.g., exhaled breath; urine, blood, and tissue sampling).
   For health outcome information, it is often difficult to distinguish a health problem of environmental or occupational origin from chronic disease. Morbidity and mortality records are often not helpful. Medical insurance or workers' compensation records may be of use. Routine screening may have occurred at the worksite. On the whole, it is important to compare exposure

with concurrent health outcome information. A good questionnaire often provides the best available information about both exposure and health status and history.

7. When evaluating an epidemiologic study result, how does one determine whether an exposure causes a health outcome?

The weight of the total amount of available information should be used in establishing an association between an exposure and a health outcome. The following causality criteria need to be considered:

1. **Strength:** a strong association between the suspected risk factor and the observed health outcome (e.g., high relative risk or odds ratio).

2. **Consistency:** the association holds up in different settings and among different groups.

3. **Specificity:** the specific exposure factor and specific health outcome are closely associated.

4. **Temporality:** the cause or exposure predates the health effect.

5. **Dose-response relationship:** as exposure intensifies, the severity of the health outcome is increased.

6. **Plausibility:** the association makes biologic sense.

7. **Coherence:** the association is consistent with what is known of the natural history and biology of the disease.

8. **Experimental evidence:** experimental studies support the hypothesis explaining the association.

9. **Analogy:** other examples with similar risk factors and health outcomes exist in the medical literature.

8. List the steps in conducting a disease outbreak investigation.

1. Confirm diagnosis of the initial case reports (called index cases).

2. Identify other unrecognized cases.

3. Establish a case definition. The case definition is tentative and may change as more information is collected; it may include symptoms, physical signs, and/or laboratory results. A trade-off between using a narrow vs. a broad case definition for epidemiologic studies should be considered, especially with respect to the effect on the rate of false-positive and false-negative cases.

4. Characterize cases by person, place, and time information (e.g., age, race, ethnicity, gender, location within a worksite or community, and timeline of the exposure and health events).

5. Create a plot of the incident cases by time (called an epidemic curve).

6. Determine whether a dose-response relationship exists (for example, people with more intense exposures have a higher prevalence than people with less intense exposures).

7. Derive an attack rate and determine whether statistical significance is achieved (attack rate = number of incident cases/number of exposed individuals). If the attack rate is statistically significant, an appropriate study can be designed with the eventual goal of making recommendations for preventive or control measures.

9. At a lead battery factory, 13 men work in the grid formation department (a known area of high lead exposure) and 26 work elsewhere in the plant. After a medical screening survey, 7 lead intoxication cases were diagnosed (6 in grid formation and 1 in another area). Calculate the attack rate and relative risk of developing lead intoxication after working in the grid formation department.

It is helpful to create a 2×2 table that relates exposure (working in grid formation) and disease (diagnosed lead intoxication).

		Lead intoxication		
		Yes	No	
Work in grid	Yes	6	7	13
formation	No	1	25	26
		7	32	

Attack rate = number of ill workers in grid formation/number who work there

$$= 6/13$$
$$= 0.46$$
$$= 46\%$$

Relative risk = $\dfrac{\text{number of ill workers in grid formation/number who work there}}{\text{number of ill workers elsewhere in plant/number who work elsewhere}}$

$$= (6/13)/(1/26)$$
$$= 0.46/0.04$$
$$= 11.50$$

10. Twenty-one cases of organophosphate intoxication are identified in an agricultural county in California. Researchers needed to determine what sort of exposure was associated with the disease. From a clinic in the area, 22 controls were selected and matched on ethnicity and age. Among the intoxication cases, 14 had worked in an almond field sprayed with pesticides; among the controls, 3 had worked in the almond field. Calculate the odds ratio of developing organophosphate intoxication if working in the almond field.

	Worked in almond field		
	Yes	No	
Cases	14	7	21
Controls	3	19	22
	17	26	43

Odds ratio of developing organophosphate intoxication if working in the almond fields $= (14 \times 19)/(3 \times 7) = 266/21 = 12.67$

Statistical significance refers to the probability that the observed difference between the two groups (either exposed and not exposed or case and control) is due to chance. The statistical significance for the above odds ratio is calculated as a 95% confidence interval of $2.35 - 83.82$. If the confidence interval does not include 1.0, statistical significance is achieved and the association is probably not due to chance.

11. For the following table showing the relationship between chronic bronchitis and the use of wood as cooking fuel, discuss the observed trend.

Years of wood use	Chronic Bronchitis	
	Case	Control
0–15	15 (17%)	38 (59%)
16–30	32 (36%)	16 (25%)
30+	41 (46%)	10 (15%)
	88	64

There is a positive dose-response relationship for using wood as a fuel and development of chronic bronchitis. For an accurate analysis, one needs to calculate an adjusted odds ratio that takes into account the potential confounding effect of smoking tobacco. For this example, the adjusted odds ratio is 3.92 with a 95% confidence interval of 1.7–9.1.

12. For a 1-year period, the number of adult asthma cases seen in a city emergency department (ED) was monitored. To determine the temporal pattern of cases, construct an epidemic curve using information in the following table.

MONTH	NUMBER OF ADULT ASTHMA CASES IN ED
January	199
February	146
March	180

Table continued on following page.

MONTH	NUMBER OF ADULT ASTHMA CASES IN ED
April	155
May	165
June	128
July	138
August	124
September	181
October	166
November	182
December	147

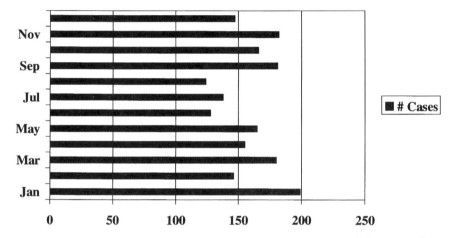

Number of persons over 14 years of age who presented with acute asthma to the hospital emergency department over a 1-year period.

The highest incidence of asthma cases occurred in January. The next graph shows the distribution of cases for the month of January.

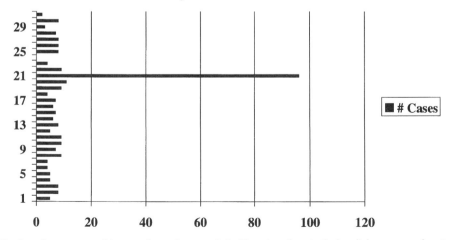

Number of persons over 14 years of age who presented with acute asthma to the hospital emergency department in January.

The shape of the graph suggests a common-source outbreak with the epidemic peak on 21 January. It was discovered that a fire in an industrial plant worsened air quality during January, which explained the increased number of asthma cases near the plant.

13. Is the association between aromatic amines and occupational bladder cancer a causal relationship?

Evaluation of the causality criteria for the relationship of aromatic amines (e.g., beta-naphthylamine and benzidine) and bladder cancer reveals that many of the criteria have been met:

1. Relative risk for factory workers exposed to aromatic amines = 3.61 (strong strength of association)

2. The relative risk increased as the duration of exposure to aromatic amines increased: no cases for exposures < 5 years duration, relative risk of 8.8 for exposures of 5–9.9 years, and relative risk of 27.2 for exposures of 10+ years (strong dose-response relationship).

3. A temporal relationship was found between onset of exposure and development of bladder cancer several years later (evidence of temporality).

4. Animal evidence shows production of tumors in two species with specific involvement of the bladder and evidence of a dose-response relationship (experimental evidence).

5. Analogous relationship to other known bladder carcinogens (analogy).

BIBLIOGRAPHY

1. Markowitz S: Problem-based Training Exercises for Environmental Epidemiology, 2nd ed. Geneva, World Health Organization, 1998.
2. Marsh G: Epidemiology of occupational diseases. In Rom WN (ed): Environmental and Occupational Medicine, 2nd ed. Boston, Little, Brown, 1992, pp 35–50.
3. Osorio AM: The environmental and occupational history. In EPA Recognition and Management of Pesticide Poisonings, 5th ed. Washington, DC, Environmental Protection Agency, 1999, pp 18–33.

2. PRINCIPLES OF ENVIRONMENTAL TOXICOLOGY

Marc Alan Lappé, Ph.D.

1. What key toxicologic principles should I know?

The major toxicologic doctrine is that the dose makes the poison. The total body burden in mg/kg of a particular chemical or its toxic metabolic byproducts is often given as a measure of the dose of a chemical or toxic agent. Often the amount of a chemical present in a sensitive or target organ system determines its damaging effect. The body's ability to metabolize, degrade, and ultimately excrete a toxic chemical is also critical to understanding toxicity. Some chemicals may become activated and hence more toxic in the course of being "detoxified." Such reactions usually take place in the liver, where enzymes such as the monooxygenases of the P450 microsomal system attack putatively toxic molecules. The body normally makes toxic molecules water-soluble or binds them to a conjugate such as glutathione to assist in detoxification. Some hormone-mimicking chemicals, such as dioxin, have toxic effects at very low doses, whereas others, such as cadmium, may have paradoxical-appearing effects. Such effects may result when a toxic chemical present in low concentrations induces its own detoxifying enzymes so that a very low dose may appear beneficial rather than toxic. Beneficial effects at ultra-low doses of toxic substances are known as "hormesis," a concept gaining increasing acceptance among toxicologists.

2. Do the general principles of toxicology apply to environmental circumstances?

Yes. The ultimate toxicity of a substance can be attributed to its concentration in susceptible living organisms in the environment. However, the effective toxicity of a chemical, such as oil residues or a toxic metal, is greatly affected by its availability. For instance, polychlorinated biphenyls (PCBs) in the sediments of the Great Lakes may be present in high concentration, but because of sequestration and slow bacterial degradation they do not pose as much of an immediate problem as do some waterborne chemicals, such as the gasoline additive methyl tert-butyl ester (MTBE), which can pose problems to water quality at low (ppb) concentrations. Similarly, chemicals such as trichloroethylene, which adsorb to soil particles, may have less effective toxicity than others that are unbound or otherwise free to migrate and concentrate in a fluid medium. In such instances, the bioavailability of a specific chemical in the environment, its persistence, and the existence of particularly vulnerable populations (elderly, young, or immunocompromised people) determine its penultimate toxicity.

3. How does the existence of different trophic levels affect the ultimate toxicity of a chemical?

Chemicals entering an ecosystem typically are first assimilated and wholly or partially metabolized by organisms at the lowest trophic levels and then passed up the food chain. Food chains may be simple or complex, depending on the number and linkages among members. Typically, the seven trophic levels begin with primary producers, traverse through primary to quaternary consumers, and end with saprophytes and decomposers. Thus, the mercury salts that entered Minamata Bay in Japan from a chemical processing plant were first methylated by anaerobic bacteria (producers) in the bay silt layer. The methyl mercury-contaminated bacteria were then assimilated by plankton and higher organisms in the next trophic level (primary consumers), until they in turn were ingested by shellfish and fin fish (secondary and tertiary consumers, respectively). When consumed by humans (quaternary consumers), the shellfish and fish, now contaminated with highly magnified concentrations of bioavailable organic mercury, exerted a profound neurotoxic effect, exceeding that predicted by the seawater levels of elemental mercury alone. Typically, toxic molecules are bioconcentrated by approximately one order of magnitude (i.e., 10-fold) with each trophic level traversed. At the highest trophic levels, notably carnivores such as polar bears and eagles, the final concentration of fat-soluble chemicals may be magnified by a million or more times above ambient environmental levels. In the instance of dichlorodiphenyltrichloroethane (DDT), water concentrations in eastern U.S. estuaries in the 1960s were typically in the range of less than 0.05 parts per billion (50 parts per trillion). In cormorants or mergansers, birds that feed on surface fish, tissue levels reached 20–25 parts per million. In the 1960s and 1970s, bald eagle populations were adversely affected through the bioaccumulation of dioxins, dibenzofurans, biphenyls, and organochlorine pesticides such as DDT and its breakdown product, DDE. Although these contaminants have been successfully reduced in some areas of the world, notably in the northwestern United States and Canada, significant levels remain elsewhere (Maine and the Great Lakes). Reproductive success of eagles has been proportionately improved in areas where organochlorine contaminants have been reduced, whereas elsewhere, such as lakes in Florida contaminated by estrogen-mimicking pesticides, reproductive damage continues.

4. What is a xenobiotic?

A xenobiotic chemical or agent is a human-made molecule not normally found in the natural environment.

5. What constitutes a "major" environmental contaminant?

Major environmental pollutants are typically measured by the magnitude of their production or release. Oil spills are commonly seen as major environmental disasters. Major environmental contaminants include ultratoxic chemicals, such as dioxin or chemicals with poor degradation characteristics that achieve ubiquitous or near-ubiquitous distribution. A classic example is DDT and its breakdown products DDE and DDD. These compounds are still found in varying proportions in the soils and sediments of 3,422 out of the 22,000 sites identified by the Environmental Protection Agency (EPA) in the National Sediment Quality Survey as posing hazards to humans or animal life.

6. Give examples of contaminants.

The major contaminants in the biosphere are generated by human activities.

1. **Sulphur oxides**, released primarily through the burning of fossil fuels, produce acidified rain (through conversion to weak sulphuric acid solutions) and have been responsible for major episodes of human toxicity. The "Donora fog" outside London in the 1960s is a classic example. Tens of thousands of people developed respiratory symptoms and illnesses after exposure.

2. **Nitrogen oxides and nitrates** comprise a second major pollution source. Nitrates accumulating from fertilizer runoff can contaminate drinking water. Children who drink water with sufficiently high concentrations (e.g., above 100 ppm) are at risk for methemoglobinemia, a condition that decreases the availability of oxygen in the blood.

3. **Mine wastes and tailings** pose both direct and indirect dangers to the environment. The direct risks stem from common heavy metals that enter contiguous ecosystems. Indirect risks stem from airborne and waterborne contaminants that pollute aquifers and water sources. A recent environmental catastrophe in Spain entailed the release of thousands of tons of heavy metal-contaminated sludge from a site near Seville. The resulting overburden of sludge contaminated at least 15,000 acres and is likely to leave the exposed farmland untillable for decades because of cadmium, lead, and other heavy metals.

4. **Pesticide contamination** is a highly diverse source of pollution. After application of persistent pesticides such as chlordane and Kepone, subsurface soils and/or waterways have been heavily contaminated, leading to fish kills and human illness. Bone marrow toxicity, liver and kidney damage, and neurotoxicity have been observed in exposed workers. Less persistent pesticides such as dibromochloropropane (DBCP) also have been involved in occupational and then environmental contamination episodes. Sperm function, motility, and production have been adversely affected among workers (e.g., at the Occidental Petroleum plant in Lathrop, California),

whereas more widespread but low-level contamination of aquifers with DBCP poses an as yet unquantified hazard. Presently, over 18,000 workers worldwide have alleged reproductive harm from DBCP. Subsoil contamination of water from DBCP used to treat soil nematodes in grape arbors and almond orchards, particularly in the Central Valley of California, has led to massive water treatment programs to eliminate pesticide residues in drinking water in the part-per-billion range. Highly water-soluble pesticides such as atrazine, which are widely used in midwestern U.S. corn fields, have led to ground water and aquifer contamination throughout the Corn Belt of the United States, with particularly ubiquitous contamination in Wisconsin.

7. How do pollutants enter ecosystems?

The traditional notion of pollution focuses on point-source origins of contamination. Point sources may be smoke stacks, outlet pipes, or sewage lines. The great preponderance of ecologically significant pollution, however, is not of point-source origin. General sources of pollution from the aggregate impact of human activities, be they cars, combustion engines generally, or wood product and agricultural burning, contribute significantly more than point sources. The present spate of carbon dioxide represents an extreme example of a relatively nontoxic gas that contributes significantly to environmental degradation. More classic sources of pollution, such as the excessive combustion of fossil fuels, remain a serious locus of contamination. For instance, in 1991 during the Gulf War, the burning of oil fields increased fourfold the mutagenic particulates in the air over Riyadh, Saudi Arabia.

8. What damages can pollutants cause?

To exposed human populations mutagens pose risks of cancer and potential reproductive damage. In general pollutants can damage ecosystems at any of several levels. Human activities as a whole, such as clear-cutting, can destabilize ecosystems, whereas toxic contaminants, such as those contributed by oil spills, tend to poison organisms at specific trophic levels. At the lowest trophic levels of primary producers, chemicals that are toxic to the metabolic machinery of bacteria and other protists or to the chlorophyll synthetic apparatus of single-cell plants, such as algae, can disrupt the energy balance of the ecosystem as a whole. Excessive copper ions in water, for instance, can be toxic to green and blue-green algae. Specific herbicides intended to poison the photosynthetic apparatus also may be toxic to single-cell organisms. Chemicals such as glyphosate or bromoxynil also have photosynthetic toxicity, but the persistence of such herbicides in the environment is fortunately short.

At slightly higher trophic levels, chemicals that impair flagellar motility or prevent the efficient incorporation of silica or calcium into dinoflagellate skeletons, including many heavy metals, are of concern. The damage produced by excessive metal ions often is manifest at low trophic levels and leads to disturbances in the available food base for higher organisms. Low-level contamination with neurotoxic chemicals, such as triclopyr, the active ingredient in Garlon herbicide, can impair swimming ability in andromadous fish such as salmon or steelhead trout at levels as low as 50 parts per billion in water.

The presence of excessive nitrogen and phosphorous may lead to overproduction of single-cell organisms, resulting in eutrophication of a marine or fresh-water ecosystem. In such circumstances, the biologic oxygen demand soars and the available oxygen is depleted, causing die-offs and further decay and oxygen depletion. At the highest trophic levels, chemical contaminants that bioaccumulate, often because of their fat solubility, can impair reproduction (e.g., PCBs, DDT) or immunologic function (e.g., dioxins, PCBs, and certain organophosphate pesticides).

9. What are the major factors limiting environmental toxicity?

Chemical or metallic xenobiotics are toxicologically limited by their persistence, accumulation, migration, and stability. The factors that determine persistence may include sunlight (photodegradation), bacterial degradation (soil microorganisms), and the presence of an ongoing source of contamination. The likelihood of bioaccumulation of any given xenobiotic is increased by its fat solubility and the number of trophic levels that it will traverse before encountering the penultimate consumer. Factors that affect the movement of a specific chemical include proclivity to bind strongly to soil particles (e.g., trichloroethylene), atomic weight (in the case of heavy metals), and molecular size. In general, the smaller the molecule, the faster its diffusion through any constant medium (Fick's law). Unstable compounds, such as organophosphate pesticides, tend to hydrolyze and degrade relatively rapidly compared to more stable compounds such as PCBs or DDT.

10. What properties of xenobiotics make them particularly harmful to the environment?

Xenobiotics that are highly reactive with organic molecules, notably the monomers commonly used in plastic manufacture, pose the greatest likelihood of toxicity to organisms in the environment. However, toxicity is often limited in time and space to the first organisms encountered because of the formation of adducts and other chemical compounds that take the chemical in question out of circulation. Examples include toluene diisocyanate (used in polyurethane production) and vinyl chloride monomer (used in making polyvinylchloride plastics). Populations residing near facilities making one or both groups of compounds have been overexposed to the monomeric components from manufacturing activities. Other xenobiotics, notably dioxins and PCBs, interact with sensitive endocrine receptors in organisms and may disrupt normal reproductive activities by interfering with proper signalling or hormonal control.

11. How does the environment recover from toxic insults?

Most if not all xenobiotics are ultimately degraded or otherwise inactivated over time through environmental factors. Toxic impacts usually occur during movement to their ultimate environmental fate. Among the most important environmental detoxifying mechanisms are the abilities of anaerobic bacteria to dechlorinate polychlorinated hydrocarbons, the reactivity of many chemicals to environmental oxidants, and the solubilization of nonpolar chemicals through the addition of polar groups. The best studied example of the first method is the dechlorination of DDT to DDE with subsequent breakdown through reductive dechlorination to DDMU, a nonchlorinated and much less toxic molecule. (Previously, it was thought that DDE could not be microbially transformed.) Many organophosphorous pesticides are first transformed into oxidation products (e.g., malathion to maloxon) before being hydrolyzed and inactivated. Such oxidized intermediates are often much more toxic than their parent compounds. To avoid this problem and ensure chemical stability, many manufacturers add antioxidants or stabilizers to their chemical products. Among the most commonly used products are 1,4 dioxane and tributyltin, both of which have important toxicologic features of their own. Dioxane is an animal carcinogen, and tributyltin has significant marine toxicity. In general, as in the body itself, most organic molecules that are taken up by environmental microorganisms are rendered more water-soluble through addition of polar molecules (e.g., the addition of OH groups to benzene rings) or more bioavailable (e.g., through methylation of mercury). The endpoint of such reactions can make the parent molecule more toxic in the short term, as exemplified by methyl mercury in Minamata Bay.

12. How do chemical pollutants move through the environment?

The most important and common pathways of environmental distribution of chemical pollutants are through air and water. Compounds such as PCBs and chemicals such as chlorpyrifos (the active ingredient in the pesticide Dursban) are globally distributed, largely by being carried as adsorbants to dust particles. Chlorpyrifos is distributed worldwide through concentration in water vapor and dissemination in fog droplets.

13. What are the principal concerns about water contaminants?

From a public health viewpoint, water contaminants pose risks to human populations when they compromise reproductive health, increase cancer risks, or impair immune function. The first two endpoints have been well documented for trihalomethanes, the major reaction products of chlorination of humic and fulvic acids in drinking water. Studies have shown that relatively high levels (> 60 ppb) of trihalomethanes in drinking water appear to increase miscarriage rates in women drinking 2 or more liters per day. Trihalomethane concentration, especially chloroform levels, also correlates with risk for bladder, rectal, and, to a lesser extent, colon cancer. The other water contaminant of major health concern is lead. At the present permissible level of 5 parts per billion, lead concentrations can accumulate in children to doses (blood leads of 15 µg/100 ml) that can impair mental functioning, attention, and normal behavior. Trichloroethylene (TCE) in drinking water at levels of 5 ppb or more have been associated with an increased risk of non-Hodgkin's lymphoma.

14. Can some environmental agents cause toxicity at ultra-low doses? Why?

Yes. Among the chemicals of greatest environmental concern, 2,3,7,8-tetrachlorodibenzodi-oxin stands out because of its ability to cause reproductive harm, immunologic damage, and possibly cancer at ultra-low doses (measured in picograms per liter). This ability is linked to dioxin's ultra-tight binding to microsomal enzymes and its concentration in the thymus and other glands of central importance for immune function.

15. What are the effects of heavy metal contaminants in the environment?

Heavy metals such as lead (Pb) and cadmium (Cd) tend to accumulate in the subsoils, where they are dispersed after airborne emission or mine tailings (Pb) or sewage sludge deposition (Cd). Soil contamination from inadvertent addition of soil amendments containing such heavy metals can ruin farmland by contaminating the soil to the point that vegetables cannot be grown without toxic accumulations. When present in soils, they may become a major source of human contamination, either through leaching into drinking water and through pica activities in which significant amounts of lead are ingested by children in contaminated materials. The resulting body burdens of Pb and Cd have their major affects on porphyrin synthesis (lead-induced porphyria), aplastic anemia (bone marrow toxicity), and neurologic functions (lowered IQ and attention deficits).

16. Can bacterial degradation of environmental pollutants be accelerated?

Yes. Bacteria can degrade both chlorinated and nonchlorinated molecules. Reductive dehalogenation occurs naturally in anaerobic subsoils and may result in the dechlorination of PCBs, chlorophenols, chlorinated solvents, and dioxins. Special strains of bacteria can be isolated from contaminated soils, propagated, and used to achieve further reductions in contaminant levels. Such an approach has been successfully used to decontaminate oil spills and TCE-contaminated soils and water.

17. What are the major fates and impacts of radioisotopes?

Radioisotopes, whether indigenous or byproducts of commercial or military activities, may pose substantial threats to human health. The two most common examples are radon gas and tritium. Radon is produced as one of the "radon daughters" in the decay pattern of radionucleotides in the radium group. Radon daughters are typically alpha particle emitters. When dispersed in the lungs, alpha particles can cause direct cell damage and DNA mutations that may lead to lung cancer. Radioactive iodine (I^{131}) is a major cause of thyroid cancer, notably in victims of the Chernobyl reactor accident.

18. How has the atmosphere been affected by environmental contaminants?

Major atmospheric pollutants (as discussed above) have varying half-lives but eventually become incorporated in biogenic cycles. Nitrous oxides are reduced to ammonia by the actions of soil bacteria that "fix" them in accessible salts or ammonia for incorporation into plants. Sulphur oxides eventually become neutralized and similarly reduced, for the most part, to sulfides and related compounds. But some atmospheric contaminants, especially the chlorofluorocarbons, have extraordinarily long half-lives in the atmosphere. Ozone destruction from these and related molecules (e.g., methyl bromide, fluorines) has produced wholesale environmental disturbance by increasing the incident ultraviolet light that impinges on the planet. Similarly, the long-term and progressive increase in carbon dioxide levels (expected to go from 300 to 1,000 ppm in the next 30 years) has a dramatic climatic impact. Through trapping of infrared wavelength radiation, the net effect of the progressive increase in greenhouse gases is to increase global temperature (global warming). This greenhouse effect may reduce biodiversity, shift growing regions, and move ecologic zones.

19. How long do environmental contaminants remain toxic?

Many pesticides and other biologic control agents are intentionally constructed to have long half-lives in the environment. Such persistence is a logical quality when the objective is to obtain long-lived protection against reinfestation. For this reason, chlordane, which has a half-life in soil of over 20 years, was an "ideal" termite control agent. But a persistent agent is an ecologic hazard when it bioaccumulates or otherwise enhances toxicity over time. Among such pesticides are dieldrin and DDT, which have protracted half-lives of 10–15 years under some environmental conditions. Their byproducts, notably DDE in the case of DDT, have even longer persistence. Some recent research suggests that the effective toxicity of such chemicals in soils diminishes over time even though their soil concentrations remain constant. A likely explanation for this paradoxic finding is that with time some xenobiotics bind tightly to soil particles and thereby become less bioavailable.

20. How can I access critical information about environmental toxicants?

Environmental information is accessed most usefully by researching individual chemicals in governmental databases, particularly those maintained by the National Library of Medicine. Among the key sources and their web sites are (1) the Agency for Toxic Substance Disease Registry (ATSDR) ToxFaqs system: [atsdr1.atadr.cec.gov.8080toxfaq.html]; (2) the Hazardous Substance Database [atsdr1.atsdr.cdc.gov:8080/hazdat.hum#A3.1]; (3) the USDA Pesticide Properties Database [www.arsusda.vog/ppdb2.html]; and (4) the Extoxnet [ace.ace.orst.edu/info/extoxnet/]. In addition the Environmental Defense Fund has established a comprehensive pesticide toxicity data base [www.scorecard.org].

21. What components of hazardous wastes are of environmental concern?

Although hazardous waste sites differ extensively in composition, several common contaminants have been reported from Superfund sites throughout the United States. Among the compounds of greatest public health concern, according to the CDC's Agency for Toxic Substance Disease Registry, are trichloroethylene, benzene, lead, and cadmium.

22. How do occupational contaminants become environmental problems?

Occupational contaminants become environmental problems through escape to the surrounding environment and, secondarily, through direct transport by workers to their homes. In the first instance, chemicals such as toluene diisocyanate can contaminate neighborhoods when emissions are inadequately controlled at factories. Similarly, dioxins escaping from pulp mills are often a major source of dioxin contamination in surrounding waterways. The EPA maintains a web site [epa.gov.] with more specific information about specific toxic sites.

23. What can be done to minimize the environmental impact of human activities?

The most effective programs to minimize environmental degradation reduce the extent or intensity of human activities or take appropriate precautions or remedial steps to minimize their impacts. Examples include programs that follow potentially toxic waste streams from cradle to grave. A case in point is the successful clean-up of the Rocky Flats nuclear facility outside of Denver, the first of 52 nuclear waste sites in 31 states to be fully decommissioned and safely converted to usable space. Other positive environmental programs capitalize on the ability of controlled microbial degradation schemes to reduce or minimize sewage waste impacts on waterways and aquifers. Secondary treatment facilities that incorporate oxygenated waste streams to permit the efficient breakdown of organic matter are becoming more and more common across the country, including new processes that rely on tiers of waste-degrading plants and algae that purify the waste. The efficiency of these organic systems is a waste stream with appreciably less biologic oxygen demand and fewer dissolved nitrates and phosphates than has been achieved with standard tank/aeration systems. The end result of the most efficient waste treatment systems is an effluent with less than 10 mg/L of total nitrogen.

As new evidence accumulates about the toxicity of chlorination byproducts, whether in pulp mills or water treatment facilities, newer systems that rely on ozone or microfiltration (pores smaller than 1/100th the diameter of a human hair) are being successfully used to treat pulp mill wastes or to filter drinking water to remove bacteria and parasites without generating harmful dioxins in pulp mills or trihalomethanes in water treatment plants.

BIBLIOGRAPHY

1. Elliott JE, Norstrom RJ: Chlorinated hydrocarbon contaminants and productivity of bald eagle populations on the Pacific Coast of Canada. Environ Toxicol Chem 17:1142–1153, 1998.
2. Hemond HF: Chemical Fate and Transport in the Environment. New York, Academic Press, 1994.
3. Klaassen CD (ed): Casarett and Doull's Toxicology: The Basic Science of Poisons, 5th ed. New York, McGraw-Hill, 1996.
4. Kosian PA, Makynene EA, Monson PD, et al: Sequestration of DDT and dieldrin in soil: Disappearance of acute toxicity but not the compounds. Environ Toxicol Chem 17:1034–1038, 1998.
5. Lappé M: Chemical Deception. San Francisco, Sierra Club Books, 1991.
6. Manahan SE: Fundamentals of Environmental Chemistry. Chelsea, MI, Lewis Publishers, 1993.
7. Rhee G-Y, Sokol RC: The fate of polychlorinated biphenyls in aquatic sediments. Great Lakes Res Rev 1:23–28, 1994.
8. Shaw IC, Chadwick J: Principles of Environmental Toxicology. Bristol, PA, Taylor & Francis, 1998.
9. Sokol RC, Bethoney CM, Rhee G-Y: Reductive dechlorination of pre-existing sediment polychlorinated biphenyls with long-term laboratory incubation. Environ Toxicol Chem 17:982–987, 1998.
10. Turnbull A: Chlorinated Organic Micropollutants. London, Royal Society of Chemistry, 1997.

3. PRINCIPLES OF OCCUPATIONAL TOXICOLOGY

Marc Alan Lappé, Ph.D.

1. What underlying principles of toxicology apply particularly to the occupational setting?

The maxim, "the dose makes the poison," applies to virtually all settings. However, the workplace is a unique environment. Unlike environmental or home-based exposures, the worker is typically exposed for 8 hours/day, 5 days/week. Contract or construction workers are a notable exception because exposures of 10–12 hours/day, 7 days/week, may be sustained for short periods. Dermal and inhalation exposures predominate, and the conditions of work often intensify exposure by increasing respiration rate, providing repetitive exposures, and permitting the build-up of dosages received over the work week. Several conditions unique to occupational settings provide unusual dosage situations: dermal or pulmonary exposures that sensitize workers may permit very low doses to have adverse effects by generating hypersensitivity. A classic example is toluene diisocyanate, which can sensitize via inhalation at the part-per-billion range. Additional factors that provide exceptions or modifications of the general rule of dose-dependent toxicity include concomitant exposures that synergize toxicity, metabolic activators of the P450 enzymes in the liver that convert nontoxic chemicals to toxic intermediates, and nonworkplace exposures to alcohol or cigarette smoke that exacerbate workplace toxins such as ketones or asbestos, respectively.

2. Give examples of exposure conditions of particular concern for worker well-being.

Classic instances of unanticipated, high-risk exposure settings include operations in confined spaces. For instances, workers who scrubbed out the interior of vinyl chloride reaction chambers were among the first to show evidence of liver angiosarcomas or brain astrocytomas. Work environments without adequate ventilation provide another setting in which exposures can be high. For example, a few, highly exposed Turkish shoemakers who worked with solvents containing high concentrations of benzene developed acute myelocytic leukemia. Other workplace settings in which high concentrations of solvent vapors, gases, or other chemicals can build up include trenching operations, tile-setting, hazardous waste clean-up, and storage tank cleaning.

3. What general regulatory principles apply to limiting potentially health-threatening exposures?

Historically, permissible workplace exposures to individual chemicals were set first by industry through the Association of Governmental Industrial Hygienists (AGIH) and later by the Occupational Safety and Health Administration (OSHA). Permissible exposure limits (PELs) were adopted. Both entities ostensibly specify air concentrations that a worker can breathe for an 8-hour shift without "material impairment" of health or physiologic functioning. TLVs are constantly reevaluated as new data become available, but PEL values used by government agencies to establish legally enforced limits often are incorporated only after protracted review and delay. General conditions of employment are based on legislation and regulations, including those of the Department of Transportation, Environmental Protection Agency (EPA), OSHA, and state agencies. Enabling statutes and regulations establish the general proposition that workplaces should be free of potentially hazardous exposures to toxic substances; that the conditions of work should not impair health; and that any potential exposure to a reproductive or carcinogenic agent should be minimized or avoided altogether. Terms used to describe the health-based limits on toxic exposure in the workplace (see table below) usually refer to exposure limits established by governmental bodies that designate safe workplace conditions. One limitation of this approach is the general lack of consideration of interactive effects. For regulatory purposes, exposures are averaged on an additive basis; the partial fraction of a TLV for chemical A may be added to the TLV for chemical B and so on, as long as the total TLV fractions do not exceed unity. For example, if the TLV for A is 200 ppm and the average exposure is 100, the fractional TLV is 100/200 or $\frac{1}{2}$; if the remaining exposures add up to TLV fractions of less than $\frac{1}{2}$, the total workplace exposure is considered within permissible limits. The weakness of this approach becomes evident when it is recognized that some chemicals exacerbate the adverse effects of others, even at concentrations below the TLV (e.g., nontoxic levels of isopropanol potentiate the liver toxicity of carbon tetrachloride).

Technical Terms Used in Occupational Health for Acceptable Exposure Levels

1. National Institute of Occupational Safety and Health (NIOSH)- or OSHA-recommended levels: advisory time-weighted averages (TWAs), usually based on an average of exposures over 1 or 8 hours.

2. OSHA permissible exposure limit (PEL): highest permitted level in an 8-hr workday.

3. NIOSH threshold limit value (TLV): maximal average encountered value during an 8-hr workday that can be safely experienced; usually the same or lower than OSHA PEL.

4. OSHA short-term exposure limit (STEL): maximal short-term concentration permitted, as reflected by a 15-minute sampling measurement; maximal permissible exposure over a 15-minute period.

5. No observable effect level (NOEL): the exposure level in humans, usually extrapolated with a safety factor of 10 from animal data, that is not expected to produce a detectable adverse effect; of no observable adverse effect level (NOAEL).

6. Lowest observable effect level (LOEL): the lowest level of exposure capable of producing a detectable effect.

7. Health-based exposure level (HBEL): an exposure level pegged to conditions necessary to ensure the maintenance of well-being.

4. How can occupational hazards be mitigated?

The general principle for reducing health-threatening exposures in the workplace is to attenuate or reduce exposure through effective mitigation measures. Toxic exposures in the workplace can be reduced or eliminated by the appropriate use of engineering controls such as ventilation, air filters, or totally enclosed operations. Occasionally, basic processes can be modified to avoid toxic intermediates. Barrier creams, respirators, and protective clothing made of impermeable material provide a secondary line of defense. Ideally, the workplace environment should be controlled through engineering so that no toxic levels of exposures are encountered.

5. What types of illnesses are commonly or uniquely experienced in the workplace?

Many respiratory diseases, such as chronic obstructive pulmonary disease (COPD) and asthma, can be induced or exacerbated by airborne toxins in the workplace. Other target organs that are commonly affected include the liver (chemical hepatitis), kidney, urogenital tract, and brain or central nervous system (CNS). Reproductive toxicity is a recently recognized addition to the traditional list of occupational diseases and illnesses. Consult a standard textbook (see bibliography) for a complete listing.

Unique workplace-related injuries or illnesses include angiosarcoma of the liver, a rare tumor experienced by vinyl chloride workers; hemorrhagic cystitis (evidenced by bloody urine) experienced by chlorinated amine workers; abnormal secondary sexual characteristics (e.g., breast enlargement) experienced by male handlers of diethylstilbestrol (DES); and azoospermia experienced by workers heavily exposed to the soil sterilizant, dibromochloropropane (DBCP).

6. How can the occupational and environmental physician prevent or reduce the likelihood of such adverse effects?

The principal role of the occupational physician (OP) is to anticipate potential occupational disease in a particular setting and to perform the requisite surveillance, monitoring, and examinations needed to ensure that no illness or disease is occurring. In conjunction with an industrial hygienist, the OP typically evaluates workplace exposures to ensure that acceptable (i.e., below TLV) levels of toxic substances are present in the breathing zone of at-risk workers; that no contact-sensitizing agents are handled without proper protection; and that exposure to potential carcinogens and reproductive toxins (e.g., certain glycol ethers) are kept to a minimum or eliminated entirely.

7. What are the diagnostic criteria for occupational exposures? How do they differ, if at all, from conventional tests of illness or disease?

Generally speaking, the hallmarks and pathognomic signs of illnesses acquired in the workplace are the same for similar or analogous diseases encountered in the outside environment. However, some highly specific diseases and disorders are relatively workplace-specific and require intensified efforts at diagnosis through testing and appropriate health assessments. For instance, asbestosis may require special x-ray and sputum analyses; angiosarcoma, special imaging; toxic brain injury, neuropsychological testing; and, reproductive effects, special biopsy and semen, sperm, endocrine, or ultrasound examinations.

8. Which exposures can be disabling or produce permanent disease?

Among the most common permanent or largely irreversible diseases produced from workplace exposure are brown-lung disease from cotton dust (byssinosis); polyneuropathies from organophosphate intoxication or prolonged chlorinated solvent exposure; emphysema from particulates or cigarette smoke; asbestosis from asbestos; occupational cancers, such as acute myelocytic leukemia from benzene exposure; and CNS effects, including secondary functional disability from protracted, high-level exposure to styrene or trichloroethylene.

9. Give examples of effective monitoring or surveillance procedures used in occupational toxicology.

Effective monitoring requires a suitable test or detection system for an incipient disease process. So-called "sentinel" diseases were used in the recent past (e.g., testicular cancer as an indicator of workplace carcinogens), but most current surveillance systems rely on biomarkers (see question 10). Monitoring for early signs of disease by using the most sensitive validated test available or measuring specific exposure markers for agents or metabolites, where appropriate, is also desirable. More refined monitoring, such as looking for serologic signs of illness or genetic damage, is also possible. Monitoring should be distinguished from screening. The target of screening is usually a specific disease entity for which there is an efficacious intervention, such as screening for early signs of liver disease in solvent workers. Monitoring implies a regular, timely testing system that examines a general population for signs and symptoms of varied diseases or disorders linked to workplace exposure. A full list of tests appropriate for dermatologic and pulmonary testing can be found in references 3 and 6.

10. What are biomarkers? How do they apply to the workplace setting?

Biomarkers are usually found in the blood. Typically, they represent evidence of a biologically significant interaction with a native component of the serum or formed blood. A typical biomarker is an adduct with DNA and the activated form of a suspected mutagen and/or carcinogen. Such biomarkers can be found after exposure to benzene and related chemicals suspected of being leukemogens.

11. What key toxic exposures must be recognized and reduced in the occupational setting?

Among the most important toxicologic factors influencing workplace illness are reactive chemicals, metals, nonbiogenic fibers and dusts, organophosphate pesticides, special pharmaceuticals, and radioactive chemicals (isotopes) and nuclides. The first category includes monomers used in the plastics industry, such as vinyl chloride. Metals of concern include lead (Pb), mercury (Hg), beryllium (Be), arsenic (As), cadmium (Cd), and, to a lesser extent, zinc (Zn). Fibers capable of producing lung fibrosis and/or malignancy include fiberglass and the various forms of asbestos. Dusts include free-crystolline silica. Organophosphate pesticides of particular concern include methyl parathion; organochlorines include chlordecone (Kepone), lindane, DDT, polychlorinated dibenzofurans (PCDFs), chlordane, and heptachlor. Radioactive isotopes used in medical imaging or therapy, such as technetium or iodine-131 pose potential hazards to technicians and medical personnel. Pharmaceuticals used in chemotherapy or immune suppression are of particular concern because of their mutagenicity, carcinogenicity, or bone marrow toxicity.

12. Give examples of dermatologic occupational diseases.

The skin is the most visible and often the most vulnerable site of occupational damage and disease. Direct effects of solvents on the skin, notably defatting, cracking, and scaling, are common workplace problems. Simple dermatitis from such chronic irritation may lead to secondary infection and more serious skin problems. For instance, chronic trichloroethylene exposure has been associated with the development of defatting and possibly scleroderma, in which the skin becomes hard and "hide-bound" often as a result of autoimmune-mediated damage to the dermis and resultant overgrowth of fibroblasts. Chronic dermatitis and inflammation also may arise from contact hypersensitivity reactions stemming from contact with known contact allergens (e.g., Rhus toxins from poison oak or ivy) or sensitizing agents such as epoxies or isocyanates used in polyurethane production.

13. How do various work environments potentially affect pulmonary function?

The lung is also a site of occupational injury and disease. Chronic exposure to small mineral or biologic fibers (e.g., fiberglass or cotton fibers, respectively) may cause lung injury, inflammation, and, in susceptible individuals (e.g., those deficient in alpha-1-antitrypsin), chronic pulmonary disease. Various forms of chemical pneumonia are common in workplace settings associated with aerosols of corrosive or highly reactive chemicals. Dusts and particulates are also a source of lung damage, leading to alveolar injury and possible emphysema. Periodic spirometry or peak expiratory flow measurements are important monitoring devices to detect the effect of these and other disease processes on lung function.

14. How do toxicologic principles from tumor biology (oncology) apply to the workplace?

Because many workers are exposed to known or suspected human carcinogens on the job, it is critical to understand the application of basic principles of tumor biology to workplace settings. Direct-acting and usually "complete" carcinogens interact directly with cellular DNA, cause genetic damage, and also may interfere with repair mechanisms. Such chemicals (and physical or energetic agents), which include vinyl chloride, benzene, and ultraviolet radiation, can reasonably be assumed to act without a threshold in the sense that their effects are exhibited at any dose level, proportional to duration and intensity of exposure. At very low doses, such agents produce tumors typically of very long latency (compare benzene-induced chronic leukemias) and low incidence. At higher doses, latencies are typically shorter and the overall cancer incidence is higher.

Other chemicals that typically induce only liver cancer in susceptible rodent species are thought to act by nongenotoxic means, either through toxicity or the phenomenon of peroxisome proliferation. Examples include some plasticizers (e.g., diethylhexylphthalate [DEHP]). Still other chemicals, such as trichloroethylene, may work through both mechanisms or a combination of effects proportional to the amount of reactive intermediates (usually epoxides) produced.

15. Which workers deserve special protections, monitoring, and/or surveillance in specific workplace settings?

By virtue of preexisting disease or illness, genetic susceptibility, age, or reproductive status many workers are at special risk from occupational toxic substances. Although it is desirable to protect all workers (both male and female) of reproductive age from exposure to any reproductive toxin (see below), such protection may be especially necessary for women in the early stages of pregnancy (first trimester). Genetically susceptible workers, such as those with alpha-1-antitrypsin deficiency, superoxide dismutase variants, xeroderma pigmentosum haplotypes, and other genetic conditions that reduce the ability to repair or defend against toxic effects of highly reactive chemicals, need to be identified and afforded appropriate protections in hazardous environments in such a way that they are not subject to employment or social discrimination or stigmatization.

16. How can occupational physicians integrate their practice with that of traditional practitioners?

Most diseases or disorders encountered in occupational settings mirror conditions or disorders encountered in everyday practice. Occupational forms of toxic substance-induced disease are typically more severe and aggressive than their spontaneous counterparts. In cases of infectious disease, such as needlestick-acquired HIV or hepatitis B, the disease process may be similar, but the latency period shorter than in traditional modes of contagion.

17. Give examples of toxicologic effects that may be particularly chronic or persistent.

Toxic insults that produce lasting and irremediable harm are of greatest concern to the occupational physician. Among the most serious irreversible effects are asbestosis and mesothelioma; emphysema (induced by smoke or particulates); permanent sensitization states (e.g., those induced by toluene diisocyanate); and permanent neurologic or neuropsychologic disability (e.g., organic solvent- or lead-induced encephalopathy).

18. What are the special concerns of the occupational physician for neurologic well-being?

The central nervous system is particularly vulnerable to irreversible damage after chronic intoxication. The OP must be vigilant for early signs of overexposure to solvents with potential for neurologic damage, such as n-hexane, chlorinated solvents, and organophosphorous pesticides with delayed effects. Early signs and symptoms, such as attention-deficit disorder, mood disturbance not related to functional causes, and disorientation, must be recognized so that early interventions can preclude further exposure to the offending chemical.

19. What databases are available to the occupational physician concerned about toxic exposures?

The occupational physician should have access to a complete set of material safety data sheets (MSDS) via hard disc and to databases on the internet. Two particularly useful guides are the *OSHA TLV Handbook* and *Chemical Exposure Guidelines*, published by the Santa Clara Center for Occupational Safety and Health (1995). Electronic databases include Toxnet (http://pmep.cce.cornell.eduprofiles/exotoxnet/) and Medline (http://www.nlm.nih.gov/databases/medline.html) as well as other National Library of Medicine databases such as Medlars and Toxline, all accessible through the internet reference above without charge.

20. How can the physician identify the particular hazardous agent in a given situation?

In most instances, workers should have been given a MSDS for the chemicals with which they work. In practice, it is likely that a given chemical will be mixed with others. To ascertain fully the nature of exposure, it may be necessary to consult an industrial hygienist, to examine company process files, and/or, in certain circumstances, to perform analyses of bulk or air samples for the concentration of suspected toxins.

21. How can the occupational physician assemble and integrate worksite exposure information in making a diagnosis?

Often the OP can assemble a meaningful exposure history from an analysis of the chemical make-up of the likely agents to which a worker has been exposed and the industrial hygienist's report. Then the OP must recreate dose and route information to arrive at a likely causative diagnosis. To do so, the OP needs actual breathing zone measurements or other analogs of exposure, a chemical analysis or cross-section of the products at issue, and a detailed worker patient history. Other workers similarly exposed may be monitored for anticipated toxic effects (e.g., a liver panel for enzyme abnormalities).

22. How can toxic exposures be differentiated from other etiologies?

It is sometimes critical to differentiate workplace exposures from exposures due to personal habits or hobbies or environmental exposures to similar or related suspect agents. A complete worker questionnaire should examine lifestyle, drug or alcohol use, hobbies, and secondary exposures from environmental and other non-job settings, as well as prior physical or psychological diagnoses or learning disabilities. Much of this evaluation will arise in the context of medicolegal issues, such as workers' compensation, but such information is also of value to the patient for differentiating and mitigating contributing exposures.

BIBLIOGRAPHY

1. Adams RM: Occupational Skin Disease, 2nd ed. Philadelphia, W.B. Saunders, 1990.
2. Agency for Toxic Substances Disease Registry: Toxicological Profile for Vinyl Chloride. Atlanta, Department of Health and Human Services, 1989.
3. American College of Occupational and Environmental Medicine Panel: Occupational and environmental competencies, v.1.0. J Occup Environ Med 40:427–440, 1998.
4. Austin H, Delzell E, Cole P: Benzene and leukemia. A review of the literature and a risk assessment. Am J Epidemiol 127:419–437, 1988.
5. Berk PD, Martin JF, Young RS, et al: Vinyl chloride-associated liver disease. Ann Intern Med 84:717–731, 1976.
6. Bowler RM, Ngo L, Hartney C, et al: Epidemiological health study of a town exposed to chemicals. Environ Res 72:93–108, 1997.
7. Hayes WJ, Laws ER (eds): Handbook of Pesticide Toxicology. New York, Academic Press, 1991.
8. Maibach HI: Occupational and Industrial Dermatology, 2nd ed. Chicago, Year Book, 1987.
9. Pope AM, Rall DP (eds): Environmental Medicine. Washington, DC, National Academy Press, 1995.
10. Rom WN (ed): Environmental and Occupational Medicine, 2nd ed. Philadelphia, Lippincott-Raven, 1992.
11. State of California Department of Health: Medical Supervision of Pesticide Workers. Guidelines for Physicians. Berkeley, CA, 1988.

4. PRINCIPLES OF INDUSTRIAL HYGIENE

Mark Goldberg, Ph.D., C.I.H., and Deborah Nagin, M.P.H., C.I.H.

1. What is industrial hygiene?

Industrial hygiene is a branch of occupational health science devoted to preventing diseases caused by workplace exposures to chemical, physical, and biologic agents. Just as physicians diagnose and treat illnesses and injuries, industrial hygienists (IHs) recognize, evaluate, and control workplace conditions that may cause adverse health effects among workers. As a public health endeavor, industrial hygiene attempts to solve problems before conditions cause ill health. Over the years, the focus of industrial hygiene has expanded beyond factories and mines to include service industries and offices. Thus, the terms *industrial* and *occupational* are often used interchangeably with the word hygiene.

2. What are the origins of industrial hygiene?

Physicians were the first to clearly recognize the relationship between workplace conditions and disease. During the early 20th century, Dr. Alice Hamilton was one of the first physicians in the United States to venture from the treatment room into the factories to deal with the root causes of certain diseases. She visited factories to learn firsthand about the conditions that caused the grave ailments associated with lead poisoning. She witnessed uncontrolled releases of dust into workroom air that was then inhaled by workers. Having "diagnosed" the problem, her training as a physician led her to the next step: finding a "cure." She was confident that lead poisoning could be prevented if the amount of dust released into the workroom air was reduced. She was thinking as an industrial hygienist—understanding the work process, identifying the source and magnitude of the exposure, and developing a solution to the problem. Industrial hygiene as it is practiced in the late 20th century did not really begin until the 1930s and 1940s, when the work of pioneers such as Alice Hamilton was integrated with engineering and chemistry.

Initially, industrial hygiene was practiced in heavy industrial sectors, such as mining, metal foundries, steel, and auto manufacturing, where recognized serious health hazards existed. The field grew slowly. Between 1910 and 1940, individual states developed small industrial hygiene units in their Departments of Labor. Professional associations of industrial hygiene were established in 1939. By the 1940s, a handful of universities granted degrees for industrial hygiene or related disciplines. However, until the 1970s the practice of industrial hygiene was limited and remained rooted principally in industry and only secondarily in government, including the federal Public Health Service. During the late 1960s and early 1970s, a confluence of social, political, scientific, and economic phenomena led to a great leap forward for industrial hygiene and for occupational health in general.

3. What sociopolitical forces and legislation moved industrial hygiene forward?

The 1960s were years of rapid social change. One of the unforeseen consequences of the upheavals wrought by the civil rights and anti-Vietnam war movements was a growing consciousness of environmental and occupational health issues. Organized labor, environmental, public health, and community organizations fought for federal standards to protect the environment and workers. In 1969, Congress established the Environmental Protection Agency (EPA), and in 1970 the Williams-Stieger Occupational Safety and Health Act (OSHAct) was passed. The OSHAct guaranteed a safe and healthful workplace for all workers.

With the passage of the OSHAct, the field of industrial hygiene blossomed. The federal Occupational Safety and Health Administration (OSHA) was created to enforce health and safety standards. Field offices responsible for enforcing these standards were opened across the U.S. The need for trained industrial hygienists to inspect workplaces and enforce regulations grew. In response to the threat of legal sanctions for violations of workplace health and safety standards, large companies began to hire industrial hygienists to ensure compliance. In addition, consulting groups flourished to meet the growing demand for workplace inspections and worker training.

The OSHAct also established the National Institute for Occupational Safety and Health (NIOSH) within the Centers for Disease Control (Department of Health and Human Services). NIOSH was assigned the task of researching the causes of occupational disease. During the 1970s, awareness of workplace diseases and the resources to deal with them increased, and the focus of industrial hygiene expanded beyond factories and mines to service industries and the corporate world. Industrial or occupational hygiene is now a discipline taught in many colleges and universities throughout the United States.

4. What are the educational requirements of an IH?

A bachelor degree is required, preferably in one of the basic sciences. Currently, most IHs have a Bachelor of Science (B.S.) or an engineering degree, and a Master of Industrial Health (M.I.H.) or a Master of Public Health (M.P.H.). The core curriculum for these degrees includes biostatistics, epidemiology, toxicology, principles of industrial hygiene, industrial processes, industrial ventilation, and physical hazards.

In addition, IHs may acquire a Certificate of Industrial Health (C.I.H.) by the American Board of Industrial Hygiene (ABIH). To be eligible to sit for the certification examination, a candidate must have a bachelor degree with 60 credits of science and 5 years of experience as a practicing IH. The examination takes place over two days and tests the candidate's knowledge in at least 10 areas of industrial hygiene science and practice.

Because the profession of industrial hygiene is not controlled by local or federal government (the ABIH is a private organization), nothing prevents a person from professionally designating him or herself as an "industrial hygienist," although the C.I.H. designation cannot be used legally in this context.

5. Where do IHs work and what do they do?

The majority of IHs work in private industry and for consulting firms. In private industry IHs manage health and safety programs, assess workers' exposures to hazards, recommend controls, and conduct employee training in health and safety issues. A smaller number work for insurance companies, local and federal government, trade unions, and as academics in colleges and universities. Governmental IHs engage in a range of activities depending on the agency for which they work and their function within the agency. Their activities may range from managing health and safety programs aimed at protecting agency employees to conducting research into possible work-related disease. Of course, the largest number of IHs in government are employed by OSHA and work mainly as compliance officers. IHs employed by trade unions conduct IH surveys for their members, develop and deliver member training, participate in contract negotiations, and represent the unions in congressional hearings and rulemaking procedures concerning relevant health and safety issues. Academic IHs teach and conduct research.

6. What are health and safety standards? How are they applied by IHs?

In general, health standards for chemical and physical agents (e.g., noise, vibration, heat, radiation) are levels of "contaminants" to which it is believed most workers may be exposed every day over a working lifetime without suffering ill health. Such levels were developed originally by private organizations of health and safety professionals and groups that recognized the importance of standards to which industry would voluntarily comply. The standards were developed mostly on the basis of human experience and animal experiments. One of the most important organizations developing occupational health standards is the American Conference of Governmental Industrial Hygienists (ACGIH). ACGIH standards, known as threshold limit values (TLVs), have gained international acceptance. In fact, when OSHA began in 1971, it adopted all of the then-current TLVs. The recommended TLVs then became permissible exposure limits (PELs)—legal limits enforceable by federal law. In addition to the PELs (exposure concentrations expressed in units of mg/mm^3 or parts of contaminant per million parts of air), some standards are more comprehensive, such as those for lead, asbestos, and vinyl chloride. Such standards contain details on methods of protecting workers with the use of proper clothing, respirators, medical tests, and training. A great deal of controversy exists concerning the levels at which the TLVs/PELs are set, with particular concern about inadequacies related to chronic disease protection. Many professionals in the public health community believe that TLVs/PELs represent a compromise between scientific knowledge and political expediency.

Because PELs are often interpreted as dividing lines between health and ill health, they play a dominant role in the practice of industrial hygiene. Although most IHs subscribe to the belief that exposures should be kept as low as feasible, the "as feasible" may often be defined by employers (i.e., from an economic standpoint). Because PELs refer to measurable quantities of contaminants, a great deal of IH practice is concerned with quantification of worker exposure. Over the past several decades, the advances in sampling and analytical methods have provided industrial hygiene with very sensitive tools for assessing occupational exposures.

7. Describe how a walk-through investigation and material safety data sheets (MSDSs) may be used by an IH to identify an exposure source.

Unless the problem is already known or is obvious (e.g., a leaking pipe), the first step is to identify the hazard. The main tool for hazard identification is the **walk-through investigation** of the worksite. During a careful inspection of all areas of the worksite, the IH searches for processes that may generate exposures such as grinding, sanding, heating, spraying, or degreasing. The hygienist observes workers on the job and focuses on questions such as:

• Are the exposures intermittent or continuous?
• Do workers in an enclosed space have adequate ventilation?
• Are workers wearing respiratory protection?
• Does the worksite reveal signs of potential problems, such as build-up of dust on machines or haze in the air?

Perhaps most importantly, the IH must talk to workers and other worksite personnel in order to identify particular problem areas or operations that are not immediately apparent.

The hygienist must attempt to determine the specific substances to which people are exposed, which may be chemical or physical hazards (e.g., noise, radiation) or biologic exposures. To evaluate potential chemical hazards, the hygienist gathers information by reading labels and **material safety data sheets (MSDSs)**. All manufacturers are required to have a MSDS on each product sold, and employers are required by OSHA to have them on file at the worksite. Although far from perfect, the MSDS provides product information, including chemical make-up, health effects, and required protective measures for handling. The information garnered from MSDSs are important clues in hazard recognition.

8. After the exposure source is identified, how is the severity of a problem evaluated and how are exposures quantified?

Quantification is accomplished by exposure assessment. There are many ways to assess exposures, and many kinds of exposures to assess. Most frequently, the IH is interested in assessing the exposure that a worker receives while he or she is performing his or her daily job during the total time spent on the job or performing a particular task. In order to measure exposure, the area surrounding the worker's mouth and nose (the "breathing zone") are assessed. Such measurements are referred to as **personal monitoring** or **assessment**. Monitoring is accomplished with the use of several simple devices: a small, belt-mounted, microprocessor-controlled sampling pump, which continuously draws air at a precalibrated flow rate through a sampling medium attached to the pump by means of a length of tygon tubing. The sampling medium, typically an adsorbent for gases and vapors such as activated charcoal and a filter for dusts, is sent to a laboratory for analysis of the particular contaminant(s) of interest. Over the past several decades, instrumentation for chemical analysis has improved greatly: it is possible to quantify contaminant concentration down to parts per billion.

IHs also have at their disposal a broad array of instruments that both sample and analyze a volume of air for contaminants. **Direct reading instruments** generally use a physical or chemical property of a contaminant to determine its concentration in air, such as its ability to conduct a current in solution, to absorb radiation of a particular wavelength, or to change color upon chemical reaction. Some direct reading instruments are used to obtain quick approximations of worker exposures during the walk-through investigation in order to determine if longer-term monitoring is necessary. Other direct reading instruments may be connected to alarms that alert workers to dangerous situations. They may be designed to test for one chemical or many. Some are so small that they can be held in the palm of the hand, whereas others require a large cart to be moved.

Hygienists also may take other types of samples that may reveal important potential sources of exposure by means other than inhalation. For instance, **wipe samples** are used to assess contamination on work surfaces or on skin. Workers may ingest contaminants if their hands come in contact with settled dust or if they eat food contaminated from contact with dusty surfaces. Additionally, settled dust may become airborne by air currents. Wipe samples of skin may help assess the presence of substances such as organic compounds (solvents) that are readily absorbed through the skin and into the systemic circulation. Occupational exposure limits refer only to airborne concentrations of substances and do not consider the potential for skin absorption. Therefore, it is important to characterize if and how much of a chemical may be deposited on the skin in order to fully assess a worker's exposure.

In addition to testing the air for contaminants, **exposures**, or more precisely, absorbed doses, may be assessed by measuring the quantity of contaminant (one of its metabolites) in the body. Most commonly, chemicals are measured in blood, urine, or exhaled air. For example, exposure to carbon monoxide may be measured by carbon monoxide in exhaled air or by measuring carboxyhemoglobin in a venous blood sample. Exposure to mercury may be assessed in urine, and exposure to benzene may be measured by phenol in urine. Although the measurement of biologic dose to assess exposure has its advantages, there are very few chemicals in common industrial use for which so-called biologic exposure indices have been developed. Also, it is not always practical or legally possible to obtain a biologic sample from a worker.

9. After the exposures have been quantified, what can be done to prevent worker exposure?

When IHs make recommendations about controlling workplace hazards, they are guided by a principle known as *hierarchy of controls*, in which engineering controls are the most desirable control methods because they eliminate or reduce the amount of hazard in the environment. **Engineering controls** include ventilation, process or equipment modification, process enclosure, substituting a safer chemical, dust reduction techniques, housekeeping, and hygiene practices. **Administrative controls** are used to reduce the number of workers exposed or to limit the length of time an individual is exposed to a hazard. However, they do not eliminate or reduce the amount of hazard in the workplace. Administrative controls include breaks and rest periods, changing the process to a different shift or location where fewer people are working, or job rotation. **Personal protective equipment** (respirators, gloves, goggles) reduce exposure for the individual worker. However, of the three types of controls they are the least desirable: they are uncomfortable, are often used improperly, and may fit poorly. When personal protective equipment must be worn in a workplace, it is important that an effective personal protective equipment program is in place so that workers are properly trained in using the equipment. Unless absolutely required by conditions, no safety and health program should be totally dependent on protective equipment.

10. How often do physicians work with IHs?

Except for occupational medicine physicians or physicians in charge of employee health at a company, most physicians do not interact at all with IHs in the course of their practice. Because physicians are not taught much about occupational diseases and have little practical experience in the area, they normally do not assess disease causation in terms of the chemical or physical hazards to which workers might be exposed. For example, if a worker sees a physician after an industrial accident and has lost an arm, the physician would probably conclude that loss of the arm is related to a machine or an adverse occupational condition. However, if a worker sees his or her physician with a kidney ailment, the physician may not think to inquire about the potential workplace exposures that may be implicated in the worker's condition.

11. Under what circumstances may an IH be of help to a physician in the diagnosis or treatment of a patient?

The following four case studies and resolutions illustrate various circumstances in which an IH may be of help to a physician:

1. A 28-year-old man visits his physician complaining of muscle aches, headaches, loss of appetite, periodic stomach cramps, and excessive tiredness. Although the patient is afebrile, the physician suspects a viral infection (flu), currently endemic to the area. Because the patient is a construction worker who works outdoors, the physician suggests bed rest and fluids for several days. The patient does improve after 3 days, and stays home another 2 days over the weekend and feels even better. On Monday, he returns to work. By Thursday the symptoms return. The physician is puzzled.

Believing that the patient's recurring illness may be related to a virus at work, the physician asked the worker whether other people he worked with are similarly stricken.The worker responded "yes," and added that one of his buddies had been tested for lead by a physician at an occupational medicine clinic. The physician has the worker tested and the results show that the worker's blood lead level is elevated. If an IH had been consulted in this case, he or she would have visited the construction worker's worksite, a bridge undergoing rehabilitation, and seen the following: during the walk-through, the IH observes iron workers performing many jobs that raise clouds of dust and plumes of smoke. The workers are using heavy pneumatic tools to remove rivets from the beams and paint from the surfaces. Some workers use oxyacetylene torches to cut through rusted beams. The IH realizes that the bridge is coated with thick layers of lead-based paint, which was commonly used for many years. The iron workers are being potentially exposed to high levels of inorganic lead dust.

In order to confirm his suspicion, the IH returns to the worksite equipped with monitoring instruments to assess the extent of worker exposure to lead. Breathing zone air samples are drawn over the course of the work shift from a number of workers performing representative tasks. The filters are sent to a laboratory for lead analysis. The results indicate that the workers are, in fact, overexposed to lead. After determining the cause of the problem, the IH recommends that the workers be fitted with the proper respiratory devices to prevent inhalation of lead, and that the contractor provide clean work clothes and wash stations for workers to wash their hands before eating to avoid taking lead dust home to their families and ingesting lead. In addition, a program of biologic monitoring for lead in blood has to be instituted in order to ensure that these measures are effective. The IH also recognizes that the problem has longer-range engineering solutions as well, such as tools equipped with vacuum cleaners to suck up generated dust before it can be inhaled.

2. A 40-year-old nurse living in a rural community visits her family physician complaining of fatigue, flu-like symptoms, and a bad cough. She is diagnosed as having the flu and bronchitis; an antibiotic and cough medicine are prescribed. The cough lasts for 2 weeks, but the fatigue persists. At one point, she suggests to her physician that she be tested for tuberculosis. However, her physician rejects the idea, saying that she exhibits none of the debilitating symptoms associated with tuberculosis (night sweats, coughing, weight loss) and that her fatigue is more likely due to her long working hours (14–16 hour days). Four months later, she is diagnosed with pneumonia. She then insists on being tested for tuberculosis. Her ppd (purified protein derivative) test is grossly positive. When the hospital infectious disease department tests the staff on her floor, nearly 40 people test positive.

Because of the public health risk, the hospital reported the problem to the Department of Health (DOH), which then investigated. In addition to experts in infectious disease, the DOH consulted two IHs, who reviewed the ventilation plans and took measurements to evaluate the ventilation patterns in the isolation room. Despite the ventilation specifications provided by the engineering department, they found that rooms are neither under negative pressure nor did they provide minimum air change rates as recommended by the Centers for Disease Control (CDC). In addition, staff had not been provided with the correct respiratory protection. The ventilation system in the newly designated "special procedures" room where sputum induction and bronchoscopies were performed was also under positive pressure, and ventilation rates were below recommended levels. Because of air flow patterns to the adjacent Geriatrics Department, the contact investigation was extended to staff and patients on that wing. Additional conversions were found. Eventually, one patient was identified (later diagnosed with multidrug resistance-TB) as the primary source of infection. The DOH recommended a complete overhaul of the hospital TB control program.

3. A 56-year-old man goes to his physician complaining of fatigue, nervousness, depression, recent lapses in memory, and almost daily headaches at work. The man's wife adds that on occasion her husband seems disoriented and unsure of where he is or what he is doing. The physician performs a clinical examination and clinically evaluates the man's mental status. The physician also orders blood and urine tests to assess possible toxic effects on the liver and kidneys and orders neuropychological testing to better characterize cognitive deficits.

Because the tests showed elevated liver enzymes and the patient did not drink alcohol, the physician suspected exposure to an exogenous agent. The neuropsychological testing battery indicated impairments consistent with a toxic encephalopathy in a number of intellectual performance areas. The physician learned that the patient has been employed for 20 years as a spray painter in a local metal fabrication shop. An IH was sent to investigate the conditions in the factory where the spray painter worked. In three large spray painting booths metal pieces were continuously sprayed by a hand-held spray gun. The spray-gun operator stood in the middle of a large booth that surrounded him on three sides. Large filters were placed on baffles at the booth interior surfaces. During spraying, paint from the gun ricocheted off of the objects being painted. The painter, the filters, and the surfaces in the interior of the booth were covered with paint. The whole area smelled of the organic compounds (solvents) used in the paints. Measurements of the ventilation system in the booth indicated that little or no ventilation was drawing the paint and its components away from the worker. Measurements of the concentration of organic vapors in the air confirmed that the operator was overexposed. It was not difficult for the physician and the IH to conclude that the patient's problems were most likely related to years of overexposure to the organic vapors.

4. Three employees who work in the same office go to a physician complaining of headaches, sore throats, and frequent bloody noses. Each employee states that the symptoms seem to get worse during the day and slowly subside after leaving work. Over the weekends the symptoms disappear completely.

To address the common complaints of the three employees, the physician notified the local health department of the problem, and the department sent an IH to investigate. The IH established that the office building in which the three employees worked was a ten-story modern structure that had been erected in the 1970s. Because the building had no windows that could be opened, all of the air supplied to the offices came through a large central air conditioning and heating system. A walk-through inspection of the patients' office revealed a newly renovated space outfitted with modern cubicle furnishings. Several of the air supply diffusers that brought air into the room were covered up. Employees in cubicles located under the diffusers said that the air was blowing directly on them, so they covered the vents with cardboard. The IH took several simple measurements with hand-held instruments: he measured the relative humidity, temperature, air velocity, and carbon dioxide in several areas of the rooms. The relative humidity readings revealed that the humidity was too low for comfort and could cause dryness of the skin and mucous membranes; the temperature readings showed that it was too warm in the room; the air velocity readings indicated that there were well ventilated areas in the room, but other areas were poorly ventilated; the carbon dioxide readings were elevated to levels associated with headaches. It did not take the IH long to determine that during the recent renovation of the office space, no thought was given to the position of the cubicles and their occupants in relation to the existing air supply and exhaust system. The IH also learned that the building management had set the air conditioning system to allow only a minimal amount of outside air to be brought into the building in order to save heating costs. Most of the air (and its contaminants) was being recirculated throughout the building. It was not difficult to fix the air conditioning problem: the system had to be adjusted to allow more air to enter from the outside. The general air supply system, however, was not as easily remedied, because the space had already been renovated, and the air supply system could not be easily moved without great disruption and expense.

12. In the case resolutions presented in question 11, the IH had access to each worksite. However, what if an IH is denied access to the worksite?

Not all employers willingly will allow an IH to investigate the workplace. Even OSHA inspectors, who are mandated by law to be admitted without delay into a workplace, are often denied entry by employers and must go to court to obtain a warrant, which is usually granted expeditiously. Ideally, the IH is able to gather the most information by observing the work environment. But much may be learned by indirect methods as well, such as talking to workers about how they do their job and what ingredients they use, asking about shared symptoms or complaints among coworkers, and reviewing product labels and MSDSs. The IH poses questions to identify high-risk processes or indicators of exposure. For example, he or she may inquire as to whether workers are engaged in activities such as grinding, sanding, chipping, or processes that generate a mist. Other questions may be aimed at learning whether surfaces are dust-laden, if and when strong or unusual odors occur, or whether workers have to shout to be heard.

13. Does the IH also participate in basic research to uncover the causes of work-related diseases?

Yes. One goal of epidemiologic studies is to determine if a correlation between an exposure to a chemical or physical agent and an adverse health outcome exists. Such studies seek to isolate the agent or agents responsible for adverse health and attempt to measure the relationship of the magnitude of exposure with the severity and/or rate of the disease. Assessment of the quality and quantity of exposure is one of the tasks of the IH. For retrospective epidemiologic studies involving exposures that have occurred in the past, the IH must reconstruct exposures from available evidence. On other occasions, the IH is part of a team studying a current disease occurrence. In this case, the IH participates in the design of exposure assessment protocols for worker monitoring. The design of such protocols is an important challenge to the IH, who often must combine a detailed knowledge of sampling and analytical methodologies, statistics, and the work process under investigation.

BIBLIOGRAPHY

1. Biological Exposure Indices: 1999 TLVs and BEIs. Threshold Limit Values for Chemical Substances and Physical Agents. Cincinnati, OH, ACGIH Worldwide, 1999.
2. Burgess WA: Recognition of Health Hazards in Industry: A Review of Materials and Processes, 2nd ed. New York, John Wiley & Sons, 1995.
3. Clayton GD, Clayton FE (eds): Paddy's Industrial Hygiene and Toxicology, 4th ed. New York, John Wiley, 1991.
4. Dinardi SR (ed):The Occupational Environment—Its Evaluation and Control. Fairfax, VA, AIHA Press, 1997.
5. Plog BA, Niland J, Quinlan PJ (eds): Fundamentals of Industrial Hygiene, 4th ed. Chicago, IL, National Safety Council, 1996.

5. A SHORT HISTORY OF OCCUPATIONAL HEALTH IN THE UNITED STATES

Michael R. Grey, M.D., M.P.H.

1. What is the essential impetus behind the history of occupational health in the U.S.?

Although the history of occupational health can be traced back to the ancients, in the United States the development of occupational disease was given enormous impetus by the Industrial Revolution. The advancement of occupational health and safety in the United States has typically been part of broader social reform movements, characterized by coalition politics and political compromise between labor and industry, catalyzed by tragic events, and spurred by heroic individuals. The medical profession has played an important role in disease definition and in framing the scientific debate, although ironically, and with some conscious effort, the evolution of a technically oriented discipline has resulted in the divergence of occupational health from mainstream medicine and medical care. As much as any medical and public health issue, the history of occupational health and safety provides clear evidence of Rudolph Virchow's observation that medicine is often politics writ small.

2. What social factors contributed to the recognition of work-related disease?

Although the sixteenth-century Italian physician, Ramazzini, is often cited as the "father of occupational medicine," occupational disease in the modern sense evolved in the aftermath of the Industrial Revolution of the nineteenth century. The nations' economy was rapidly transformed from dependence on small shops controlled by skilled guildsmen to a highly mechanized economy powered by an increasingly unskilled labor force with little influence over the conditions of work. Industrial growth was powered by successive waves of immigrants, urbanization, and the amassing of great fortunes in the hands of a new and influential capitalist class. This mechanization invariably generated workplace hazards that far exceeded those that were possible before wide-scale industrialization.

Along with these socioeconomic developments, a new medical and public health paradigm emerged. The bacteriologic revolution led to a deemphasis on environmental factors in health and disease in the belief that all disease could be linked to microbes. Before the spectacular successes of the bacteriologic revolution, according to medical historian Charles Rosenberg, "the body was seen, metaphorically, as a system of dynamic interactions with its environment. Health or disease resulted from a cumulative interaction between constitutional endowment and environmental circumstance." Despite the ascendancy of the biomedical model, however, labor and its allies continued to view occupational disease as an indication of a flawed social welfare system, thereby setting the stage on which political debate about occupational health and safety issues has been fought throughout the twentieth century.

3. What historical factors contributed to the creation of the workers' compensation system in the U.S.?

In the United States and abroad, occupational health and safety reform has characteristically advanced as part of larger social reform movements catalyzed at times by work disasters such as the deadly 1911 fire in New York City's Triangle Shirtwaist Factory. The movement toward occupational health and safety first gained significant momentum as part of the reformist spirit of the Progressive Era, an era imbued with a sense of volunteerism and benign paternalism mixed with antipathy toward the immigrant classes that swelled the nations' cities and created the urban slums. Immigration reached its peak at the turn of the century, and by 1900 nearly half of the population lived in cities compared with a mere 19% at the time of the Civil War. The segregation of immigrants in slums at best generated paternalism among social reformers who hoped to inculcate democratic values among the laboring classes. Not infrequently, however, such developments generated an intense backlash of fear that foreigners were an infecting nest of moral decay and disease.

During this era political and social forces coalesced along a broad range of social reforms. Ill-health was only part of a reform spirit focused on labor, education, suffrage, tenement reforms, and sweatshops. Reformers believed in better government by enlightened citizens and advocated legislative efforts at the state level on behalf of maternal and child health, child labor laws, pure food laws, and industrial health and safety. Inspired by Taylorism, the belief in the efficient use of resources within the capitalist system, many industrialists and patricians worked to remedy the most egregious excesses in industry in an effort to preserve the social order and maintain a healthy workforce. Although most reforms were national in scope, they were typically local in implementation. The federal government played a limited role; municipalities, local charities, and the growing list of industrial philanthropists worked in public and private partnership for social reform.

The advancement of occupational health and safety has frequently made strange bedfellows. For example, after the Triangle Shirtwaist Factory fire, a coalition of business, media, unions, and progressives formed a strong political force that merged radical and conservative elements to reform disastrous working conditions. The horrific working conditions of America's urban slum dwellers also provided ample opportunity for "muckraking" journalists to splash graphic descriptions of working conditions in newspapers across the land, spurring a sense of outrage among the middle classes and radicalism among the working classes in turn-of-the-century America.

Rarely have reform movements rested solely on humanitarian and moral grounds. Instead, the economic necessity of conserving human resources grew alongside the broader movement toward national conservation, as evidenced in President Theodore Roosevelt's creation of the National Parks System. Thus workers' safety and maternal and child health were linked to the early environmental movement, each viewed as a national treasure to be conserved out of both moral and economic necessity. Although socialists and other radical groups opposed the weight given to economic justifications, they worked successfully with less ideologically driven groups for incremental reforms such as workers' compensation.

By the turn of the century, the national economy truly was forged by urbanization and the growth of railroads. Workers had little protection if they were injured on the job and could resort only to the tort system to obtain redress for work-related conditions. However, the attention given by social reformers and the media to occupational issues led to increasing successes when workers sued their employers. Juries began to reject the historical precedent of individual culpability and gave huge awards to worker plaintiffs. Against this backdrop workers' compensation laws began to develop on a state-by-state basis from 1910 onward.

In 1900 there were no state-based workers' compensation laws, but within 15 years nearly all states had enacted such laws. The development of workers' compensation was a classic story involving coalition politics, yellow journalism, and compromise. Industrialists, upset at the growing public perception of industry as a death-dealing environment and feeling the economic coercion of unfavorable lawsuits, formed the National Safety Council in 1912 to establish minimal standards for industrial safety. Although the National Safety Council focused on individual responsibility and safety as opposed to the work environment and disease, it was a step forward. On the other end of the political spectrum, the American Association for Labor Legislation (AALL) was a coalition of labor leaders, corporate liberals, social reformers, and academics whose somewhat moderate goal was to achieve consensus between labor and capital in regard to health and safety legislation. The AALL adopted the motto, "Social Justice is the Best Insurance against Social Unrest," and played an important role in promoting workers' compensation laws and forcing the matchmaking industry to eliminate phosphorus, thereby stemming the epidemic of disfiguring "phossy jaw" among matchmakers. The AALL not only led the fight for workers' compensation but also fought to enact state-based universal health insurance programs. The latter effort foundered in the aftermath of the anti-German sentiment accompanying World War I and with the American Medical Association's withdrawal of support. The AALL also worked on behalf of the 8-hour work day and 6-day work week; child labor laws; a uniform reporting system for work injuries to collect accurate statistics; improved factory inspections; and, because of the strong association of tuberculosis with the laboring class, augmented efforts to control "the white plague" by improving home and work environments.

It was also an era of increased attention to food sanitation, as exemplified in the muckraking classic by Upton Sinclair, *The Jungle*, and the eventual passage of the Food and Drug Act. In 1910, New York City bakers went on strike to protest unsanitary working conditions. The union successfully linked unsanitary products with unsanitary conditions, generated enormous public sympathy, and rallied middle-class support for workplace reforms. The buying public needed little reminding about the possibility of infection by goods produced in slums; looking for the union label took on real meaning because union shops were viewed as more hygienic.

This important coalition broke down after the passage of workers' compensation, which was one of the few legislative efforts clearly in the best interest of both industry and labor. Workers' compensation was designed to limit employers' liability and to provide timely recompense for injured workers. Unfortunately, the appreciation of occupational disease was less than the appreciation of occupational injuries; to this day workers' compensation laws remain more accessible in injury cases.

4. What has been the historic role of industry in occupational health and safety?

For internal reasons American industry has been involved with medicine beyond its periodic participation in larger social reform movements and coalition politics, as demonstrated by the numerous and extensive development of both medical care and occupational medicine programs in numerous corporations dating before the turn of the century. The horrific injury rate in the booming railroad industry spawned a number of medical care plans and benefit associations. Similar efforts existed in many mining, manufacturing, and service companies, such as U.S. Steel, the Anaconda Mining Company, and Macy's, to name a few.

The important role played by the nascent insurance industry in the control of certain high-profile occupational disease provides a rare glimpse of the unfulfilled potential of the insurance industry in identifying and preventing occupational disease and injury. For example, in the 1920s and 1930s diligent field work by progressive actuaries working for Metropolitan Life and Prudential documented that silicosis remained prevalent despite the institution of "safe" dust levels. The epidemiologic evidence gathered by insurance company field workers helped to elucidate the complex interaction of silicosis with tuberculosis and defined a prototypical example of the multicausal etiology of chronic lung diseases among industrial workers.

Throughout the 1940s and 1950s occupational medicine matured into a full-fledged scientific discipline. Corporate medical departments and residency and fellowship training programs bloomed, and ancillary disciplines such as occupational health nursing, industrial hygiene, and vocational rehabilitation continued to evolve. Momentum was increased by the remarkable growth of the military-industrial complex and the development of the nuclear industry.

5. Why have the contributions of occupational and environmental factors to disease received so little attention in American medical education?

Changes in medical education and medical practice were gathering force in the aftermath of World War I. Increasing residency positions coincided with increasing centralization of care in hospitals and with specialty domination of medical practice in the hospital environment. The war gave impetus to such changes, which continued throughout the remainder of the century. In regard to occupational health and safety, the evolving dominance of specialists took the diagnosis of occupational disease out of the hands of general practitioners. Medical practitioners educated in the Progressive Era were certainly influenced by the attention given to occupational health issues and did not shy away from making occupational diagnoses in their patients. As Rosner and Markowitz demonstrated in their social history of silicosis, *Deadly Dust*, both industry and specialists tended to discount diagnoses made by general practitioners. Such attitudes were reflected in the medical literature about occupational disease, which virtually disappeared from journals most accessible to generalists. Instead, it increasingly appeared in specialty journals and was "remarkable in the dramatic difference in tone, argument, terminology, for its inaccessibility to lay people, its lack of clear class base, its abstractions from the human suffering it generally described, and its impersonality." Ironically, the profound economic collapse during the 1930s resulted in a "blurring of the line between health and welfare, disease and dependence." Thus, while Labor attempted to use occupational health issues as a means of achieving social welfare objectives, physicians, industry, and the newly emerging profession of industrial hygiene adopted increasingly technical definitions of industrial disease.

The medicalization of occupational disease during this period had other consequences as well. For example, this shift promoted a change in the manner in which research and prevention regarding occupational health and safety issues were funded. Beginning in the 1930s, occupational health programs were transferred out of departments of labor and into departments of health, where they typically remain today—a symbol that occupational disease is viewed primarily as a medical issue.

6. Who was Alice Hamilton? Why is she important?

Alice Hamilton (1869–1970) was a pioneering physician who first delved into the problem of occupational disease in 1908 when the governor of Illinois asked her to investigate industrial diseases in Illinois. Hamilton was a resident of Chicago's well-known Hull House and a friend of the famous social reformer, Jane Addams. Through her lifetime work of visiting industrial sites, evaluating workers, convincing management and legislators to take action, teaching and conducting research as the first woman faculty at Harvard Medical School, Hamilton played a critical role in the study and prevention of a wide range of industrial conditions, including the elimination of phosphorus in matches and the reduction of lead, mercury, benzene, trinitrotoluene, carbon dioxide, and carbon monoxide poisoning. Hamilton's profound influence on the nascent discipline of industrial hygiene (most early hygienists were, in fact, physicians and not engineers) and the importance of toxicology to occupational disease is eloquently detailed in her 1943 autobiography, *Exploring the Dangerous Trades*.

7. What was the impact of World War II on occupational medicine?

The profound impact of WWII on American society and industry cannot be overstated. The wage freeze enacted by Congress, the manpower shortages caused by the war, and prolabor legislation supported by President Franklin D. Roosevelt spurred the growth of unions, diversified the workforce, and forced industry to consider alternative means of attracting and maintaining its workforce. One consequence was the tremendous growth of employer-based health insurance, gained as part of the collective bargaining process. Although occupational health per se was not the generative force in this important development, the widespread availability of insurance—at least theoretically—has made it possible to advance the recognition and treatment of occupational diseases and injuries. Of greater importance, the severe labor shortages caused by the war forced both industry and the government to pay significantly more attention to occupational health issues than ever before. Indeed, the historical roots of current understanding of ergonomic issues can be traced directly to this period when protecting workers (be they bomber pilots or Rosie the Riveter) was at a premium.

8. What is OSHA? What factors led to its creation?

The tumultuous years of the 1960s saw the commencement of yet another push on behalf of worker health and safety, one that would eventually culminate in the 1971 passage of the Occupational Safety and Health Act (OSHAct). Once again, occupational health and safety advanced in the wake of both a broader reform spirit and tragedy. The reform movement of the 1960s initially embraced civil rights but in turn included the environmental, consumer, antiwar, and occupational health and safety movements. As with the infamous Triangle Shirtwaist Factory fire some 70 years earlier, occupational health catapulted into national consciousness after an explosion in a West Virginia coal mine that left 200 workers dead. The public furor that followed, along with a concerted and powerful push by the United Mine Workers of America and the AFL-CIO, prompted the rapid passage of the Coal Mine Health and Safety Act in 1969. Fresh from these successes, organized labor and public health and medical progressives, among others, organized a successful push for the 1971 OSHAct. Although frequently criticized on both ends of the political spectrum, Congress sweepingly declared that its purpose and policy was "to assure as far as possible every working man and woman in the nation safe and healthful working condition." OSHAct remains a landmark piece of social legislation and created the framework within which occupational health and safety issues are approached to the present day. The OSHAct also created the National Institute of Occupational Safety and Health (NIOSH) within the U.S. Public Health Service, which has a research and technical advisory role for OSHA. Lastly, the development in the 1970s of the Committees on Occupational Safety and Health (COSH) was part of a broader grassroots movement that touched on a number of other areas, including environmental, women's, and consumer issues.

9. What are the important agencies involved in environmental health issues? What factors led to their creation?

The 1970s and 1980s have seen the ascension of environmental concerns over workplace health issues by a public mobilized to demand a healthier environment. Catastrophic events such as Love Canal, Three Mile Island, Bhopal, and Chernobyl have heightened the public's awareness of the interconnection between work, environmental contamination, and health. In the 1970s Congress took an active role in environmental regulation with the passage of the Clean Air Act (1970) and the Clean Water Act (1972), which set standards for airborne emissions and air pollution and industrial effluents and drinking water, respectively. The Resource Conservation and Recovery Act (RCRA, 1976), and the Comprehensive Environmental Response, Compensation and Liability Act (CERCLA, 1980)—sometimes referred to as the Superfund act—are the two main federal laws responsible for dealing with land disposal practices and clean-up. From the CERCLA legislation, the Agency for Toxic Substances and Disease Registry (ATSDR) was created to prevent or mitigate adverse human health effects from environmental hazards. Both NIOSH and ATSDR have taken active roles in supporting educational efforts for medical and public health professionals.

BIBLIOGRAPHY

1. Hamilton A: Exploring the Dangerous Trades: The Autobiography of Alice Hamilton. Boston, Little, Brown, 1943.
2. Rosner D, Markowitz G: Deadly Dust: Silicosis and the Politics of Occupational Disease in Twentieth Century America. Princeton, NJ, Princeton University Press, 1991.
3. Sellars CC: Hazards of the Job: From Industrial Disease to Environmental Health Science. Chapel Hill, NC, University of North Carolina Press, 1997.

II. Hazards

6. HEALTH HAZARDS OF SOLVENTS

Elizabeth A. Katz, M.P.H., C.I.H., and James E. Cone, M.D., M.P.H.

1. What are solvents?

The term *solvents* generally refers to organic compounds that are effective in dissolving other substances. They exist as liquids and gases (the gases are termed *vapors* if the solvent is liquid at room temperature). Most, but not all, have significant volatility, odor, and toxicity. Solvents are available as individual compounds, mixtures (such as gasoline and paint thinner), and constituents of tradename products. Many solvents are organic hydrocarbons, which are lipophilic. As a result, the most common manifestations of toxicity involve the skin, liver, and peripheral and central nervous systems.

2. What types of work involve significant solvent exposure?

Solvents are widely used in industry, including manufacturing, agriculture, construction, and service work. They are frequently found in paints, inks, and other coatings; adhesives; spray products; pesticide formulations; and cleaners, paint strippers, and degreasers. Liquid fuels, chlorofluorocarbon refrigerants, anesthetic gases, and dry-cleaning fluids are composed of solvents. Significant solvent exposure is often found in the following industries:

- Painting
- Printing
- Carpet and tile laying
- Furniture assembly and refinishing
- Vehicle, ship, and machinery repair
- Dry cleaning
- Maintenance
- Various manufacturing and assembly jobs

Serious confined-space incidents often involve volatile solvents. When workers enter tanks or holds in order to clean, paint, or empty them of remaining contents, they may be overcome by high levels of solvent vapor.

3. What health effects are associated with solvent exposure?

Short-term, low-level airborne exposure to most common organic hydrocarbon solvents may cause symptoms such as mild skin irritation, headache, dizziness, feeling of intoxication, nausea, visual disturbances, and/or eye, nose, and throat irritation. Higher-level exposure may cause disorientation, confusion, difficulty in concentrating, diarrhea, vomiting, shortness of breath, and fatigue. At very high levels, solvents may reduce the threshold for seizure activity and cause cardiac arrhythmias and/or central nervous system depression, leading to coma and ultimately death.

Long-term dermal exposure to organic hydrocarbon solvents has been associated with an increased risk of defatting and cracking of skin, rashes, and more rapid absorption of other chemicals. The effects of long-term inhalation or ingestion of organic hydrocarbon solvents are listed in the table below.

Health Effects of Solvent Exposure

ORGAN SYSTEM	MANIFESTATION	EXAMPLES
Central nervous system	Memory loss, confusion, difficulty in concentrating, fatigue, and chronic headache	Toluene, xylene, jet fuel, naphtha

Table continued on following page.

Health Effects of Solvent Exposure

ORGAN SYSTEM	MANIFESTATION	EXAMPLES
Peripheral nervous system	Numbness and tingling of extremities	*n*-Hexane, methyl ethyl ketone, 1,1,1-trichloroethane
Cranial nerves	Facial numbness Acquired loss of color vision Blindness	Trichloroethylene Styrene Methanol (by ingestion)
Gastrointestinal system	Fatty liver, chemical hepatitis	Xylene, 2-nitropropane
Renal system	Glomerulonephritis	Aromatic hydrocarbons
Hematologic system	Aplastic anemia, leukemia Anemia	Benzene Ethylene glycol ethers
Reproductive systems	Miscarriages Fetal alcohol syndrome	Glycol ethers Ethanol (by ingestion)

4. What is chronic toxic encephalopathy?

Chronic toxic encephalopathy (CTE) refers to the persistent symptoms of headache, dizziness, fatigue, difficulty in concentrating, confusion and short-term memory loss associated with long-term exposures to toxic agents such as organic hydrocarbon solvents and lead or other heavy metals. It also may be called painter's syndrome if diagnosed in a solvent-exposed worker. CTE caused by exposure to solvents involves three recognized stages, as described by the World Health Organization:

Type I: Symptoms alone
Type II: Symptoms and either mood disturbance (Type IIA) or cognitive changes noted on neuropsychological testing (Type IIB)
Type III: Frank dementia

Physical examination of a person suspected of having CTE should include a careful mental status examination with, at a minimum, serial 7s, digit span, and short-term memory testing. If symptoms of memory loss, difficulty in concentrating, headache, or fatigue are accompanied by any abnormality in mental status testing, formal neuropsychologic testing is most likely necessary.

5. What is the prognosis for CTE due to solvent exposure?

Some patients with CTE due to solvents may report symptomatic improvement with avoidance of further neurotoxic exposure, although often they show persistent decline in cognitive function as measured by standard neuropsychological tests. Cognitive retraining (a method of improving memory function through specific exercises) may be helpful in some cases.

6. What medical conditions may increase the risk from exposure to solvents?

• Preexisting ischemic heart disease (methylene chloride is metabolized to carbon monoxide)
• Alcoholism, alcoholic hepatitis
• Acute or chronic hepatitis
• Chronic cardiac arrhythmias
• Seizure disorder

7. Can other substances be substituted for hazardous solvents?

Yes. The popularity of latex paints, as substitutes for traditional paints using solvent vehicles, has greatly decreased organic solvent exposure among painters and construction workers. Water-based inks are widely used by printers, and various water-based adhesives, degreasers, coatings, and paint strippers are available. Besides water-based formulations, alternative, presumably safer solvents are often used to replace highly flammable or toxic solvents. However, there is a real danger that the substitute material will introduce new hazards. Examples include glycol ethers used in many latex-based paints (hematologic and reproductive toxin), d-limonene (allergic contact dermatitis), and caustic paint strippers (skin and eye burns). Historically, chlorinated solvents replaced flammable hydrocarbons; then chlorinated solvents became undesirable because of toxicity problems. Studies continue to discover health effects of traditional and newly popular solvents. Therefore, substitute materials should be evaluated carefully for physical hazards and toxic properties of solvent and nonsolvent ingredients.

8. Can ventilation be used to control exposures?

Local mechanical ventilation is a highly effective method of controlling solvent vapors. General mechanical ventilation may be effective, depending on the volume of air that may be exhausted and directional flow away from workers' breathing zones. Advantages of mechanical ventilation compared with respirators generally include much higher reliability of vapor control; greater worker comfort and efficiency; fewer worker compliance problems; and fewer regulatory requirements. In field work (e.g., construction, shipyard work) portable blowers may be helpful.

9. What training and information should be made available?

Clear labeling of containers, readily accessible material safety data sheets, and regular safety meetings are essential for solvent workers. Proper work methods, use of protective equipment, health hazards, and flammability hazards should be communicated.

10. What protective clothing can be used?

Glove materials must be selected for resistance to specific solvents and other chemicals that are handled. Sources of glove performance data include the glove manufacturer and the *American Conference of Governmental Industrial Hygienists Guidelines for the Selection of Chemical Protective Clothing*. Goggles, aprons, and coveralls may be necessary for some solvent jobs.

11. How useful are respirators for protection against solvent exposure?

Use of respirators for solvents is subject to many potential pitfalls, including improper selection of equipment, leakage and fit problems, and poor maintenance. In addition, certain problems apply specifically to the use of filter respirators for solvents:

1. Casual use of organic vapor solvent respirators purchased at hardware stores by small businesses or construction workers is often ineffective.

2. Organic vapor filters, made of activated charcoal, are often assumed to be appropriate for all types of organic solvent vapors. In fact, they are useful for a broad range of solvents but ineffective for methanol and methyl chloride. Organic vapor filters are also ineffective for formaldehyde (sometimes considered to be a solvent), except those specifically labeled for such use. In addition, solvents with poor warning odor are unsafe to use with filter respirators; an odor is essential to warn the user of cartridge breakthrough or face-seal leakage. Commonly used solvents with poor warning odor include methylene chloride, styrene, and chlorofluorocarbons.

3. Olfactory fatigue is an insidious problem in solvent work. Failure to detect solvent odor leads to continued use of poorly functioning respirators.

4. The life of an organic vapor filter is variable and difficult to predict from the manufacturer's data. High humidity (> 50%) substantially decreases filter capacity. Furthermore, filters last longer in an unchanging test environment than in a typical work environment, where vapor concentrations vary substantially over time. Breathing resistance does not change noticeably when the filter is saturated with moisture or solvent.

12. What are the reproductive effects of solvents?

Toluene abuse (glue sniffing or huffing) and heavy alcohol use during pregnancy are associated with specific birth defect syndromes. We do not know whether safe levels of exposure to organic hydrocarbon solvents during pregnancy can be determined. Occupational reproductive toxicity of solvents (with the exception of glycol ethers) has not been conclusively demonstrated in the absence of maternal toxicity, although it has been shown that pregnant women absorb 50% compared with 10% absorption by nonpregnant women. Solvent exposure, therefore, should be minimized during pregnancy because of epidemiologic evidence suggesting that prevalent levels of maternal and paternal occupational solvent exposure may increase the risk of fetal harm.

Glycol ether solvents appear to increase the risk of miscarriage in women, even when no toxic symptoms are present. They have been shown to cause birth defects in animals. The table below lists the chemical names, abbreviations, and synonyms of industrially important glycol ethers. In general, these compounds are easily absorbed through the skin.

Common Glycol Ethers

COMMON NAME	ABBREVIATION	CHEMICAL NAME
Ethylene glycol monomethyl ether	EGME	2-Methoxyethanol
Ethylene glycol monomethyl ether acetate	EGMEA	2-Methoxyethyl acetate
Ethylene glycol monoethyl ether	EGEE	2-Ethoxyethanol
Ethylene glycol monoethyl ether acetate	EGEEA	2-Ethoxyethyl acetate
Ethylene glycol monopropyl ether	EGPE	2-Propoxyethanol
Ethylene glycol monobutyl ether	EGBE	2-Butoxyethanol
Ethylene glycol dimethyl ether	EGDME	1,2-Dimethoxyethane
Ethylene glycol diethyl ether	EGDEE	1,2-Diethoxyethane
Diethylene glycol	DEG	
Diethylene glycol monomethyl ether	DEGME	2-(2-Methoxyethoxy)ethanol
Diethylene glycol monoethyl ether	DEGEE	2-(2-Ethoxyethoxy)ethanol
Diethylene glycol monobutyl ether	DEGBE	2-(2-Butoxyethoxy)ethanol
Diethylene glycol dimethyl ether	DEGDME	Bis(2-methoxyethyl)ether
Triethylene glycol dimethyl ether	TEGDME	
Propylene glycol monomethyl ether	PGME	1-Methoxy-2-propanol
Propylene glycol monomethyl ether acetate	PGMEA	
Dipropylene glycol	DPG	
Dipropylene glycol monomethyl ether	DPGME	

13. Which solvents are carcinogenic?

Only benzene has been shown to be a human carcinogen (causing leukemia). Based on animal data, several other solvents are suspected human carcinogens, including methylene chloride, carbon tetrachloride, chloroform, dioxane, perchloroethylene, and dimethylformamide.

BIBLIOGRAPHY

1. Aksoy M: Leukemogenic and carcinogenic effects of benzene. Ad Mod Environ Toxicol 16:87–99, 1989.
2. Baker EL: A review of recent research on health effects of human occupational exposure to organic solvents. J Occup Med 36:1079–1092, 1994.
3. Bolla KI, Schwartz BS, Stewart W, et al: Comparison of neurobehavioral function in workers exposed to a mixture of organic and inorganic lead and in workers exposed to solvents. Am J Indust Med 27:231–246, 1995.
4. Broadwell DK, Darcey DJ, Hudnell HK, et al: Work-site clinical and neurobehavioral assessment of solvent-exposed microelectronics workers. Am J Indust Med 27:677–698, 1995.
5. Burton RC, Upfal MJ: Screening for occupational-related diseases. Primary Care 21:249–266, 1994.
6. Crump KS: Rick of benzene-induced leukemia: A sensitivity analysis of the Pliofilm cohort with additional follow-up and new exposure estimates. J Toxicol Environ Health 42:219–242, 1994.
7. Katz EA, Shaw GM, Schaffer DM: Exposure assessment in epidemiologic studies of birth defects by industrial hygiene review of maternal interviews. Am J Indust Med 26:1–11, 1994.
8. Morrow LA, Steinhauer SR, Ryan CM: The utility of psychophysiological measures in assessing the correlates and consequences of organic solvent exposure. Toxicol Indust Health 10:537–544, 1994.
9. National Institute of Occupational Safety and Health: Worker Deaths in Confined Spaces. A Summary of Surveillance Findings and Investigative Case Reports. Cincinnati, National Institute of Occupational Safety and Health, U.S. Department of Health and Human Services, DHHS(NIOSH) Publication No. 94–103, 1994.
10. Sallmen M, Lindbohm M-L, Kyyronen P, et al: Reduced fertility among women exposed to organic solvents. Am J Indust Med 27:699–713, 1995.

7. FUNDAMENTALS OF PESTICIDES

John E. Midtling, M.D., M.S.

1. What is a pesticide?

Pesticides are defined under the Federal Insecticide, Fungicide, and Rodenticide Act (FIFRA) as "any substance or mixture of substances intended for preventing, destroying, repelling or mitigating any pest."

2. What are the clinically most important pesticides?

Inorganic compounds
- Methyl bromide

Botanicals
- Cypermethrin
- Permethrin
- Pyrethrum
- Rotenone

Chlorinated hydrocarbons
- DDT (dichlorodiphenyltrichlorethane)
- Dieldrin
- Methoxychlor

Organic phosphorous compounds
- Chlorpyrifos
- Demeton
- Diazinon
- Dichlorvos
- Malathion
- Mevinphos
- Parathion
- Phosphamidon
- Trichlorphon

Carbamates
- Aldicarb
- Carbaryl
- Carbofuran
- Thiodicarb

Phenols
- DNOC (dinitroorthocresol)
- Pentachlorophenol

3. Which is a better test of acute toxicity of organophosphates: red blood cell (RBC) cholinesterase or serum cholinesterase?

Organophosphate and carbamate pesticides bind and lower cholinesterase. Serum cholinesterase is affected by liver disease. RBC cholinesterase is subject to much less variation than plasma cholinesterase. Serum cholinesterase is the first to be elevated in acute poisoning. When pesticide exposure is suspected, sequential values of red blood cell cholinesterase should be obtained to determine a return to individual baseline levels and therefore evidence of depression; a high degree of variability in red blood cell cholinesterase may be seen within a normal range. Return of RBC cholinesterase to baseline levels following acute exposure may take several weeks.

4. Which pesticide metabolites can be measured in urine? When would this be useful to check?

DDA (dideoxyadenosine), a metabolite of DDT, was the first excretory product of pesticides detected in urine. Dieldrin, as well as a wide range of the chlorinated hydrocarbon insecticides, also is detectable in urine. Organophosphate metabolites also may be detected in urine by measuring for alkylphosphate metabolites. Although not metabolically specific, these metabolites can be used to determine the degree of exposure to organophosphates. Carbamate metabolites, including malathion, also may be detected in urine.

5. When did the organophosphate pesticides originate?

Organophosphate pesticides were developed as toxic nerve gases to be used during World War II.

6. What are the symptoms of acute organophosphate poisoning?

Signs and symptoms of acute organophosphate poisoning are secondary to cholinesterase inhibition. Symptoms include headache, difficulty concentrating, nervousness, blurred vision, weakness, nausea, cramps, and diarrhea. Signs include sweating, miosis, tearing, salivation, and vomiting. Severe signs include cyanosis, papilledema, muscle twitching and weakness, convulsions, and coma.

7. What are the potential delayed effects of acute organophosphate poisoning?

Delayed effects may include anxiety, depression, sleep disturbance, disturbance in memory and concentration, and visual disturbance, including alteration in color vision.

8. What are the chronic effects of acute organophosphate exposure?

Some pesticides, such as chlorpyrifos, can cause polyneuropathy secondary to demyelination and axonal degeneration.

9. How do the symptoms and signs of carbamate poisoning differ from those of organophosphate poisoning?

The symptoms and signs of carbamate poisoning are similar to organophosphate poisoning, but are generally milder and less prolonged.

10. When should atropine and/or pralidoxime be administered in cases of acute organophosphate poisoning?

In serious cases of organophosphate poisoning, atropine (2–4 mg) is given intravenously and repeated at 5–10 minute intervals until atropinization occurs. Pralidoxime (1 gm) is given by slow intravenous route if the patient does not respond satisfactorily to atropine.

11. Often pyrethrins are mixed with other agents for their synergistic effects. Are the health effects also synergistic on humans?

Pyrethrins, extracts of the chrysanthemum flower, are generally combined with a synergist and used in sprays and aerosols against a variety of flying insects. Certain compounds may increase the toxicity of pyrethrins to insects by as much as 100 times. In terms of historical development, current use, and the number of active compounds, the methylenedioxyphenolic compounds are of greatest importance as synergists. Some synergists act by enhancing or prolonging insect flight, making aerosol use more effective. Others interfere with the detoxification of the pesticide by insects; they may act through inhibition of microsomal enzymes.

Inhibition of microsomal enzymes may inhibit the ability of mammalian species to detoxify carcinogenic substances. Synergists such as piperonyl butoxide have their own toxic effects, such as anorexia, watery eyes, irritability, prostration, cancer, and even death. Synergized pyrethrins are more likely to cause necrosis of liver cells.

12. Which pesticides are a common cause of occupational asthma?

Pyrethrins are a common cause of asthma. Other common agents include DDVP-Baygon, dieldrin, as well as a variety of petroleum distillate vehicles.

13. Who is at greatest risk for pesticide-related dermatitis? Which pesticides are most likely to cause dermatitis?

Pesticide-related dermatitis is an occupational hazard for mixers, applicators, manufacturers, and formulators. Common agents that cause dermatitis include pyrethrins, nicotine, quassia, chloropicrin, randox, dazomet, acrylonitrile, rotenone, lindane, captan, captafol, maneb, zineb, PCNB (pentachloronitrobenzene), benomyl, dinobuton, dithrinone, nitrofen, p-chlorobenzene and delt.

14. Which pesticides have been linked with reproductive toxicity?

Reproductive toxicity has been linked to benzene hexachloride (BHC), lindane, aldrin, dichlorodiphenyldichloroethylene (DDE), DDD, DDT, methyl parathion, dichlorophenoxyacetic acid (2,4-D), trichlorophenoxyacetic acid (2,4,5-T), and 2,3,7,8-Tetrachlorodibenzo *p*-dioxin (TCDD).

15. What solvents are commonly used in combination with pesticides?

Common solvents include carbon tetrachloride, dichloromethane, dichlorodifluoromethane, 1,3-dichloropropene, epoxyethane, tetrachloroethylene, trichloroethane, trichloroethylene, xylene, and benzene.

16. How do the health effects of combined solvent and pesticide exposure typically present?

In some cases the pesticidally inert ingredient constitutes the major hazard to human health. Depression of bone marrow, sudden death from cardiac arrhythmias or narcosis are problems consistent with solvent exposure. Fullness of the head, headache, blurred vision, dizziness, unsteady gait, nausea, nervous twitching, and collapse are signs of narcotic-like action and solvent exposure.

17. Which herbicides were contaminated with dioxins?

Herbicides such as 2,4,5-T and 2,4-D were contaminated with dioxin.

18. Which pesticide residues on foods may adversely affect children?

Organochlorine pesticides are of particular concern; they have a long half-life and tend to accumulate in fatty tissue and bone.

19. Which U.S. federal and state agencies regulate pesticides?

The United States Food and Drug Administration (FDA) enforces pesticide residue tolerances established by the Environmental Protection Agency (EPA) for food products. The EPA was given the authority to set standards of public protection under the Federal Insecticide, Fungicide, and Rodenticide Act (FIFRA). FIFRA established a system for pesticide registration. A 1972 amendment established consideration of risk offered by each material a prime requirement for registration. FIFRA established worker safety guidelines, including "re-entry times," for various pesticides. The Occupational Safety and Health Act (OSHAct) is designed to ensure that every workplace is free from recognized hazards that are likely to cause death or serious physical harm. An executive order established that the EPA is also responsible for agricultural worker protection.

With the exception of Alaska, all states require registration of pesticides prior to their use. For example, California has a program that joins county agricultural commissioners with the California Department of Food and Agriculture to oversee the pesticide use. The Birth Defect Prevention Act (CA, 1984) requires the California Department of Food and Agriculture to review chronic toxicity studies that support the registration of pesticides. The California Department of Health Services is an advisory agency with respect to pesticides. The Structural Pest Control Board is responsible for the licensing and regulation of commercial structural pest control operators. The Department of Industrial Relations enforces health and safety guidelines.

20. What influence do international regulatory bodies have on pesticide regulation?

The United Nations Food and Agriculture Organization (FAO) has published a set of guidelines for legislation that outline processes for registration of pesticides. These recommendations were reviewed and endorsed by the International Labor Office (ILO) and the World Health Organization (WHO). Through the Agency for International Development (AID), the United States has attempted to promote training in developing countries that use pesticides.

21. What are the active ingredients of common household pesticides?

Pesticides are commonly used in homes and gardens. Carbamates and pyrethrins are commonly used for home flea control and garden use.

22. How toxic are household pesticides to children? How common are pesticide poisonings in the home?

When improperly used or stored, household pesticides can be quite toxic to children. Poisonings that result from improper application, accidental ingestion, or improper storage are increasingly commonplace. Proper use, storage, and disposal of home-use pesticides are essential.

BIBLIOGRAPHY

 1. Adams RM: Pesticides and other agricultural chemicals. In Adams RM (ed): Occupational Skin Disease. New York, Grune and Stratton, 1983.
 2. Barnett PG, Midtling JE: Educational intervention to prevent pesticide induced illness of fieldworkers. J Fam Pract 10:123–125, 1984.
 3. Clayton GD, Clayton FE (eds): Patty's Industrial Hygiene and Toxicology, Vol. 2. New York , John Wiley & Sons, 1982.
 4. Coye MJ, Barnett PG, Midtling JE: Clinical confirmation of organophosphate poisoning of agricultural workers. Am J Ind Med 10:339–409, 1986.
 5. Coye MJ, Barnett PG, Midtling JE: Clinical confirmation of organophosphate poisoning with sequential cholinesterase analyses. Arch Intern Med 147:438–442, 1987.
 6. Duncan RC, Griffith J: Monitoring study of urinary metabolites and selected symptomatology among Florida citrus workers. J Toxicol Environ Health 16:509–521, 1985.
 7. Environmental Protection Agency (EPA): Chemicals Registered for the First Time as Pesticidal Active Ingredients under FIFRA. Office of Pesticide Programs, U.S. EPA, Washington, D.C.,1988.
 8. Hayes WJ, Laws ER (eds): Handbook of Pesticide Toxicology. San Diego, Academic Press, 1991.
 9. Jacobziner H: Causes, control and prevention of accidental poisonings. Public Health Rep 81:31–42, 1966.
10. Klaasen CD (ed): Casarett and Doull's Toxicology: The Basic Science of Poisons, 5th ed. New York, McGraw-Hill, 1996.
11. Loumis TA: Essentials of Toxicology. Philadelphia, Lea & Febiger, 1978.
12. Midtling JE, Barnett PG: Clinical management of fieldworker organophosphate poisoning. West J Med 142:14–18, 1985.
13. Midtling JE: Acute poisoning following exposure to an agricultural insecticide. MMWR 34:464–471, 1985.
14. Midtling JE: Comments on persistence of symptoms after mild to moderate acute organophosphate poisoning. J Toxicol Environ Health 13:91, 1984.
15. Romero P, Midtling JE: Congenital anomalies associated with maternal exposure to oxydemeton-methyl. Environ Res 50:256–261, 1989

8. CHLORINE AND ORGANOCHLORINE COMPOUNDS

Mary A. Ross, Ph.D., and Peter Orris, M.D., M.P.H.

1. Discuss the importance of exposure to chlorine and chloramines.

Chlorine is widely used in household cleaners, disinfection, and industrial chemical production; it is one of the most common exposures in both the workplace and nonoccupational settings. In 1982, the World Health Organization (WHO) estimated an annual global industrial use of about 25 million tons of chlorine and a predicted annual growth rate of 4.5%. According to recent estimates, 69% of industrial chlorine was used for chemical production, 18% in the pulp and paper industry, and 6% in sanitation. Chlorine gas exposure also may occur in swimming pools or households when bleach is mixed with acidic cleaners, such as sodium acid sulfate (acid drain cleaner). Chloramine gas can be produced by mixing bleach with basic cleaners (such as lye-based drain cleaner).

Exposure to chlorine or chloramines is one of the most common complaints in poison centers. A compilation by the American Association of Poison Control Centers of reports from 65 poison control centers in 39 states includes almost 204,000 cases of human exposures to cleaning products in 1994, which represent 10% of all reported poisoning incidents. In one survey of workers at a pulp mill in Canada, 257 workers reported an average of 24 exposure episodes to chlorine and derivatives over a 3–6 month period.

2. What are the acute health effects of exposure to chlorine or chloramines?

The signs and symptoms of chlorine or chloramine exposure include cough, shortness of breath, throat irritation, chest pain, wheezing, dizziness, vomiting, ocular irritation, nasal irritation, and abdominal pain. Pulmonary parenchymal damage may occur within 10 minutes of exposure, and hyperchloremic acidosis may result. The effects of chlorine-related exposure are usually temporary and can be treated with fresh air and liquids; symptoms typically resolve within 6 hours. In a survey of 216 patients, only 16 had symptoms for more than 6 hours after exposure; 1 patient with a preexisting chronic respiratory problem was admitted for continued respiratory distress. The symptoms from occupational exposures are similar to those in household exposures; however, 60% of pulp mill workers described a flulike syndrome that lasted for an average of 11 days and was exacerbated by new bouts of exposure.

3. What are the chronic health effects associated with exposure to chlorine or chloramines?

Although exposure to chlorine or chloramines results primarily in acute symptoms that resolve within a matter of hours, persistent respiratory symptoms have been reported as a result of occupational or household uses, particularly in persons with preexisting respiratory diseases. These persistent respiratory effects include asthma and reactive airways dysfunction syndrome as well as several case reports of emphysema.

The use of chlorine or chloramines for disinfection of drinking water supplies or swimming pools also results in the formation of halogenated compounds, such as chloroform, that are suspected to be carcinogenic. Numerous studies have indicated associations between consumption of chlorinated drinking water and cancers of the bladder, rectum, or colon. In a recent metaanalysis, consumption of chlorinated water was significantly associated with a 1.21-fold increase in risk of bladder cancer (for both mortality and incidence studies). Exposure to chloroform and similar compounds in chlorinated water may occur via the skin or inhalation during showers or baths as well as through ingestion of chlorine-treated water; according to some studies, the total internal dose from showering or bathing exceeds that from tap water ingestion.

4. Define organochlorine compounds.

The group of chemicals commonly known as organochlorines is a subset of all chlorinated hydrocarbons. The term is used to describe chlorinated hydrocarbons that are lipophilic and thus accumulate in the environment and in biota. Common examples are polychlorinated dibenzodioxins (dioxins or PCDDs), polychlorinated dibenzofurans (furans or PCDFs), polychlorinated biphenyls (PCBs), and some pesticides, such as dichlorodiphenyltrichloroethane (DDT), dieldrin, and chlordane.

5. Discuss the significance of dioxins and furans.

Dioxins and furans are produced as byproducts from the manufacture or combustion of organic compounds with chlorine; they have no known industrial use. Dioxins were a contaminant of the herbicide 2,4,5-T, a component of Agent Orange, which was used to defoliate forested areas during the Vietnam War. Dioxins and furans are produced when chlorine is used in the bleaching process in pulp and paper mills, and furans are generated during the combustion of PCBs. Incineration of municipal, medical, and hazardous wastes may also result in dioxin or furan production; global emissions from these combustion processes are estimated at 3000 kg/year. There are 75 different PCDDs and 135 PCDFs. The prototype of the dioxins is 2,3,7,8-tetrachlorodibenzo-p-dioxin (TCDD), which is considered to be the most toxic of the dioxins. Scientists have derived a toxic equivalent (TEQ) method to relate the toxic effects of other dioxinlike chemicals to those of TCDD. Using data from the National Human Adipose Tissue Survey (NHATS), Orban et al. (1994) found a mean level of 5.38 ppt TCDD in the U.S. general population and a mean level of dioxinlike compounds, expressed as TEQs, of 27.9 ppt (ng/kg).

6. Discuss the significance of PCBs.

Commercial production of PCBs began in the U.S. in 1929; an estimated 1.2 million tons of PCBs have been produced worldwide. The 209 different PCBs were sold as mixtures under trade names such as Arochlor and Kanechlor. Their chemical stability, low flammability, and insulating properties resulted in their widespread use in electrical transformers and capacitors, as flame retardants and lubricating and hydraulic oils, and for many other industrial uses. However, concern about health effects and the longevity of PCBs in living organisms and the environment prompted reinvestigation, and in 1976 the U.S. Congress banned the use of PCBs with passage of the Toxic Substances Control Act. PCB concentrations in ambient air range from 0.8–10 ng/m^3; in soil or sediment average levels are less than 10–40 mg/kg, although soil levels up to 500 mg/kg have been found in polluted areas. Because of their potential to accumulate in fatty tissues, PCBs can be found in food items at levels of 20–240 µg/kg in animal fat, 5–200 µg/kg in cow's milk, or 10–500 µg/kg in the fat of fish.

7. Discuss the significance of organochlorine pesticides.

Organochlorine pesticide production began in the 1940s with DDT and similar compounds and increased dramatically through the 1950s. These insecticides were used commonly because they were inexpensive to produce, had low acute mammalian toxicity, and were effective in killing insects. However, concern about their persistence in the environment, damage to wildlife species, and potential harm to human health caused public health officials to reevaluate their uses. In the U.S., most of the persistent organochlorine pesticides have been banned from use or voluntarily removed from the market by their manufacturer—DDT in 1972, dieldrin in 1974, benzene hexachloride in 1978, aldrin in 1987, and chlordane in 1989 (except for ant control). Lindane (gammahexachlorocyclohexane), however, is sold as an over-the-counter agent for head lice control, and methoxychlor remains in use as a general insecticide. Although their use is banned in most developed countries, organochlorine pesticides such as DDT are still used in developing countries; WHO continues to recommend their use for indoor structural applications in malaria control programs.

8. What is the distribution of organochlorine compounds in the environment?

Even the organochlorines that are no longer in use are still present in the environment because of their persistence and tendency to accumulate in biota. Researchers at the University of

Indiana measured concentrations of organochlorines in 209 bark samples from 90 sites throughout the globe. Concentrations of dieldrin ranged from 10–1000 ppb in lipids, whereas hexachlorocyclohexanes (including the pesticide lindane) were found in concentrations exceeding 10,000 ppb in lipids. The distribution of the compounds supported a global distillation hypothesis: semivolatile compounds (such as lindane) are readily distilled to colder, higher latitudes, whereas less volatile compounds (such as endosulfan and DDT) tend to remain near the original region of use.

9. Who is at risk of exposure to organochlorine compounds?

All living organisms carry some organochlorines in their tissues, but some subpopulations have had larger exposures. Workers in the chlorophenoxy herbicide or chlorophenol industry, as well as chlorophenoxy herbicide sprayers, have been exposed to higher levels of dioxins than the general population. Some workers in the pulp and paper industry also have been exposed to higher levels of dioxinlike chemicals. In addition, acute exposures to organochlorine compounds have occurred in several communities, including Seveso, Italy, where an explosion at an herbicide manufacturing plant resulted in very high dioxin exposures to residents, and communities in Taiwan and Japan, where residents used cooking oil contaminated with PCBs and PCDFs. Mean concentrations of 4.1 mg/kg PCBs and 184.2 mg/kg dioxinlike compounds have been found in the fat of a population of Inuits living near the Arctic Circle and whose diet is high in animal fat.

Environmental exposures to organochlorines occur mainly through dietary consumption of foods contaminated with organochlorine compounds. In the United Kingdom, Duarte-Davidson and Jones (1994) estimated that the general population exposure of PCBs is 0.53 µg/person/day; food consumption constitutes 97% of the exposure. Fish, milk and dairy products, meat, eggs, and vegetables/root crops accounted for 39%, 30%, 16%, 6%, and 4% of the dietary exposure, respectively.

10. What acute health effects are associated with exposure to organochlorine compounds?

Organochlorine insecticides. The organochlorine insecticides, including DDT, dieldrin, and chlordane, are central nervous system stimulants; their mode of action is interference with transmission of impulses along nerve cell membranes, which causes neuronal irritability. General signs and symptoms of acute overexposure include headache, dizziness, nausea, vomiting, muscle weakness, ataxia, and eventually epileptiform convulsions. If seizures develop, they generally do so within several hours; they are often self-limited but may recur. Large exposures may result in respiratory failure and death. An estimated dose of 10 mg/kg DDT will cause signs of poisonings in humans, and there have been a few reports of fatalities with DDT. Studies of workers exposed to DDT found few acute health effects other than an apparent reversible stimulation of liver enzyme function. In contrast, a number of fatalities have been associated with exposure to cyclodienes (aldrin/dieldrin, heptachlor, chlordane, toxaphene). Even at low doses, these insecticides tend to induce convulsions before less serious signs of illness occur.

Dioxins, furans, and PCBs. One health effect of PCDD, PCDF, and PCB exposure is chloracne, a skin disorder ranging in severity from comedones alone to pustules and a classic acne vulgaris-like presentation. Although the development of chloracne is considered to be evidence of exposure to organochlorines, investigators studying community exposure to dioxins in Seveso, Italy, found that people with high serum dioxin levels do not always develop chloracne. Some evidence indicates hepatic effects of PCBs in highly exposed groups. Studies in workers indicate some changes in liver function as well as increased urinary porphyrin excretion; however, the clinical significance of these effects is not known. In 1978–1979, approximately 2000 Taiwanese people were affected by Yu-Cheng disease, or oil disease, as a result of consuming contaminated rice bran oil. The oil had been contaminated with PCBs as well as PCDFs and quarterphenols, which were formed during the cooking process. A similar outbreak occurred in Japan in 1968; the resulting disease was called Yusho disease (Japanese for oil disease). The acute signs and symptoms of Yu-Cheng or Yusho disease are as follows:

1. Dermatologic symptoms include (1) keratotic changes, such as follicular accentuation, horny plugs, comedo formation, acneform eruptions, meibomian gland enlargement, keratotic plaques, and deformity of nails, and (2) pigmentation changes of mucosa, skin, and nails, particularly a brownish-gray coloring of the nails.

2. Ocular signs include increased discharge, eyelid swelling, soreness, and easy fatigue of the eyes.

3. Increased infections of the respiratory system and skin. Clinical tests found decreases in serum IgA and IgM; decreases in total T-cells, active T-cells, and helper T-cells (but not suppressor T-cells or B-cells); and enhanced spontaneous proliferation of lymphocytes.

4. Subjective constitutional complaints include general malaise or fatigue, headache or dizziness, and reduced appetite.

5. Significant reproductive effects (see question 11).

PCB concentrations ranged from 1–347 ppb initially, although the range of disease severity did not vary directly with the blood levels. When samples were collected 3 years later, a mean PCB concentration of 53.6 ppb was found in the blood.

11. What chronic health effects are associated with exposure to organochlorine compounds?

The effects of dioxins and dioxinlike chemicals are largely mediated through the aryl hydrocarbon (Ah) receptor. The natural function of the Ah receptor remains unknown, but research indicates that interaction of dioxinlike chemicals with this receptor results in induction of mRNA for a number of proteins. The non–dioxin-like chemicals, such as orthochlorinated PCBs, have been shown to have neurologic and developmental effects that are not related to Ah receptor induction.

Cancer. Dioxin has been found to be carcinogenic in all animal species tested, and TCDD has been classified as a known human carcinogen by the International Agency for Research on Cancer (IARC). Studies in rats, mice, and hamsters found tumors in multiple sites after low levels of exposure. Epidemiologic studies have had varied findings, yet analysis of several well-controlled studies found that dioxin exposure in workers was associated with increases in soft-tissue sarcoma. Furthermore, multiple myeloma, lung cancer, Hodgkin's disease, and non-Hodgkin's disease have been linked to dioxin exposure. Recent analyses of data from multiple groups of workers indicate an association between PCB exposure and cancer, particularly hepatobiliary tumors. PCBs, as a group, have been classified as probable human carcinogens by IARC and the U.S. EPA based on results of animal studies.

Developmental effects. In a follow-up study of Yu-Cheng children exposed to high levels of PCBs or PCDFs in utero, Guo et al. reported persistent developmental effects:

1. Persistent delay in growth. Yu-Cheng children are 7% lighter (p < 0.05) and 2.3% shorter (p < 0.01) than controls.

2. Delayed development, as measured with the Bayley Scale of Infant Development (p < 0.05) and Stanford-Binet Intelligence Scale for Children, Revised (5 points lower than controls).

3. Increased behavioral problems were found at 3–9 years of age, as measured with the Rutter's Child Behavior Scale A, and increased activity was found with the Werry-Weiss-Peters Activity Scale (Yu-Cheng children scored 8–53% higher than controls).

4. More frequent reports of bronchitis, upper respiratory infections, and ear infections.

5. Higher total porphyrin excretion (95 vs. 81 mg/L) and increased frequency of urinary porphyrin concentrations above 200 mg/L (11% vs. 3%).

6. Reduced penile length in boys aged 11–14 years.

Developmental effects also have been found in children exposed to organochlorines at environmental levels. Studies in Michigan and Oswego show that children born to women whose diets rely heavily on Great Lakes fish have reduced physical growth and neurobehavioral development. In the most recent report from the Michigan cohort, the most highly exposed children were 3 times more likely to have low average IQ scores and twice as likely to be at least 2 years behind in reading comprehension. This association was found with estimates of in utero exposure but not with exposure from breastfeeding. In a study in North Carolina, where women were not selected for unusual dietary organochlorine exposure, poorer gross motor function and depressed neonatal behavior were associated with PCB levels in umbilical cord serum.

Neurologic effects. The cohort studies described above have measured some neurobehavioral changes in children exposed prenatally to organochlorine compounds, particularly PCBs. Animal studies also have shown neurologic effects of the non–dioxin-like compounds. The PCBs that are chlorinated in the ortho or ortho, para positions are most potent in causing neurologic changes; interference with dopamine production is one proposed mode of action.

Effects on the immune system. Animal studies have indicated an immunosuppressive action of the dioxins and the dioxinlike PCBs, and some human studies have reported increased rates of infection in exposed subjects. The literature reveals little evidence for immunotoxic effects of the organochlorine insecticides; however, some organochlorine pesticides have a dioxin-like structure and may have immunosuppressive properties similar to those of dioxin.

Reproductive effects. Animal studies in which exposure to PCBs, dioxins, or furans occurred in utero or via lactation revealed evidence of decreased reproductive function (reduced sperm production and ejaculation, impairment of sex organ and urogenital tract development, reduced reproduction capacity of the offspring). Recent human studies show some evidence of a proposed link between deterioration in semen quality, which may affect adult reproductive performance, and environmental factors (such as organochlorine exposure) acting before or just after birth. A recent metaanalysis confirmed findings of declining sperm densities in men in "Western" countries. Because of the wide geographic variation in sperm count and quality, however, more data are needed before conclusions can be drawn.

Endocrine system effects. In people with relatively high exposure to dioxinlike compounds (but lower than occupationally exposed people), evidence indicates altered levels of circulating thyroid hormones and decreases in circulating testosterone levels. Animal studies also show that organochlorine exposure is associated with decreased androgen concentrations and feminization of male offspring as well as decreased levels of the thyroid hormones, triiodothyronine and thyroxine.

12. What is the proposed mechanism for effects of organochlorine compounds on the developing fetus?

Many organochlorine compounds have been found to act as endocrine disruptors. The chemical structure of many organochlorine compounds is sufficiently similar to the structure of steroid hormones to allow chemical contaminants to interfere with natural hormonal function (i.e., blocking or mimicking their actions). In animal studies, exposure to dioxins or PCBs has been found to alter levels of thyroid hormones and reproductive hormones as well as levels of some neurotransmitters, particularly dopamine. Animal studies also have provided evidence of adverse reproductive effects in adult animals exposed to low levels of organochlorines in utero. Neurobehavioral changes seen in childhood or adverse reproductive effects in adulthood may be associated with exposure to low levels of environmental pollutants during the susceptible period of fetal development.

13. What are the environmental effects of organochlorine compounds?

A growing body of evidence indicates that organochlorine contaminants in the environment cause adverse health effects in wildlife species. Environmental contamination by dioxins, furans, PCBs, or organochlorine pesticides has been associated with reduced reproductive function in numerous species of birds, fish, shellfish, and mammals as well as disrupted sexual development, such as demasculinization. Alteration of immune function observed in birds and mammals has been attributed to environmental contamination. In a Florida lake contaminated with the insecticides DDT and Dicofol, highly significant changes were found in estradiol and testosterone levels and morphology and organization of reproductive organs in both male and female alligators compared with alligators from nearby, uncontaminated lakes.

14. What is the risk to a member of the general population?

For a person without an unusual environmental or occupational exposure to organochlorine compounds, there is concern but no proof that reproductive or developmental effects may be associated with dietary organochlorine exposures. In a recent review, DeVito et al. compared the estimated body burden of dioxinlike chemicals in the U.S. general population with the levels associated with health effects in animal studies. The authors used an estimate of 13 ng/kg as the general population body burden of dioxin equivalents (TEQs), whereas Orban et al. had estimated an average concentration of dioxinlike chemicals of 28 ng/kg. Populations with high environmental or occupational exposures have body burdens of 96–7000 ng TEQ/kg body weight. Induction of cancer in animals has been reported at body burdens of 944–137,000 ng TCDD/kg body weight, whereas noncancer effects in animals occur at body burdens of 10–12,500 ng TCDD/kg body weight. These estimates indicate that effects are seen in animal studies at levels sometimes close to the levels in the general population. In particular, studies in rhesus monkeys found developmental delays in young monkeys with exposure levels only approximately 3 times higher than the level found in the general population. Endometriosis (in rhesus monkeys) and decreased sperm count (in rats) was seen with body burdens only five-fold higher than the burden in the unexposed general population.

Researchers at the Harvard School of Public Health recently assessed the general population health risk from dietary exposures to a number of metals and pesticides. Depending on the method used to address below-detection-limit measurements in food items, the percentage of the U.S. population predicted to be exposed to pesticides at levels that produce an excessive lifetime cancer risk greater than 10^{-4} ranged from 10–85% for dieldrin and 0–20% for heptachlor epoxide (heptachlor metabolite).

15. What are the guidelines or standards for chlorine and organochlorine exposures?

A number of regulatory agencies or organizations have established guidelines or standards for levels of contaminants in the environment, workplace, or food items. The Environmental Protection Agency (EPA) establishes regulatory limits on the levels in drinking water (40 CFR 141) and some food items. The Food and Drug Administration (FDA) regulates the amount of some contaminants allowed on raw food crops or edible seafood (21 CFR 314). The Occupational Safety and Health Administration (OSHA) sets standards for allowable concentrations in the workplace, based on a worker's 8-hour exposure (29 CFR 1900).

Regional health authorities also establish health advisories for sport fish or wildlife. State health authorities monitor sport fish for contaminant levels and issue advisories that recommend against consumption of particular fish species/sizes for individual waterbodies. The advisories are generally posted in public areas near the lake or stream or may be obtained from regional health agencies. The health practitioner should urge patients who engage in sport fishing or hunting to be aware of health advisory recommendations.

Chlorine. The workplace exposure standard established by OSHA is 3 mg/m^3, and the NIOSH recommends an 8-hour exposure limit of 1.45 mg/m^3. WHO reports an irritation threshold level of 0.06–5.8 $\mu g/m^3$ (0.02–2 ppb) and an upper level of 11.6 mg/m^3 (4 ppm) above which odor and irritation become intolerable. WHO recommends that ambient levels of chlorine be kept below 0.1 mg/m^3 (0.034 ppm) for the protection of the general public.

Organochlorine compounds
1. PCDDs/PCDFs
   - The EPA established a drinking water standard of 5×10^{-8} for 2,3,7,8-TCDD.
   - NIOSH classifies TCDD as a potential occupational carcinogen and recommends that exposure be limited to the lowest feasible concentration.
2. PCBs
   - The EPA established limits of 0.004 mg/L (adults) or 0.001 mg/L (children) in drinking water.
   - The FDA requires limits of 0.2–3 ppm PCBs in meat or dairy items and infant foods.
   - OSHA requires an 0.5 mg/m^3 (54% chlorine) or 1 mg/m^3 (42% chlorine) workplace limit for 8-your exposures, whereas NIOSH recommends that workers not breathe air containing more than 0.001 mg/m^3 PCBs.

3. Pesticides
- The EPA established the following drinking water standards: 0.0002 mg/L lindane; 0.002 mg/L chlordane, 0.0004 mg/L heptachlor, 0.005 mg/L toxaphene, and 0.4 mg/L methoxychlor.
- OSHA established the following workplace standards (8-hour exposure): 0.5 mg/m^3 chlordane, 1 mg/m^3 DDT, 0.25 mg/m^3 dieldrin, 0.5 mg/m^3 heptachlor, 0.5 mg/m^3 lindane, and 15 mg/m^3 methoxychlor.
- NIOSH established the following recommended exposure limits (8-hour exposure): 0.5 mg/m^3 chlordane and 0.5 mg/m^3 lindane.
- NIOSH classifies DDT, dieldrin, TCDD, heptachlor, and methoxychlor as potential occupational carcinogens and recommends that exposure be limited to the lowest feasible concentration.

16. What should a health practitioner do when a patient has been exposed to chlorine release or mixed household cleaners?

As described previously, symptoms of chlorine/chloramine exposure include cough, shortness of breath, throat irritation, chest pain, wheezing, dizziness, vomiting, ocular irritation, nasal irritation, and abdominal pain. Most patients recover within 6 hours with rest, fresh air, and liquids. However, some patients, especially those with a preexisting respiratory problem, may be at risk of continued respiratory problems (primarily bronchospastic) that require supportive care, including extended bronchodilator therapy. Severe exposure requires follow-up in a few days and in 6 months to assess pulmonary function, especially airway reactivity.

17. What are the signs and symptoms of organochlorine pesticide poisoning? How can it be treated?

The organochlorine compounds kill insects by interfering with the function of nerve cells; thus, high level exposure to organochlorine pesticides may result in nervous system effects. The signs and symptoms are similar for all organochlorines except DDT, for which tremor may be the initial manifestation. For other organochlorine insecticides, seizures may be the first manifestation of toxicity. Other signs and symptoms include nausea, vomiting, headache, dizziness, myoclonus, opsoclonus, leg weakness, agitation, and confusion. Seizure may be controlled promptly with diazepam followed by phenobarbital; more aggressive procedures such as general anesthesia or neuromuscular blockage can be used if initial treatment is inadequate. Cholestyramine is a nonabsorbable, bile acid-binding anion exchange resin that should be administered to all symptomatic patients. Gastric lavage is appropriate if ingestion occurred within several hours, and activated charcoal may be used after or in place of gastric lavage. Other emergency treatment to maintain breathing and adequate circulation may be necessary, and skin should be decontaminated.

18. What advice can be offered to a worker with known or likely exposure to organochlorine compounds?

A detailed occupational history should be taken. PCDD, PCDF, and PCB levels can be measured in the blood, but they are not usually clinically indicated. No treatment is known for the disease caused by chronic organochlorine exposure, and no therapy is available to reduce existing organochlorine concentrations. Identification of the exposure source and prevention of further exposure are crucial; studies of exposed populations indicate that acute symptoms often abate with time after removal from exposure.

19. What advice can a health practitioner offer a patient with concerns about potential environmental exposures?

Because of the long environmental half-lives of organochlorine compounds, people may be exposed via scenarios such as the following:

1. The patient's family has lived in their home for many years and recently learned that a nearby industrial facility is contaminated with PCBs and PCDFs.

2. A leaking electric transformer has left an oily spot near the patient's home, and the patient is concerned for the health of children playing nearby.

3. A woman who has regularly eaten sport fish has become pregnant and is concerned about the health of her child and the advisability of breast-feeding.

Local sources of organochlorines are certainly possible; PCB-contaminated soils near leaking electric transformers are fairly common in many communities. Obviously, the appropriate health or environmental agency officials should be consulted to determine whether contamination has occurred and to initiate remediation, if needed.

In general, exposure to organochlorine compounds from dietary sources exceeds exposure from other sources in the environment. Because organochlorine pollutants concentrate in the food chain, health practitioners should be aware of the sport fish advisories or other recommendations by health authorities and alert patients to the need to avoid consuming fish or wildlife with high pollutant levels. Patients should be reassured that, even with moderately prolonged exposure, they are at low, although elevated, risk for developing exposure-related chronic disease, including cancer.

The risk may be greater to the fetus during pregnancy; thus the need to avoid exposure to foods likely to be contaminated by organochlorines is probably most important for women of child-bearing age. Studies such as the Lake Michigan fish-eaters study indicate that organochlorine exposure in the pre- or perinatal period may result in subtle neurobehavioral effects. Because organochlorine compounds tend to accumulate in fatty tissues, their concentrations may be elevated in breast milk. Estimated daily intakes of dioxinlike chemicals (in TEQs) range from 5–900 pg/kg/day in breast-fed infants from several countries. In contrast, WHO's recommended allowable daily intake for dioxins is 10 pg/kg/day, and the Agency for Toxic Substances and Disease Registry has proposed a minimal risk level of 7 pg/kg/day for infants (intermediate duration of breastfeeding). Clearly, breast milk may be a significant source of organochlorine compounds; however, breast-feeding remains the recommended option for feeding young infants because of its many other widely-recognized benefits.

To prevent accumulation of organochlorine chemicals, health professionals can recommend avoiding consumption of foods most highly contaminated with organochlorines, especially fish or wildlife species on health advisory lists. Fatty foods, such as butter or meat, are also likely to have higher levels of chlorinated compounds; reducing fat intake has health benefits in addition to reducing organochlorine exposure. PCBs were once commonly used in capacitors or electric transformers and other equipment, and patients may be advised to determine whether they work with equipment that contains PCBs (their use was banned in the U.S. in 1976). Prevention of further exposure, risk communication, and reassurance are appropriate areas of discussion.

Unfortunately, there is no effective cure for organochlorine exposure and no effective means of reducing organochlorine levels in the body. The toxicokinetic half-lives of the organochlorine compounds vary from a few months to almost 30 years; the PCBs, in combination, are considered to have a half-life of 7 years. Thus, the best means of reducing potential health effects from organochlorine compounds is to prevent exposure in the first place. On a global scale, the use of long-lived organochlorine compounds should be eliminated. To reduce individual exposures, health practitioners can make patients aware of the need to follow health advisories about sport fish or wildlife consumption and to reduce intake of fatty foods that are more likely to have elevated levels of organochlorine compounds.

Disclaimer: No official support or endorsement by the Environmental Protection Agency or any other agency of the Federal Government is intended or should be inferred.

BIBLIOGRAPHY

1. Agency for Toxic Substances and Disease Registry: Toxicological Profiles for Aldrin/Dieldrin; Chlordane; DDT, DDE, DDD; Heptachlor, Heptachlor Epoxide; Methoxychlor; Mirex and Chlordecone; PCBs; Toxaphene. Agency for Toxic Substances and Disease Registry, Atlanta, 1996.

2. Agency for Toxic Substances and Disease Registry: Public Health Implications of Persistent Toxic Substances in the Great Lakes and St. Lawrence Basins. Agency for Toxic Substances and Disease Registry, Atlanta, 1997.

3. Ayotte P, Dewailly E, Ryan JJ, et al: PCBs and dioxin-like compounds in plasma of adult Inuit living in Nunavik (Arctic Quebec). Chemosphere 34:1459–1468, 1997.

4. Birnbaum LS: The mechanism of dioxin toxicity: Relationship to risk assessment. Environ Health Perspect 102(Suppl 9):157–167, 1994.

5. Brouwer A, Ahlborg UG, Van den Berg M, et al: Functional aspects of developmental toxicity of poly-halogenated aromatic hydrocarbons in experimental animals and human infants. Eur J Pharmacol 293:1–40, 1995.

6. Brzuzy LO, Hites RA: Global mass balance for polychlorinated dibenzo-p-dioxins and dibenzofurans. Environ Sci Technol 30:1797–1803, 1996.

7. Colborn T, vom Saal FS, Soto AM: Developmental effects of endocrine-disrupting chemicals in wildlife and humans. Environ Health Perspect 101:378–384, 1993.

8. Courteau JP, Cushman R, Bouchard F, et al: Survey of construction workers repeatedly exposed to chlorine over a three to six month period in a pulpmill. I: Exposure and symptomatology. Occup Environ Med 51:219–224, 1994.

9. DeVito MJ, Birnbaum LS, Farland WH, Gasiewicz TA: Comparisons of estimated human body burdens of dioxinlike chemicals and TCDD body burdens in experimentally exposed animals. Environ Health Perspect 103:820–831, 1995.

10. Duarte-Davidson R, Jones KC: Polychlorinated biphenyls (PCBs) in the UK population: Estimated intake, exposure and body burden. Sci Tot Environ 151:131–152, 1994.

11. Goldfrank LR, Flomenbaum NE, Lewin NA, et al: Goldfrank's Toxicologic Emergencies, 4th ed. Norwalk, CT, Appleton & Lange, 1990.

12. Guo YL, Lambert GH, Hsu C-C: Growth abnormalities in the population exposed in utero and early post-natally to polychlorinated biphenyls and dibenzofurans. Environ Health Perspect 103(Suppl 6):117–122, 1995.

13. International Agency for Research in Cancer: Statement released February 14, 1997. IARC Monograph 69, 1997.

14. Jacobson JL, Jacobson SW: Intellectual impairment in children exposed to polychlorinated biphenyls in utero. JAMA 335:783–789, 1996.

15. Kimbrough R: Selected other effects and TEFs. Teratog Carcinog Mutagen 17:265–273, 1997/98.

16. Klaassen CD (ed): Casarett and Doull's Toxicology: The Basic Science of Poisons, 5th ed. New York, McGraw-Hill, 1996.

17. Litovitz TL, Felberg L, Soloway RA, et al: 1994 Annual report of the American Association of Poison Control Centers Toxic Exposure Surveillance System. Am J Emerg Med 13:551–597, 1995.

18. Lonky E, Reihman J, Darvill T, et al: Neonatal behavioral assessment scale performance in humans influenced by maternal consumption of environmentally contaminated Lake Ontario fish. J Great Lakes Res 22:198–212, 1996.

19. MacIntosh DL, Spengler JD, Ozkaynak H, et al: Dietary exposures to selected metals and pesticides. Environ Health Perspect 104:202–209, 1996.

20. Morris RD, Audet AM, Angelillo IF, et al: Chlorination, chlorination by-products and cancer: A meta-analysis. Am J Public Health 82:955–963, 1992.

21. Mrvos R, Dean BS, Krenzelok EP: Home exposures to chlorine/chloramine gas: A review of 216 cases. South Med J 86:654–657, 1993.

22. National Institute for Occupational Safety and Health: Pocket Guide to Chemical Hazards. U.S. Department of Health and Human Services, Centers for Disease Control and Prevention. NIOSH, Cincinnati, 1994.

23. Orban JE, Stanley JS, Schwemberger JG, Remmers JC: Dioxins and dibenzofurans in adipose tissues of the general U.S. population and selected subpopulations. Am J Public Health 84:439–445, 1994.

24. Pohl HR, Hibbs BF: Breast-feeding exposure of infants to environmental contaminants—a public health risk assessment viewpoint: Chlorinated dibenzodioxins and chlorinated dibenzofurans. Toxicol Indust Health 12:593–611, 1996.

25. Simonich SL, Hites RA: Global distribution of persistent organochlorine compounds. Science 269:1851–1854, 1995.

26. Swan SH, Elkin EP, Fenster L: Have sperm densities declined? A reanalysis of global trend data. Environ Health Perspect 105:1228–1232, 1997.

27. Toppari J, Larsen JC, Christiansen P, et al: Male reproductive health and environmental estrogens. Environ Health Perspect 104(Suppl 4):741–803, 1996.

28. World Health Organization: Environmental Health Criteria 101: Chlorine and hydrogen chloride. World Health Organization, Geneva, 1982.

9. LEAD POISONING

Karen L. Hipkins, R.N., N.P.-C., M.P.H., and Michael J. Kosnett, M.D., M.P.H.

1. Is lead poisoning a common problem in the United States?

Although the toxic effects of lead have been known for centuries, lead poisoning is still widespread in the United States and throughout the world. Nonoccupational lead poisoning occurs in adults and children, but adults are exposed to lead primarily in the workplace. Lead affects multiple body systems and can cause permanent damage. Exposures that were thought to be without harm in the past are now considered hazardous as new information emerges about lead toxicity, particularly its effects on behavior, reproductive outcomes, and blood pressure.

Lead is not an essential element and serves no useful purpose in the body. Efforts to reduce lead in the environment, primarily by eliminating lead from gasoline, have resulted in lowering the overall geometric mean blood lead level (BLL) in the United States from approximately 13 μg/dl in the late 1970s to < 3 μg/dl by 1991. However, although the average BLL has markedly declined, NHANES III survey data (1991–1994) indicated that 4.4% of U.S. children had BLLs ≥ 10 μg/dl. Additionally, thousands of workers in high-risk industries are still overexposed, and their children may be at risk for "take-home" lead exposure.

Clinicians caring for lead-exposed patients need to be informed about the health effects of lead, employer and physician responsibilities, and worker rights. Lead poisoning, if undetected, often results in misdiagnosis and costly care. When the diagnosis of lead poisoning is initially missed, it is frequently the result of a failure to take a detailed occupational and environmental history.

2. Which industries and environmental sources are associated with lead exposure?

General industry

- Lead production or smelting
- Brass, bronze, or lead foundries
- Scrap metal handling
- Firing ranges
- Machining or grinding lead alloys
- Manufacture of radiation shielding
- Ship building/repairing
- Mining
- Battery manufacturing or recycling
- Automotive radiator repair
- Lead soldering
- Ceramic manufacturing
- Cable stripping
- Brass polishing
- Rubber manufacturing
- Plastics manufacturing

Construction industry

- Renovation, repair, or demolition of structures with lead paint
- Welding or torch-cutting painted metal
- Sanding, scraping, burning, or disturbing lead paint
- Use or disturbance of lead solder, sheeting, flashing, or old electric conduit
- Plumbing, particularly in older buildings

Environmental sources

- Home remodeling or painting, peeling paint
- Folk remedies (e.g., azarcon, greta, pay-loo-ah, kandu)
- Pica (e.g., ingestion of lead-contaminated soil or ceramics, plaster or paint chips)
- Retained lead bullet or fragment in or near a synovial joint
- Melting lead for fishing weights, bullets, or toys
- Imported vinyl miniblinds
- Recreational target shooting
- Lead-glazed table or cookware
- Lead-contaminated drinking water supply
- Using lead glazes for ceramics

- Lead came and solder in stained-glass artwork
- Lead-soldered cans
- Lead-contaminated candies
- Backyard scrap metal recycling
- Moonshine (liquor from a homemade still)
- Antique pewter plates, mugs, utensils; imported brass or bronze kettles
- Leaded crystal tableware
- Mine tailings
- Beauty products such as kohl eye make-up, certain hair dyes

3. How is lead absorbed? How is it excreted?

Routes of exposure for inorganic lead are inhalation and ingestion. Lead fume and soluble respirable dust are almost completely absorbed by inhalation. Adults absorb approximately 15% of an ingested dose through the gastrointestinal (GI) tract in contrast to 50% GI absorption in children. GI absorption is generally inversely proportional to particle size and directly proportional to solubility of the lead compounds. Once absorbed, lead is found in all tissues, but eventually > 90% of the body burden is accumulated (or redistributed) into bone, where it remains with a half-life of many years. Lead is excreted primarily through the urine (> 90%); lesser amounts are eliminated via feces, sweat, hair, and nails.

4. What symptoms should make a clinician think of lead poisoning?

Because lead interferes with the function of enzymes and essential cations (particularly calcium) in cells throughout the body, lead poisoning is usually associated with multisystemic signs and symptoms. Clinically, the most significant are the neurologic, hematopoietic, GI, cardiovascular, renal, and reproductive systems. Wide variation exists in individual susceptibility to lead poisoning with a corresponding range in the spectrum of clinical findings. Symptoms sometimes appear in adults with blood lead concentrations as low as 25 µg/dl; more commonly, however, overt symptoms emerge in patients whose peak blood lead concentration has exceeded 40–60 µg/dl. Subacute or chronic intoxication is more common than acute poisoning.

Early symptoms are often subtle, nonspecific, and/or subclinical, involving the nervous system (listlessness, fatigue, irritability, sleep disturbance, headache, difficulty in concentrating, decreased libido), GI system (abdominal cramps, anorexia, nausea, constipation, diarrhea), or musculoskeletal system (arthralgia, myalgia). Other less common conditions include tremor, toxic hepatitis, or acute gouty arthritis (saturnine gout). In general, the number and severity of symptoms worsen with increasing BLL. A high level of intoxication may result in delirium, coma, and seizures associated with lead encephalopathy, a life-threatening condition.

Signs and Symptoms of Lead Toxicity in Adults

MILD TOXICITY	MODERATE TOXICITY	SEVERE TOXICITY
Mild fatigue or exhaustion	Headache	Colic (intermittent,
Emotional lability	General fatigue or somnolence	severe abdominal
Difficulty in concentrating	Muscular exhaustion, myalgia, arthralgia	cramps)
Sleep disturbances	Tremor	Peripheral neuropathy
	Nausea	Convulsions
	Diffuse abdominal pain	Encephalopathy
	Constipation or diarrhea	
	Weight loss	
	Decreased libido	

From Hipkins KL, Materna BL, Kosnett MJ, et al: Medical surveillance of the lead exposed worker: Current guidelines. Am Assoc Occup Health Nurs 46(7):330–339, 1998.

5. What are the possible effects of low-level lead exposure on blood pressure?

Research shows multiple systemic health effects at levels once believed safe. Several animal and epidemiologic investigations suggest that lead may elevate blood pressure in susceptible adults at blood concentrations as low as 10 μg/dl. A recent study of 590 men aged 48–92 years, with predominantly nonoccupational lead exposure and a mean BLL concentration of 6.3 μg/dl, found that increases in bone lead concentration were associated with an increased risk of hypertension. Because hypertension is a significant risk factor for heart disease, lead exposure may exert an important effect on cardiovascular mortality.

6. What are the possible effects of low-level lead exposure on renal function?
Early kidney damage may be difficult to detect. Urinalysis is often unremarkable, and blood urea nitrogen (BUN) and creatinine may not reach abnormal levels until loss of renal function is substantial. Recent epidemiologic studies have associated low levels of lead exposure with decrements in renal function. A 10-μg/dl increase in BLL has been associated with a 10.4-ml/min decrease in renal creatinine clearance rate in a population with an average BLL of 8.1 μg/dl. In a population of older men with mean BLL concentration of 8.6 μg/dl (range: 0.2–54.1), a 10-fold increase in BLL predicted an increase of 0.08 mg/dl in serum creatinine concentration, roughly equivalent to 20 years of aging. The extent to which such low blood lead levels were a cause of decreased renal function rather than a result of subclinical renal insufficiency is not known.

7. What are the possible effects of low-level lead exposure on the nervous system?
Subclinical slowing of nerve conduction velocity has been reported at BLLs as low as 30 μg/dl, but overt peripheral neuropathy usually requires blood lead concentrations in excess of 100 μg/dl for months to years. Neuropsychological studies in workers with blood lead concentrations of 30–50+ μg/dl have detected subtle adverse effects on reaction time, visual-motor coordination, and mood. Lead and other heavy metals may be slow to enter and leave the brain tissue. Consequently, central nervous system effects may have a delayed onset and sometimes persist well after the BLL has dropped below the action levels required by the lead standards. Such effects may negatively affect job performance and safety.

8. What are the possible hematopoietic effects of low-level lead exposure?
Frank anemia usually does not occur until BLLs are > 50–60 μg/dl. In people without frank anemia, however, bone lead levels were significantly correlated with a decrease in hemoglobin and hematocrit, even though BLLs were low (mean: 8.3 μg/dl); this finding may reflect a subclinical effect of bone lead stores on hematopoiesis.

9. What are the possible reproductive effects of low-level lead exposure?
Abnormal sperm morphology and decreased sperm count have been observed at blood lead concentrations in excess of 40 μg/dl. Lead readily crosses the placenta and may be present in breast milk. Impaired cognitive development has been observed in children with prenatal lead exposure; however, prospective longitudinal studies of low-level lead exposure (e.g., < 20 μg/dl) suggest that postnatal exposure between ages 2–3 years rather than prenatal exposure is correlated with impaired cognitive function and academic performance in the teenage years. Such effects in young children occur without an apparent dose threshold.

10. What are the lead standards of the Occupational Safety and Health Administration (OSHA)?
Two federal OSHA lead standards, the 1978 general industry (29 CFR 11910.1025) and the 1993 construction industry (29 CFR 1926.62) standards, require employers and physicians to follow specific guidelines for protecting lead-exposed workers. Depending on the level of workplace exposure, lead-using businesses may be required to have a medical surveillance program with a licensed physician as medical supervisor. Physicians should be completely familiar with the standard's requirements before implementing such a program. The standards predate newer knowledge about the health effects of lead, particularly at lower levels. Therefore, as noted below, the standards may not adequately protect workers' health. Copies of the lead standards can be obtained from the OSHA website (http://www.osha.gov).

11. How should an adult be evaluated for suspected lead exposure?

Medical evaluation for lead exposure includes a general and lead-specific history and physical exam with special attention to the body systems noted above. Laboratory tests to diagnose lead poisoning and to assess end-organ damage are indicated.

The single best diagnostic test for lead exposure is the BLL. Although it reflects the amount of lead currently found in blood and soft tissues (and hence key target organs), it is not a reliable indicator of prior or cumulative exposures or total body burden. Lead in the blood reflects both the current exogenous external exposure and the endogenous slow release of lead that may have accumulated in the bones over a period of years. When interpreting the BLL, three key questions to keep in mind are whether the exposure is (1) acute or chronic, (2) recent or remote, and (3) high or low. BLLs performed under the OSHA lead standards must be conducted by laboratories that meet certain proficiency requirements.

Erythrocyte protoporphyrin (EP) or zinc protoporphyrin (ZPP) is sometimes used as an indirect measure of lead exposure. An increase indicates that lead is affecting the heme synthesis pathway. The effect may begin at a BLL as low as 25–30 µg/dl in some adults, but the test is not > 90% sensitive until blood lead concentration exceeds 50 µg/dl. An increase in EP or ZPP usually lags behind an increase in BLL by 2–6 weeks. Therefore, a normal EP or ZPP in the presence of an elevated BLL suggests recent lead exposure. Of other disorders that may cause an elevated EP or ZPP, the most common are iron deficiency anemia and inflammatory conditions. Screening for other causes is recommended if the EP or ZPP is > 50 µg/dl and the BLL is below the threshold of heme effect.

Other tests required by the OSHA standards, depending on the magnitude of lead exposure, include complete blood count with red cell indices and peripheral smear, serum creatinine, blood urea nitrogen, and complete urinalysis. Evaluation of reproductive status, including sperm analysis or a pregnancy test, may be pertinent for some workers and should be provided upon the employee's request. If a respirator is used, spirometry is recommended as part of the medical clearance required by OSHA. The physician may perform other tests as deemed necessary based on sound medical practice. The physician also may make recommendations to the employer for employee protections that may be more stringent than the specific provisions of the standards.

12. Which workers must be monitored?

Medical monitoring requirements under the OSHA standards are determined by a worker's exposure to lead in the air, by a worker's BLL, and, in the construction trades, by work involving certain high-exposure "trigger tasks." Higher BLLs require more frequent monitoring of BLL and ZPP. The employer must perform personal air sampling if employees are exposed to lead at work. OSHA defines the action level (AL) as an airborne lead concentration of 30 µg/m^3. The AL triggers certain other requirements of the standards. Air monitoring does not necessarily reflect the actual amount of exposure, particularly when significant exposure occurs through hand-to-mouth activities, such as eating, drinking, or smoking in the workplace, that contribute to lead ingestion. Routine BLL and ZPP monitoring of lead-exposed workers provides important additional information to guide prevention efforts.

13. How soon after exposure does a person manifest signs or symptoms of lead poisoning?

The onset of signs or symptoms after lead exposure is highly variable and depends in part on the intensity of exposure as well as individual host factors. For example, an intense high dose that increases blood lead concentration above approximately 80–100 µg/dl over the course of 1–3 days may result in the onset of neurologic symptoms, such as headache, fatigue, or irritability, and GI symptoms, such as constipation or colic, within a few days to 1 week. The person may have minimal or no signs or symptoms within the first 24 hours.

When symptoms of intense high-dose lead exposure first appear, they may be accompanied by laboratory abnormalities such as hemolysis and mild-to-moderate elevations in liver transaminases. With subacute or chronic exposure to lead (e.g., blood lead concentrations rising above 40–60 µg/dl over the course of weeks to months), the onset of multisystemic signs and symptoms is often insidious and may not be apparent until the BLL remains in this range for several weeks.

In people with long-term, high-dose exposure who have accumulated elevated amounts of lead in bone, pathologic processes that rapidly accelerate bone turnover may release the lead into the soft tissues. As a result of this abrupt redistribution, they may develop the appearance or recrudescence of overt lead poisoning years after the last known external lead exposure has ended. Although relatively rare, delayed lead poisoning of this nature has been described in people who developed high bone turnover in association with thyrotoxicosis and immobilization osteoporosis. Compared to lead absorbed directly in the circulation from external routes, lead redistributed to the circulation from skeletal stores may result in a higher fraction of lead in the plasma component of whole blood. Plasma may be responsible for diffusing into intracellular targets in the soft tissues. However, because more than 99% of blood lead is normally found in erythrocytes, significant increases in the plasma fraction may not be readily apparent.

Lead bullets retained in the body after a gunshot wound may dissolve and release large amounts of lead into the circulation years to decades after the original injury. Systemic exposure to the retained lead becomes more likely if the fragments lodge or mechanically migrate into a joint space, where physical friction and the action of joint fluid hasten the dissolution process. People with retained lead bullets should be cautioned that they are at risk for the abrupt (or insidious) appearance of lead poisoning even years after they recover from the initial gunshot trauma.

14. Why do some people appear to be more susceptible to lead poisoning than others?

A high degree of interindividual variability in susceptibility to overt lead intoxication is a common observation in clinical occupational medicine. Within the same workforce, some workers may remain completely free of symptoms at the same exposure levels and blood concentrations that cause other workers to be overtly ill or impaired. The mechanisms behind this variability are not completely understood. Lead-binding proteins elaborated by the body in response to lead exposure may afford protection against some of the pathologic effects of lead in tissues such as brain, liver, and kidney. Genetic polymorphisms that affect the expression of these proteins may influence susceptibility to some of lead's toxic effects.

Nutritional factors that affect the GI absorption of lead also may influence susceptibility to lead intoxication. Clinical studies have shown that GI lead absorption is increased in people with iron deficiency. Ingested lead is also more likely to be absorbed in people who maintain a low calcium diet or whose lead exposure occurs on an empty stomach. Although measures to prevent lead exposure assume highest priority, efforts to address such nutritional factors, particularly in children with poorly characterized environmental lead exposure, may have an adjunctive role in diminishing the impact of lead ingestion.

15. What treatment is currently recommended for adult lead poisoning?

Primary management of lead poisoning is source identification and removal from exposure. Recommendations for medical treatment of children and adults differ significantly. Treatment decisions should be made on an individual basis in consultation with a physician knowledgeable about medical management of lead poisoning.

Management Guidelines for Blood Lead Levels in Children

BLOOD LEAD (µg/dl)	SIGNIFICANCE	MANAGEMENT
< 10	Background	Guidance and well-child care
10–14	Low	For 10 or higher, tiered management according to
15–19*	Mild	CDC guidelines[†]
20–44	Moderate	For 20 or higher, public health and medical evaluation and treatment (see CDC guidelines)[‡]
45–69	High	For 45 or higher, chelation recommended
≥ 70	Severe	Medical emergency

* Capillary blood lead ≥ 15 µg/dl should be confirmed with venous test before referral or treatment.
† Screening Young Children for Lead Poisoning: Guidance for State and Local Public Health Officials. Atlanta, U.S. Department of Health and Human Services, 1997.
‡ For details and resources, contact local health department lead poisoning prevention program.

Management Guidelines for Blood Lead Levels in Adults*

BLOOD LEAD (µg/dl)	MANAGEMENT
< 10	No action needed
10–24	Identify and minimize lead exposure
25–49	Remove from exposure if symptomatic; monitor blood lead and ZPP
50–79	Remove from work with lead; immediate medical evaluation indicated; chelation *not* indicated unless significant symptoms due to lead poisoning are present
≥ 80	As above; chelation may be indicated if symptomatic; important to consult on individual case basis

* Consult OSHA General Industry and Construction Lead Standards for occupational exposure. For more information, call state health department or nearest university-based occupational and environmental health clinic.

16. How does a physician implement removal from a workplace exposure?

Under the OSHA lead standards, the physician must recommend to the employer that an employee be removed from lead exposure and enter a **medical removal protection (MRP)** program if any of the following conditions are met:

General industry standard

1. A single BLL is ≥ 60 µg/dl, *or*

2. An average of the last three BLLs or all BLLs over the previous 6 months (whichever covers a longer period) is ≥ 50 µg/dl, *or*

3. The employee has a "detected medical condition" that places him or her at increased risk of "material impairment to health" from lead exposure. (The OSHA lead standards do not define these terms; thus, the physician is given the discretion to make such a determination on an individual basis.)

Construction industry standard (applicable to workers engaged in the construction, demolition, or renovation of residential or commercial buildings, ships, storage tanks, or similar structures)

1. A single BLL is ≥ 50 µg/dl, *or*

2. The employee has a detected medical condition that places him or her at increased risk of material impairment to health from lead exposure (see above.)

A physician can remove an employee with a BLL below the specified MRP levels on the basis of relevant medical findings, such as symptoms commonly associated with lead toxicity or conditions not arising from lead poisoning that nonetheless increase the patient's vulnerability. Pregnancy or the desire to become pregnant may form the basis for medical removal. Whenever an employee is placed on MRP because of an elevated BLL, the frequency of biologic monitoring must be increased to at least once per month. After two consecutive BLLs are 40 µg/dl or less, the physician may recommend to the employer that the employee return to the previous work if the employer has taken steps to control lead exposure and the employee's symptoms or any other clinical manifestations of toxicity have resolved. It is recommended that the blood tests be at least one month apart to allow for mobilization and excretion of the lead burden.

During the time an employee is removed from work with lead by a physician's recommendation, the employee must retain earnings, seniority, and other benefits. The physician may allow an employee on MRP, if physically able, to work in an area free of lead exposure. The OSHA standards permit a worker on MRP to work in any area where the 8-hour time-weighted average (TWA) air lead concentration is less < 30 µg/m^3. However, because significant lead exposure may occur even when air lead levels are not elevated (e.g., by hand-to-mouth ingestion), the supervising physician should carefully review the safety of any lead-related work for an employee on MRP. The standards require the employer to continue to pay the employee's usual wages and benefits during the removal period, whether or not the employee is working. If workers' compensation disability benefits are used to pay a portion of the salary, the employer is responsible for paying the balance. On return to work, the employee is guaranteed his or her former job status. It is important to realize that when the specific "trigger" for medical removal was a BLL of 50 or 60 µg/dl and 40 µg/dl for return to lead exposure were incorporated into the OSHA lead standard for general industry in the late 1970s, the background (nonoccupational) contribution to blood lead was considered to be 19 µg/dl. Because background blood lead concentrations in the late 1990s now average < 3 µg/dl and recent findings suggest adverse affects of lead < 40 µg/dl, it may now be both prudent and feasible for workplaces to maintain employee BLLs below 20 µg/dl.

17. How should a clinician manage a lead-exposed worker who is pregnant or has concerns about reproductive issues?

Exposure to lead is known to have serious adverse reproductive effects for both men and women. In addition, bone lead stores may be mobilized during pregnancy and lactation, particularly in women on low-calcium diets. The Centers for Disease Control and Prevention (CDC) has established 10 µg/dl as a blood lead level of concern in children. Because fetal blood contains approximately 80% of the blood lead concentration of the mother, the mother's BLL ideally should be kept below 10 µg/dl before and during pregnancy. A woman with occupational exposure to lead who is or plans to become pregnant may need to be placed on MRP by the physician to maintain a BLL < 10 µg/dl. In the absence of effects on sperm count or concentration, the impact of paternal lead exposure on reproductive outcome is uncertain and remains an important research question.

18. When is chelation therapy indicated for adults?

As noted earlier, the primary therapy for lead poisoning is cessation of exposure. Prophylactic chelation therapy solely to prevent the rise of blood lead levels is a violation of the OSHA lead standards. Before initiation of diagnostic or therapeutic chelation therapy, workers must be notified in writing as to why they should receive the therapy.

No randomized, blinded clinical trials of lead chelation in adults indicate that chelation therapy has an effect on clinical outcome. The use of chelation therapy generally should be reserved for adults with significant symptoms or signs of toxicity and should be undertaken only under strict and skilled clinical supervision. Occasionally, adults with a high BLL (e.g., 90 µg/dl) may remain asymptomatic. They should be removed from exposure and followed carefully, but chelation therapy may not prove necessary. Levels > 100 µg/dl are usually associated with significant symptoms that may warrant chelation. Chelation is contraindicated in pregnancy. Chelation guidelines are empirical and may change as new agents and information become available.

Chelation therapy primarily reduces lead in the blood and soft tissues, such as liver and kidney but not the generally larger fraction of lead in bone. In people with substantial bone lead stores who undergo chelation, reequilibration of lead from bone into blood and soft tissues may result in a rebound effect with a rise in the BLL after an initial drop. Symptoms associated with lead toxicity may recur. However, the clinician should consider whether the rise in blood lead concentration after cessation of chelation may be the result of renewed lead exposure.

19. Is the chelation challenge test useful?

The term "chelation challenge test" refers to a procedure, first introduced in the early 1960s, that measures the quantity of lead excreted into the urine during a designated period (usually 24 hours) after administration of a single challenge dose of a chelating agent. However, chelation challenge tests have not been found to be a valid predictor of health effects, nor are they a reliable reflection of body lead burden or long-term lead exposure. Chelatable lead may reflect little of the large fraction of body lead burden found in bone. Currently, no data indicate that the chelation challenge test can identify people who may derive a therapeutic benefit from chelation. A more promising indicator of bone stores and consequently total lead body burden is noninvasive x-ray fluorescence (XRF) of the bone.

20. What is bone XRF? When should it be used?

Noninvasive in vivo (K shell) x-ray fluorescence measurement of the concentration of lead in bone (KXRF) has found increasing application as a biomarker of long-term, cumulative lead exposure. Epidemiologic studies of the effects of chronic lead exposure show correlations between lead measured in cortical and/or trabecular bone and history of exposure. Availability of KXRF may facilitate clinical investigation of dose-response relationships for adverse health effects attributed to lead in adults—such as neuropsychological dysfunction, nephropathy, and hypertension—for which the association between extent of exposure and onset of disease has yet to be determined.

Apart from epidemiologic studies, KXRF measurement of bone lead may have value as an adjunct to biologic monitoring or clinical evaluation in individual workers. For example, in a worker whose blood lead concentration is slow to decline after removal from high-level lead exposure, a high bone lead concentration may confirm redistribution of internal skeletal stores as a significant contributing factor. Conversely, the finding of a normal or low bone lead concentration increases the likelihood of significant external exposure. However, the clinician should be aware that external exposure may be a source of significant lead exposure regardless of bone lead stores.

21. What is "take-home" lead exposure?

Household members are at risk for lead poisoning if lead is carried home on a worker's body, clothes, or shoes ("take-home" exposure). The lead dust then settles on the furniture, floors, and carpeting. Lead contamination of a worker's personal vehicle also may pose a risk to family members. Employers may face civil liability for health damage to household members caused by an improperly protected worker who takes lead home. Children under 6 years old and the fetus are at increased risk. Many "take-home" exposures are initially identified when a child is found to have an elevated BLL on routine screening.

22. Is lead poisoning preventable?

Yes. By asking about possible lead exposure within the occupational and home environment, clinicians in occupational and primary care practices can play an important role in the identification, intervention, and prevention of lead poisoning for adults and children. Lead poisoning rarely occurs in isolation. The finding of lead poisoning in one patient should trigger an inquiry into potential hazardous exposure to others who share the patient's work or home environment or may have similar sources of exposure.

Workplace medical surveillance is a tool to identify excessive lead exposure and to direct and evaluate exposure reduction efforts. The ultimate goal is to reduce worker BLLs to those of the general population. The key is exposure reduction through proper engineering controls and work practices. Employers may need to obtain technical assistance in controlling exposures. By working together, the employer and clinician can use biomedical information to identify problems and evaluate improvements in the workplace.

BIBLIOGRAPHY

1. Agency for Toxic Substances and Disease Registry: Toxicological Profile for Lead (Update). Atlanta, U.S. Department of Health and Human Services, Public Health Service [draft edition 1997; final edition due in Spring 1999].
2. Cake KM, Bowins RJ, Vaillancourt C, et al: Partition of circulating lead between serum and red cells is different for internal and external sources of lead. Am J Indust Med 29:440–445, 1996.
3. Centers for Disease Control and Prevention (CDC): Screening young children for lead poisoning: Guidance for state and local public health officials. Atlanta, U.S. Department of Health and Human Services, Public Health Service, 1997.
4. Centers for Disease Control and Prevention (CDC): Update: Blood lead levels—United States. 1991–1994. MMWR 46:141–145, 1997.
5. Hipkins KL, Materna BL, Kosnett MJ, et al: Medical surveillance of the lead exposed worker: Current guidelines. Am Assoc Occup Health Nur 46(7):330-339, 1998.
6. Hu H, Rabinowitz M, Smith D: Bone lead as a biological marker in epidemiologic studies of chronic toxicity: Conceptual paradigms. Environ Health Perspect 106:1–8, 1998.
7. Jackson RJ , Cummins SK, Tips NM, Rosenblum LS: Preventing childhood lead poisoning: The challenge of change. Am J Prev Med 14(3S):84–86, 1998.
8. Kosnett MJ: Lead. In Olson KR (ed): Poisoning and Drug Overdose, 2nd ed. Norwalk, CT, Appleton & Lange, 1994, pp 196–200.
9. Landrigan PJ, Todd AC: Lead poisoning. West J Med 161(2):153–159, 1994.
10. Schwartz J: Lead, blood pressure and cardiovascular disease in men. Arch Environ Health 50:31–37, 1995.

10. MERCURY

Perrine Hoet, M.D., M.I.H., M.Sc.

1. What is mercury?

Mercury (Hg) is a metal that occurs naturally in the environment and exists in different forms, including elemental, inorganic, and organic compounds. There are three oxidation states. Metallic (elemental) mercury is a shiny, silver-white, odorless liquid that is found, for example, in mercury thermometers. Metallic mercury evaporates at room temperature to form mercury vapor, a colorless, odorless gas. The mercurous and mercuric states combine with other elements, such as chlorine, sulfur, or oxygen, to form inorganic mercury compounds or "salts," such as mercurous chloride or calomel (Hg_2Cl_2), mercuric chloride or sublimate ($HgCl_2$), mercuric oxide (HgO), and mercuric sulfide or cinnabar. Mercury can bind covalently to at least one carbon atom to create a large number of organomercurial compounds such as methylmercury or phenylmercury. Like inorganic mercury compounds, they also exist as salts (for example, phenylmercuric acetate).

2. What are the most common occupations involving mercury exposure?

Approximately 70,000 workers in the United States are regularly exposed to mercury.

Metallic mercury: production of chlorine gas and caustic soda (chloroalkali plants); extraction of gold from ore concentrates or recycled gold articles; jewelry; manufacture of thermometers, manometers, barometers and precision instruments; production of mercury battery cells; production of fluorescent tubes and mercury vapor lamps; preparation of dental amalgams; histologic staining. In the past, production of felt hats from rabbit fur represented an important source of exposure.

Inorganic mercury compounds: synthesis of other mercury compounds; reagents in analytical chemistry. Numerous mercury-containing compounds have been used as germicides, insecticides, mildewcides, fungicides, and topical antiseptics.

Organic mercury compounds: laboratory reagents, preservatives and antifungals in latex paints or inks and adhesives; slimcides in paper mills; catalysts for the manufacture of certain polyurethanes; contraceptive gels and foams; disinfectants; laundry and diaper services. Numerous compounds also are used to protect seeds from fungal infections. This last use and the use of phenylmercuric compounds as antifungal agents in paints have been banned in many countries. Methylmercury is produced mainly by microorganisms in the environment rather than by human activities. Methylation of metallic and mercuric mercury is likely to occur in bacteria in sediments of sea- and lakebeds.

3. What are the most common sources of exposure to mercury in the home?

1. Some mercury compounds are still used as topical antiseptic/disinfectant agents (Mercurochrome, thimerosal) in eye drops, eye ointments, nasal sprays, and vaccines. Mercurous chloride was widely used at one time in medicinal products, such as laxatives, worming medications, and teething powders. In addition, herbal preparations may be contaminated with mercury.

2. The mercury in food is generally present in the form of methylmercury. The average daily intake is estimated by assuming that intake from non-fish sources is negligible in comparison with that from fish or shellfish. The average daily intake of total mercury has been calculated to be about 3 mg, of which 80% is ingested as methylmercury and 20% as inorganic mercury (0.6 mg/day, of which 10% is absorbed). In cases of severe environmental contamination and ingestion of fish from polluted water, as occurred in Minamata and Niigata in the 1950s–1960s, the daily intake may reach toxic levels. Concentrations of 1–20 mg/kg of methylmercury in fish have been reported to result in a maximal daily intake of about 5 mg in persons with fish consumption

of 200–500 gm/day. In Iraq in the 1970s, toxic levels were reached after eating bread prepared from wheat treated with a methylmercury-containing fungicide. Similar outbreaks of methylmercury poisoning have occurred in Iraq, Pakistan, Ghana, and Guatemala.

3. Intoxications have been observed after use of mercury-containing creams and soap by some dark-skinned people to achieve a lighter skin tone.

4. Is exposure to organic mercury compounds used as fungicides in latex paints associated with a risk of mercury poisoning?

Several studies have shown that mercury vapor can be released from the mercury-containing paint on interior house walls.

5. What other sources may lead to high levels of mercury exposure?

Sources of higher exposure to mercury also may include inhalation of mercury vapors released from metallic mercury spills, incinerators, and facilities that burn mercury-containing fuels (for example, coal or other fossil fuels). Exposure near hazardous waste sites is likely to occur by inhaling contaminated air, entering in contact with contaminated soil, or drinking contaminated water.

6. Compare the routes of absorption of organic, inorganic, and metallic mercury.

Route of absorption	Organic	Inorganic	Metallic
Gastrointestinal tract	Very high	Low (10%)	Very low (0.1%)
Skin-mucosa	Possible	Possible	Very low
Respiratory tract	Easy	Depends on compound	Very high

7. What factors are important in the pharmacokinetics of the various forms of mercury?

Inhalation represents the main route of uptake of metallic mercury vapor; approximately 80% of the amount of mercury inhaled as vapor is absorbed at the alveolar level. Thus, most of the inhaled vapor enters the bloodstream and distributes rapidly to other parts of the body. When mercury vapor is inhaled, it is oxidized rapidly in red blood cells and tissues, mainly the liver and brain, to form the divalent cation. This reaction, however, is not rapid enough to prevent a significant fraction of the dissolved vapor from reaching the blood-brain barrier. Hence, the lipophilic vapor crosses the blood-brain barrier, is oxidized into the divalent form of mercury, and remains trapped. The oxidized form is assumed to be the proximate toxic species accounting for the effects of mercury vapor on the central nervous system. The gastrointestinal (GI) absorption of liquid metallic mercury is quite low (approximately 0.1%); most of the metallic mercury that a person swallows in liquid form does not easily enter the bloodstream and is eliminated in the feces. Inorganic mercury compounds are probably absorbed from the human GI tract at a level of less than 10% on average, but absorption varies considerably with the compound. Moreover, the corrosive action of some compounds (mercuric chloride) may alter the permeability of the GI tract, enhancing absorption. The rate of absorption of inhaled inorganic mercury aerosol and particles depends on the size and solubility of the compound.

To a certain extent, inorganic mercury also can enter the bloodstream directly through the skin. Organic mercury compounds are easily absorbed by all of the usual routes. Methylmercury in the diet is almost completely absorbed into the bloodstream and distributed to all tissues within about 4 days.

In blood, inorganic mercury is equally distributed between plasma and red blood cells, whereas organic mercury is found mainly in red blood cells. Methylmercury is highly stable and resistant to biotransformation, but derivatives such as phenylmercury compounds easily liberate inorganic mercury. The principal sites of deposition after exposure to metallic mercury vapor are the kidneys and brain; after exposure to inorganic mercury salts, the principal site of deposition is the kidney. Some mercury may stay in the body for weeks or months.

Because of its high lipophilicity, metallic mercury can be transferred readily through the placenta to the fetus and through the blood-brain barrier to the central nervous system. Inorganic compounds can reach most organs; however, their low lipophilicity reduces their ability to penetrate barriers and to accumulate in the brain and fetus. The distribution of methylmercury is similar to that of metallic mercury; a relatively large amount of Hg can accumulate in the brain and fetus (compared with inorganic Hg) because of its ability to cross the blood-brain and placental barriers. Mercury concentration in saliva has been investigated; however, this analysis is not routinely done and is not a significant predictor of exposure.

8. How are the various forms of mercury eliminated?

After exposure to metallic mercury, elimination occurs mainly through the urine and feces, although some elemental mercury is exhaled. Inorganic mercury is eliminated through the urine and feces. Organic mercury compounds are excreted predominantly in the feces. Both inorganic and methylmercury are excreted in breast milk.

9. Why does mercury seem to persist in urine long after cessation of occupational exposure?

Because mercury accumulates in the kidneys and brain, small amounts are constantly released from both depots. Thus urinary elimination of mercury persists for a long period after cessation of occupational exposure. Biologic half-lives ranging from 69 to 109 days have been reported in urine. Part of the mercury stored in the brain is eliminated slowly and has a biologic half-life that may exceed several years.

10. What are the acute effects of short-term inhalation of mercury vapor?

In cases of short-term inhalation of high levels of metallic mercury vapor, the target organ is the respiratory tract; the most commonly reported symptoms include cough, dyspnea, and chest tightness. In more severe cases pneumonitis, pulmonary edema (alveolar and interstitial), lobar pneumonia, fibrosis, and desquamation of the bronchiolar epithelium (with ensuing bronchiolar obstruction, alveolar dilatation, emphysema, and pneumothorax) have been observed. Exposure to high concentrations of elemental mercury vapors can produce a syndrome, similar to metal fume fever, characterized by asthenia, fever, chills, myalgia, and elevated leukocyte count. Acute inhalation of mercury vapor also may cause stomatitis, nausea, vomiting, or diarrhea and has resulted in effects ranging from mild transient to frank proteinuria, hematuria, and oliguria as well as acute renal failure with degeneration or necrosis of the proximal convoluted tubules.

11. What are the chronic effects of prolonged inhalation of mercury vapor?

The central nervous system is the most critical target tissue after prolonged exposure to elemental mercury vapor. The classical symptoms of chronic mercurialism are intentional tremor, erethism (personality and behavioral changes, shyness, irritability, insecurity, loss of memory, insomnia), and stomatogingivitis (inflammation of mouth and gums). They may occur alone or in combination. The tremor may begin in the eyelids, lips, and fingers; it increases with intentional movements, is aggravated by emotional stress, and disappears during sleep. Severe cases may result in generalized tremor with violent spasms. Changes in vision or hearing also may occur. The neurologic manifestations of mercury poisoning may include symptoms (weakness, numbness, paresthesia, muscle cramps) and signs (muscle atrophy, fasciculations, sensory loss) associated with damage to the peripheral nervous system. However, levels of occupational exposure have been reduced in recent years, and clinical toxic effects are rarely observed today.

The kidney is the second major target organ. All forms of mercury can cause kidney damage if large amounts are absorbed. However, renal alterations of clinical relevance are rare, despite the fact that the kidney represents the major organ of deposition during chronic exposure; cases of nephrotic syndromes have been described only after severe intoxication.

Many studies have investigated the early subclinical neurologic effects (alterations of intellectual functions and emotional state; disturbances of the motor system; such as tremor and psychomotor incoordination; peripheral neurotoxicity, such as nerve conduction velocity) and renal effects (urinary proteins of low or high molecular weight, enzymes, tubular antigens) of long-term exposure to relatively low concentrations of mercury. The most sensitive indicators remain to be identified.

Inorganic mercury salts are teratogenic in experimental animals. Because of considerable gaps in knowledge, limit values proposed for occupationally exposed populations should not be considered protective against the possible embryo-fetotoxic effects of metallic and inorganic mercury in humans.

12. If a child breaks a household oral thermometer in his or her mouth and swallows a small amount of mercury, what treatment, if any, is recommended?

Liquid metallic mercury is poorly absorbed after ingestion. Hence, if a child swallows the mercury content of a thermometer, the risk of systemic intoxication is low. Most of the mercury is excreted in the feces. If the parents are anxious, the mercury concentration in blood may be measured to exclude significant absorption.

13. What methods should be used to clean up a broken thermometer in the home?

A greater risk comes from metallic mercury spilled in small drops after a thermometer is broken. Mercury may be recovered from tiled floors with an eye dropper, but may be difficult to retrieve from hardwood floors. Mercury may contaminate cracks in the floors and vaporize over time. Carpets are particularly difficult to clean after mercury spills. Cases of intoxication have been described despite diligent attempts to clean the carpet. A vacuum cleaner that aspirates mercury may be the origin of recontamination after each future use. When mercury is thrown in a wash basin, care should be taken that no drops are left in the basin or pipe. The safest way to eliminate mercury is to trap it in water (to limit evaporation) and take it to the pharmacist.

14. What is acrodynia?

Acrodynia (pink disease) is rare but has been reported in children after use of mercury derivatives in teething powder or ointments applied to the skin. Diapers rinsed in a mercury-containing solution, mercury dispersed from fluorescent bulbs, long-term injection of gammaglobulin preserved with ethylmercurythiosalicylate, and inhalation of mercury vapor from latex paint also have been responsible for pink disease.

15. What are the symptoms of acrodynia?

Affected children become irritable and generally miserable and have difficulties in sleeping. Profuse sweating, conjunctivitis, photophobia, and generalized rash follow, accompanied by itching, flushing, and swelling. The extremities become cold, painful, red, and swollen, and the skin (mainly of palms and soles) desquamates. In most cases increased levels of mercury in urine were reported.

16. What is the primary target organ of methylmercury?

The nervous system is the principal if not the only target tissue for effects of methylmercury in adults. Signs and symptoms of intoxication do not appear until several weeks after absorption. Sensory, visual, and auditory functions and coordination are commonly affected. The earliest effects are paresthesia, malaise, and blurred vision, followed by concentric constriction of the visual field, deafness, dysarthria, and ataxia. The general population does not face a significant risk from methylmercury. However, people who have eaten fish contaminated by large amounts of methylmercury (Japan) or seed grains treated with methylmercury or other organic mercury compounds (Iraq) have experienced permanent damage. The effects of methylmercury on adults differ both qualitatively and quantitatively from the effects of prenatal or possibly early postnatal exposure. The fetus is at particular risk. Exposure to methylmercury interferes with brain development, affects normal neuronal development, and leads to altered brain architecture, heterotopic cells, and decreased brain size; it also may affect cell division at critical stages during the formation of the central nervous system. Exposure to methylmercury is also likely to be more dangerous for young children than for adults. The inhibition of protein synthesis is one of the earliest detectable biochemical effects in the adult brain, but the sequence of events leading to overt brain damage is not yet understood.

17. What elements of the history are important in evaluating a suspected case of occupational or environmental mercury poisoning?

Questions that are important to ask in history-taking include the following:
- What is your occupation?
- Do you wear protective uniforms, footgear, or other protective devices? Do you take them home?
- Where do you live? (Near an incinerator, hazardous waste site, sewage sludge, or area where a mercury-containing pesticide is used?)
- How long have you lived in your current home? (Possibility of latex paint?)
- Describe your diet. (Fish consumption?)
- Have you recently been treated by a dentist? How many amalgams do you have?
- What medications do you use? (Nose drops, antiseptics, gargle or mouthwash?)
- Do you use skin-lightening cream or soap?
- Have you recently broken a thermometer, any precision instrument containing mercury, or a mercury lamp?

18. What biomarkers are used to quantify exposure to mercury?

The mean total mercury levels in blood and urine of the general population are generally below 1 µg/100 ml and 5 µg/gm creatinine, respectively. Intra- and interindividual differences in biomarkers may be due to dental amalgam (blood, urine) and ingestion of contaminated fish (blood).

Urine is the most commonly used medium for monitoring occupational exposure to metallic mercury vapor and inorganic forms of mercury; organic mercury represents only a small fraction of urinary mercury. In newly exposed workers, urinary excretion does not immediately follow the onset of exposure; during the latency period the body accumulates a certain quantity of mercury. In a steady-state situation, urinary levels reflect the amount of mercury stored in the kidneys. Blood levels are measured less frequently. However, because blood levels of mercury peak sharply during and soon after short-term exposure, suspicion of temporary high exposure to mercury vapor can be confirmed by immediate blood sampling. Urinary mercury levels are less informative.

According to the World Health Organization, at a urinary excretion level of 100 µg/gm creatinine, the probability of developing classical neurologic signs of mercurial intoxication (tremor, erethism) and proteinuria is high. An exposure resulting in 30–100 µg/gm creatinine increases the incidence of less severe toxic effects that do not lead to overt clinical impairment. In a few studies, tremor has been recorded electrophysiologically at low urine concentrations (25–35 µg/gm creatinine). Other studies found no such effect at low exposure levels.

19. Which more accurately reflects the degree of mercury deposited in the brain—urinary or blood levels?

Neither urinary levels nor blood levels reflect the degree of mercury deposited in the brain.

20. How is dietary exposure differentiated from occupational exposure?

When levels of occupational exposure are low, the presence of amalgams or fish consumption may mask occupational absorption. When dietary intake of mercury is suspected as a possible source of exposure, speciation may be performed to exclude the influence of methylmercury from the diet. Another possibility is to analyze plasma and blood cells separately, because methylmercury accumulates primarily in blood cells. However, such analyses are not routine. The American Conference of Governmental Hygienists suggests the following biologic exposure indices for workers exposed to elemental and inorganic mercury; 35 µg/gm creatinine in urine (sampling time: preshift) and 15 µg/L in blood (sampling time: end of shift, end of work week).

21. What is the role of hair analysis in the monitoring of mercury exposure?

Hair analysis has become the most widely used means of biologic monitoring in populations suspected of exposure to methylmercury through fish consumption. It is specially useful to recapitulate maternal blood concentrations during pregnancy. The short segments of hair reveal recent exposure (i.e., blood levels within the past month or so). The longest hairs on the head recapitulate previous exposure. In view of the risk of external contamination by mercury, hair does not seem to be a satisfactory biologic material for evaluating exposure to mercury vapor.

22. What parameters are used to assess the effects of exposure to mercury?

Renal dysfunction. Several parameters have been evaluated for assessing early renal damage: markers of decreased function, such as increase in serum creatinine and serum beta$_2$ microglobulin or urinary proteins; markers of renal cytotoxicity, such as increases in urinary excretion of antigens and enzymes; and biochemical markers, including thromboxane, fibronectin, and kallikrein. None of these markers is specific for mercury intoxication.

Neurologic dysfunction. Neuropsychological and neurophysiologic effects can be investigated by psychomotor tests, cognitive function tests, mood-state scales, psychomotor coordination, and electrophysiologic investigations. None of these tests is specific for mercury intoxication.

23. What regimens are useful for treatment of mercury poisoning?

1. Immediate withdrawal from exposure.

2. Close pulmonary monitoring after acute inhalation of metallic mercury vapor.

3. Gastric lavage after ingestion of inorganic salts. Inclusion of salt-poor albumin or sodium formaldehyde sulfoxylate in the lavage fluid has been suggested. Oral administration of charcoal also has been proposed. Emesis should not be induced after ingestion of potentially caustic compounds such as mercury oxide.

4. Symptomatic treatment includes chelation therapy for mobilization of mercury from the body. Progress can be monitored by measuring the concentrations of mercury in blood and urine. Several chelating agents have been recommended:

- British antilewisite (BAL; 2,3-dimercaptopropanol), an effective chelator for inorganic mercury salts, has two sulfhydryl groups that can bind mercury and compete with its binding to sulfhydryl groups in body tissues. Approximately 50% of the dimercaprol-mercury complex is excreted through the kidneys; the remainder is eliminated in bile and feces. Significant reabsorption of mercury from bile may occur. Toxic side effects have been observed, including urticaria, elevated blood pressure and heart rate, nausea, vomiting, headache, conjunctivitis, lacrimation, and paresthesia. BAL appears to be effective in patients with high exposure levels and symptomatic patients but less effective in cases of chronic intoxication. BAL should be avoided in cases of methylmercury poisoning because it has been shown to increase brain levels of mercury in animal studies.

- D-penicillamine or its derivative, N-acetyl-D-penicillamine, also may be used in cases of elemental and inorganic mercury exposures. It can be taken orally. It is excreted only by the kidneys and should be used with extreme caution when renal function is impaired. It may be used alone or after treatment with BAL. Acute allergic reactions may occur.

- Newer derivatives appear promising, but experience is limited. Data suggest that DMSA (2,3-dimercaptosuccinic acid) and DMPS (2,3-dimercaptopropane-sulfonate) produce fewer side effects, but experimental studies have shown that they mobilize mainly mercury stored in the kidneys and seem less effective at mobilizing mercury accumulated in the brain.

- Hemodialysis with infusion of a chelator (cysteine, N-acetylcysteine) has been reported to be effective in cases of severe poisoning with renal failure. Because methylmercury undergoes enterohepatic recirculation in experimental animals, the administration of a nonabsorbable, mercury-binding substance (e.g., polythiol resin) into the gastrointestinal tract has been suggested.

CONTROVERSIES

24. To what extent should clinicians be concerned about dental amalgam containing mercury? What about mercury hypersensitivity?

Besides the consumption of fish contaminated with methylmercury, the other most likely form of exposure for the general population is absorption of mercury vapor released from dental fillings. Dental amalgam is a mixture of mercury with a silver-tin alloy. Most classical silver-colored amalgams consist of about 45–50% mercury, 25–35% silver, 2–30% copper, and 15–30% tin. Short-term exposure to high concentrations of elemental mercury vapor may occur during dental treatment (removal of old fillings; carving and polishing of new fillings). Long-term exposure to lower mercury concentrations occurs when the metal is released in the form of vapor from the occlusal fillings as a result of corrosion. The rate of release is increased when the amalgam surface is stressed by chewing, grinding, and brushing. Significant data show that such exposure can lead to an increased concentration of mercury in urine, blood, and several organs, including the central nervous system and kidneys. The average daily uptake of mercury vapor from a moderate number of fillings has been estimated to range from 3.8–21 µg/day, with corresponding retentions of 3–17 µg/day. Lower rates have been recently reported. Insufficient evidence supports a relation between the number of amalgam fillings and increased prevalence of complaints and symptoms such as paresthesia, tremor, irritability, and anxiety. The exceptions are individual cases of allergies, in which such symptoms occasionally have been reported in relation to amalgam fillings. In most cases the main symptoms are facial dermatitis, sometimes with erythematous and urticarial rashes. The possible causal role of dental amalgams also has been suggested in cases of oral lichen planus and generalized dermatitis. Hypersensitivity to mercury can be confirmed by patch tests.

25. What are the most effective ways of reducing or preventing mercury exposure?

Mercury is an element and therefore cannot be broken down. Incineration is not recommended as a disposal method. Recycling of mercury-containing compounds is an important method of disposal.

Prevention is certainly the best management of toxicity in the occupational setting. Wherever possible, mercury should be handled in hermetically sealed systems, and extremely strict hygiene conditions should be applied at the workplace. Local exhaust ventilation systems should be installed, and filtration of the ventilated air before release may be required in some cases. When mercury is heated, even stricter controls are required. When mercury is spilled, it easily infiltrates crevices and gaps in the floor and workbenches. Because of its vapor pressure, a high atmospheric concentration may result from even seemingly negligible contamination. Therefore, the work area where mercury is used should be easily cleanable and have a nonporous, nonabsorbent surface, slightly tilted toward a collector. Alternatively, a metal grill may be placed over a gutter filled with water to collect any drops of mercury that fall through the grill. Working surfaces should be cleaned regularly. Commercial decontaminating powders or solutions as well as mercury collectors are available and may be of some help. Spills are collected by pressing the foam-padded lid of the collector against the drops. Collected drops are released by pressure against the perforated disc when the container is recapped. Vacuum cleaners equipped with special filters adsorbing mercury vapors are also available. Ambient air monitoring should be done to ensure adequate clean-up. Workers should wear nonporous protective clothing without pockets. Work clothing should never be taken home.

BIBLIOGRAPHY

1. Agency for Toxic Substances and Disease Registry: Toxicological Profile for Mercury. Atlanta, U.S. Department of Health and Human Services, 1994.
2. Alessio L, Crippa M, Lucchini R, Roi R: CEC Criteria Document for Occupational Exposure Limit Values. Inorganic Mercury. Commission of the European Communities, Joint Research Centre, 1993.
3. Berlin M: Mercury. In Friberg L, Nordberg G, Vouk V (eds): Handbook on the Toxicology of Metals, 2nd ed. Amsterdam, Elsevier, 1986, pp 387–445.
4. Clarkson TH, Hursh J, Sager P, Syversen T: Mercury. In Clarkson TH, Friberg L, Nordberg G, Sager P (eds): Biological Monitoring of Toxic Metals. New York, Plenum Press, 1988, pp 199–246.
5. Lauwerys R: Mercury. In Parmeggiani L (ed): ILO Encyclopaedia of Occupational Health and Safety. Geneva, 1983, pp 1332–1334.
6. Lauwerys R, Hoet P: Industrial Chemical Exposure. Guidelines for Biological Monitoring. Boca Raton, FL, Lewis Publishers, 1993, pp 74–82.

7. World Health Organization: Environmental Health Criteria 101. Methylmercury. Geneva, World Health
    Organization, 1990.
8. World Health Organization: Environmental Health Criteria 118. Inorganic Mercury. Geneva, World Health
    Organization, 1991.

11. CADMIUM AND COBALT

John R. Balmes, M.D., Lynda Sisson, M.D., M.P.H.,
and Cornelius H. Scannell, M.D., M.P.H.

CADMIUM

1. What are the most common occupations involving cadmium exposure?

Cadmium is not mined. It is refined as a byproduct of the smelting of other metals, such as zinc, copper, and lead. Cadmium is used most commonly in electroplating of iron and steel to improve corrosion resistance. Another common use of cadmium is to make pigments for paints and plastics. Cadmium stearate is added to plastics as a stabilizer and to copper alloys to improve mechanical properties. Alkaline batteries are often of the nickel-cadmium type. Because cadmium has a relatively low boiling point (765° C), the use of cadmium-containing solder or welding electrodes or welding on cadmium-plated materials can generate cadmium fumes. Occupational exposure has been documented in all of these processes.

2. What is itai-itai disease?

In Toyama Bay, Japan, there was an epidemic of renal disease in people, especially postmenopausal women, exposed to cadmium from eating rice grown in fields irrigated with cadmium-containing effluent from a mine. The renal disease was characterized by proteinuria and osteomalacia. Affected women complained of bone pain; hence, the name itai-itai (ouch-ouch) disease.

3. By what routes of absorption does cadmium exposure occur?

Skin absorption is negligible. Gastrointestinal absorption is usually only about 5% of an ingested dose, but this rate may increase up to 20% in people with iron or calcium deficiency. Certain grains, such as rice and wheat, concentrate cadmium present in soil or water so that environmental exposure usually results from eating contaminated foods. Pulmonary absorption, which is the main route of occupational exposure, is higher (up to 50%).

4. What are the acute effects of cadmium exposure?

Inhalational exposure to cadmium fumes, usually associated with welding or using silver solder, may result in initial symptoms—fever, chills, and metallic taste—that resemble the symptoms of metal fume fever. Unlike the relatively benign flulike illness of metal fume fever, cadmium pneumonitis may be a severe illness, involving shortness of breath, hypoxia, and frank respiratory failure due to noncardiogenic pulmonary edema. Such respiratory effects may be delayed for up to 24 hours after exposure. The severity of the respiratory effects of cadmium fume inhalation depends on the intensity of exposure. With mild exposure, recovery is usually complete after several days. With intense exposure, death or permanent pulmonary impairment may result. Ingestion of large amounts of cadmium salts may directly irritate the gastric muscosa, leading to nausea, vomiting, abdominal cramps, and diarrhea. Symptoms develop rapidly after such an ingestion.

5. What is the critical target organ of chronic cadmium exposure?

The kidney is the organ most affected by chronic cadmium exposure. Absorbed cadmium is transported in the blood to the kidneys, liver, and muscle. Cadmium stimulates the production of metallothionein, a protein that binds the metal in blood and tissue. Cadmium-metallothionein complexes in the plasma are filtered by the glomeruli but are efficiently reabsorbed in the proximal renal tubules. If the cadmium concentration in renal tubular cells accumulates to a certain threshold (100–300 µg/gm of tissue), renal toxicity occurs. As a result, proximal renal tubular reabsorption is decreased as manifested by loss of proteins, such as beta-2 microglobulin or retinol-binding protein, in the urine. 1-Hydroxylation of 25-hydroxyvitamin D, which occurs with renal tubular cells, is impaired. When tubular toxicity is severe, other components of the glomerular filtrate are lost in the urine (e.g., calcium, phosphate, amino acids), and eventually glomerular function becomes compromised, leading to an elevated serum creatinine. Osteomalacia, osteoporosis, and bone pain tend to occur in persons with decreased dietary calcium intake and/or hormonal effects, such as postmenopausal women.

6. What other chronic effects are associated with cadmium exposure?

Other chronic effects of cadmium exposure include emphysema (with inhalational exposure), anemia (usually mild), liver dysfunction (often subclinical elevation of transaminases in serum), and increased risk of prostate and lung cancers.

7. How should one approach the diagnosis and management of acute inhalational exposure to cadmium?

When a patient presents with acute symptoms after inhalation of metal fumes, it is important to ask whether cadmium was present. Unfortunately, the patient may not be aware of its presence because cadmium is often only a trace component. As noted above, the initial presentation after cadmium fume inhalation may be confused with a benign condition, metal fume fever. Measurement of cadmium in the blood may show an elevated level that documents exposure. Therapy is supportive. Chelation is problematic because cadmium mobilized from pulmonary and other tissues is likely to be deposited in the kidneys and thus may precipitate renal dysfunction.

8. What are the pharmacokinetics of cadmium in the human body?

With chronic exposure, cadmium levels in whole blood increase several-fold during the first few months and then plateau. With cessation of exposure, cadmium in whole blood decreases following a two-component model. An initial rapid clearance phase (half life = ~ 100 days) is followed by a much slower phase (half-life = ~ 10 years). Thus, measurement of cadmium during ongoing exposure may be misleading because an increased blood level may occur with a relatively low body burden (after a few months), and an unimpressive blood level may be observed after prolonged removal from exposure despite a high body burden. (In persons not occupationally or environmentally exposed to cadmium, the whole blood cadmium level is typically well below 1 µg/100 ml). Smokers tend to have slightly higher blood cadmium levels because each cigarette contains from 1–2 µg of cadmium; approximately 10% is absorbed.

Cadmium is excreted primarily through the urine. In persons not occupationally or environmentally exposed, urine cadmium levels are typically below 2 µg/gm of urinary creatinine. With ongoing exposure, most filtered cadmium is reabsorbed in the proximal tubules so that urinary cadmium may not be much elevated. When binding sites within renal tissue become saturated, urinary cadmium increases because reabsorption decreases. After renal dysfunction has developed, urinary cadmium markedly increases, reflecting loss of cadmium sequestered in proximal tubular cells. Even if exposure ceases, urinary cadmium remains elevated; as more cadmium is lost in the urine, more is redistributed to the kidneys from other tissues. Persons with cadmium-induced renal toxicity usually have a urinary cadmium level > 10 µg/gm of urinary cadmium.

9. How should workers with chronic occupational exposure to cadmium be monitored?

Because the kidneys are the target organ of chronic cadmium dysfunction, workers should be monitored to prevent the development of renal dysfunction. The critical parameter correlating with toxicity is the renal burden of cadmium, which at present cannot be easily measured. Thus, other biologic parameters that tend to correlate with renal cadmium burden are measured instead. The earliest marker of cadmium-induced renal toxicity is increased excretion of low-molecular-weight proteins that normally are reabsorbed in the proximal tubules. The most commonly measured protein is beta-2 microglobulin (normal level = < 200 µg/gm of urinary creatinine). Measurement of retinol-binding protein is a reasonable alternative.

Exposed workers also should undergo periodic pulmonary function tests to detect evidence of emphysema and screening tests for prostate cancer (e.g., digital rectal examination and prostate-specific antigen [PSA] measurement) after the age of 50 years.

10. How should cadmium-induced chronic health effects be prevented?

Occupationally exposed workers with elevated blood or urinary cadmium should be removed from further exposure. If possible, other materials should be substituted for cadmium. If substitution is not possible, engineering controls should be used to minimize exposure, and workers need to be trained to avoid cadmium exposure. Administrative measures, such as banning eating, drinking, and smoking in cadmium-containing areas, also may reduce exposure.

11. An ironworker presents to the emergency department (ED) at 10:00 PM with fever, chills, myalgias, burning substernal chest pain, and cough after welding earlier that day on a steel structure that he thought was galvanized. His physical exam reveals a respiratory rate of 24, and bilateral inspiratory crackles at the bases that do not clear with cough. His arterial oxygen saturation is 90% on room air, his white blood count is elevated, and his chest radiograph reveals diffuse, patchy infiltrates. Why should you suspect cadmium fume inhalation? How should you determine whether your suspicion is correct?

Although the patient's history of welding on what he thought was galvanized steel suggests metal fume fever, the severe respiratory symptoms and objective evidence of respiratory dysfunction do not support such a diagnosis. As noted above, respiratory symptoms and signs after metal fume inhalation should always prompt consideration of possible cadmium exposure. This patient was originally sent home from the ED but returned several hours later when his symptoms worsened. Intubation was avoided, but he required supportive care, including supplemental oxygen and inhaled bronchodilator therapy. He also developed mild renal insufficiency. The correct diagnosis of acute cadmium pneumonitis was made after a call to the regional poison control center (PCC). Based on the patient's presentation, the PCC suggested cadmium inhalation, which was confirmed with a urinary cadmium level of 17 µg/gm urinary creatinine.

COBALT

12. What are the most common occupations involving cobalt exposure?

Cobalt is produced as a byproduct of the mining and processing of copper and nickel ore. Cobalt is both hard and magnetic. It is used to make alloys such as high-strength steel and permanent magnets. Cobalt is the binder in "hard metal," a cemented tungsten carbide that is used in the manufacture of machine tools, saw blades, and drill tips. Cobalt is also found in other types of cemented carbides, such as abrasives used to polish diamonds. Cobalt compounds are used as pigments in glass manufacture and the ceramic industry; as drying agents in paints, lacquers, and inks; as catalysts in the oil and chemical industries; as additives in animal feeds; and as foam stabilizers.

13. What are the most common environmental exposures?

Food and beverages containing cobalt are the main sources of environmental exposure. Concentrations of 0.1–5.0 mg/l have been found in drinking water. Traces of cobalt are found in cement and various household products. However, there is no indication that cobalt metal or cobalt compounds constitute a health risk to nonoccupationally exposed populations. In fact, cobalt is an essential nutrient for humans, and vitamin B_{12} (hydroxocobalamin) contains cobalt.

14. What are the pharmacokinetics of cobalt in the human body?

Cobalt is primarily absorbed from the pulmonary and gastrointestinal tract. Although skin absorption may occur, it does not appear to lead to systemic toxicity. The rate of absorption depends on the solubility of the compound, which, in turn, is determined primarily by the presence of other substances, such as the components of tungsten carbide with exposure to hard metal. In the body, the highest concentrations of cobalt are found in the liver and kidneys. Cobalt is not a cumulative toxin, and the total body cobalt content tends to remain stable at a level of 1.5 mg. It is excreted in the urine and to a lesser extent in the feces. Urinary excretion of cobalt is characterized by an initial rapid clearance phase of a few days' duration followed by a slower second phase that lasts for several years.

15. What is the mechanism of cobalt toxicity?

Although the exact mechanism of cobalt toxicity is not fully understood, the general consensus is that it can induce abnormal immune responses in the skin and respiratory tract. Another postulated mechanism is that cobalt is capable of generating free radicals through an oxidant effect that, in turn, injures tissues.

16. What are the target organs of cobalt toxicity?

1. **Respiratory tract.** Exposure to cobalt or hard metal dust may cause allergic asthma with recurrent episodes of cough, wheezing, and shortness of breath. The latent period between onset of exposure and development of asthmatic symptoms ranges from a few months to a few years. The presence of specific IgE antibodies to cobalt-conjugated human serum albumin has been reported in patients with cobalt-induced occupational asthma. Asthma caused by cobalt may resolve after cessation of exposure or persist if the affected worker is not promptly removed from further exposure. Some workers exposed to cobalt develop giant cell interstitial pneumonitis, which, in the setting of hard metal dust exposure, is usually called hard metal disease. Repeated episodes of pneumonitis may lead to pulmonary interstitial fibrosis. A subgroup of workers with cobalt-induced pneumonitis develop a rapidly progressive and potentially fatal form of pulmonary fibrosis. Symptoms and signs identical to those found with other types of pulmonary fibrosis are typically present in workers with cobalt-induced pulmonary fibrosis, including nonproductive cough, shortness of breath, tachypnea, poor lung expansion, crackles on auscultation, and finger clubbing. Chest radiographs in such workers show nonspecific evidence of interstitial disease, and pulmonary function tests show nonspecific changes consistent with restrictive and diffusion impairments. Bronchoalveolar lavage and lung biopsy may reveal characteristic multinucleated giant cells.

2. **Skin.** Cobalt exposure may lead to allergic contact dermatitis. It also may have direct irritant effects. Cobalt-induced contact dermatitis is associated with a specific cell-mediated immune response involving sensitization of T lymphocytes. Patch testing and lymphocyte transformation testing have been used to confirm the diagnosis.

3. **Hematopoietic system.** Cobalt is a potent stimulus for red blood cell production. In fact, cobalt salts were once used for the treatment of sickle cell anemia and other congenital anemias. The mechanism appears to be increased erythropoietin production as a result of local hypoxia. However, polycythemia does not appear to have been a problem recognized among cobalt-exposed workers except in those who have interstitial pulmonary fibrosis with chronic hypoxemia (i.e., secondary polycythemia).

4. **Myocardium.** Cobalt has been linked to the development of cardiomyopathy. This association, observed among heavy consumers of beer that contained cobalt as a foam stabilizer, is potentially confounded by alcohol use. Cobalt has been shown, however, to be a direct cardiotoxin capable of causing cardiac muscle dysfunction. Nonetheless, it is not clear whether occupational exposure to cobalt is capable of causing clinical cardiomyopathy.

5. **Thyroid gland.** Decreased thyroid function with goiter is a known side effect of cobalt therapy for anemia. One study showed reduced uptake of radiolabeled iodine with administration of cobalt. In the occupational setting, subclinical hypothyroid effects have been reported, but no evidence suggests that it is a clinical problem among cobalt-exposed workers.

17. How should workers with occupational exposure to cobalt be monitored?

Biologic monitoring of cobalt exposure is somewhat problematic given the pharmacokinetics of its elimination from the body. The biphasic elimination rate of cobalt in urine makes it difficult to correlate exposure levels and urine concentrations. Some studies have demonstrated a reasonable linear relationship between cumulative exposure and urinary concentration. Therefore, it has been proposed that exposure to cobalt should be monitored by obtaining two urinary levels: the first at the end of a work week and the second at the end of the first period of work after a prolonged period off work. The two levels should reflect cumulative and current exposure, respectively. A linear relationship between exposure and blood concentration also has been demonstrated, but only when ambient levels are high (i.e., > 0.05 mg/m^3, the current threshold limit value [TLV] of the American Conference of Governmental Industrial Hygienists).

Environmental monitoring of cobalt levels provides a reasonable assessment of worker exposure, although in a workplace where hard metal dust is the source of cobalt exposure, measurement of airborne cobalt concentration can be difficult. Regular monitoring of urine cobalt concentrations has been used to monitor relatively low-level exposures. A medical surveillance program for occupational asthma and interstitial lung disease, including review of respiratory symptoms, spirometry, diffusing capacity, and chest radiographs, should be instituted for workers who are clearly at increased risk of cobalt-induced respiratory tract disease (e.g., hard metal grinders and diamond polishers). Symptomatic workers without evidence of interstitial lung disease should be evaluated for occupational asthma with cross-shift spirometry, serial peak expiratory flow measurements, or challenge for nonspecific airway responsiveness. Pulmonary function tests and chest radiographs are somewhat insensitive tests for interstitial lung disease, and normal results do not preclude the diagnosis. Referral to a pulmonary specialist should be considered if one suspects the diagnosis even with a normal chest radiograph and normal pulmonary function.

18. What treatments are available for cobalt-induced health effects?

Initial treatment of cobalt-induced occupational diseases usually requires removal of the worker from further exposure. Symptoms of cobalt-induced asthma should be treated according to the National Asthma Education Project guidelines. Interstitial lung disease is initially treated with prednisone, but other agents, including cyclophosphamide, have been successfully used in individual cases after failure to respond to prednisone. Workers with irritant dermatitis should be protected from skin exposure, and those with a positive cobalt patch test or lymphocyte transformation test should avoid all skin contact with cobalt-containing compounds. Various antidotes for acute cobalt intoxication have been suggested, but none can be specifically recommended.

19. How should cobalt-induced health effects be prevented?

High levels of airborne cobalt can be successfully lowered with engineering controls such as local exhaust ventilation systems and dust suppression techniques. The application of such controls in recent years appears to have lowered the prevalence of cobalt-induced interstitial pulmonary fibrosis compared with historic rates.

20. A woman applying for a job as a hard metal tool grinder presents with a history of a recurrent skin rash related to jewelry wear and a positive patch test for cobalt by her dermatologist. Is she at increased risk of cobalt-induced respiratory tract disease? Should she be excluded from the job?

No clear correlation has been observed between cobalt dermatitis and cobalt-induced respiratory tract disease, either asthma or interstitial lung disease. As noted above, cobalt contact dermatitis involves delayed hypersensitivity. Prudence dictates avoidance of further exposure to cobalt in persons with dermatitis diagnosed by positive patch test or lymphocyte transformation testing. The woman should be offered a job without cobalt exposure. Persons with cobalt-related irritant dermatitis can work in jobs involving cobalt, but steps should be taken to reduce skin contact.

BIBLIOGRAPHY

1. Balmes JR: Respiratory effects of hard metal exposure. Occup Med State Art Rev 2:327–344, 1987.
2. Barnhart S, Rosenstock L: Cadmium chemical pneumonitis. Chest 86:789–791, 1984.
3. Davison AG, Taylor AJN, Darbyshire J, et al: Cadmium fume inhalation and emphysema. Lancet i:663–667, 1988.

4. Jarup L, Elinder CG: Dose-response relations between urinary cadmium and tubular proteinuria in cadmium-exposed workers. Am J Indust Med 26:759, 1994.
5. Nemery B, Casier P, Roosels D, et al: Survey of cobalt exposure and respiratory health in diamond polishers. Am Rev Respir Dis 145:610–616, 1992.
6. Scansetti G, Lamon S, Talarico S, et al: Urinary cobalt as a measure of exposure in the hard metal industry. Int Arch Occup Environ Health 57:19–26, 1985.
7. Shaikh ZA, Tohyama C, Nolan CV: Occupational exposure to cadmium: Effect on metallothionein and other biologic indices of exposure and renal function. Arch Toxicol 59:360–364, 1987.
8. Sprince NL, Oliver LC, Eisen E, et al: Cobalt exposure and lung disease in tungsten carbide production. Am Rev Respir Dis 138:1220–1226, 1988.

12. BERYLLIUM

Kathleen Kreiss, M.D.

1. What industries and jobs involve beryllium exposure?

Beryllium is an extremely lightweight metal (atomic weight of 9) that is transparent to x-rays and gives up neutrons. These properties led to its use as a lens in x-ray machines and in nuclear weapons as a neutron moderator. As a 1–2% alloy of beryllium-copper, it confers properties of strength, resistance to fatigue and impact, and freedom from deformity due to strain (elastic drift). Thus, beryllium-copper is used in springs and scientific equipment. Beryllium oxide (beryllia) is used to make ceramics, which are excellent heat conductors and high-temperature insulators; hence, beryllia ceramic chips are metallized with circuits for many semiconductor applications, including ignition switches in automobiles.

Industries using beryllium or its compounds include the primary production industries, high-technology ceramics, and alloys for special applications in nuclear weapons, aerospace, dentistry, golf clubs, and tools. Within these industries, virtually all job descriptions may involve beryllium exposure. In addition, beryllium exposure may occur but be unsuspected in reclamation of precious metals.

Exposure in the primary extraction industry involves soluble beryllium salts, and the fumes in extraction furnace operations appears to confer high risk of sensitization and disease in comparison with other processes in metal and alloy production. Elsewhere in the industry, exposure primarily involves dust or beryllium aerosols, as in machining of beryllium-copper alloy, beryllium metal, or beryllia ceramics. Machining processes have been shown to confer excessive risk in both metal and ceramic segments of the industry. Approaches to exposure control include enclosing operations with exhaust ventilation and provision of respiratory protection.

2. What diseases does beryllium cause?

The principal target organs for beryllium-related health effects are the skin and lungs. When workers are exposed to beryllium or its compounds, a small percentage develop granulomatous lung disease, known as chronic beryllium disease. In the beryllium extraction industry, a large percentage of workers develop contact dermatitis and/or beryllium skin ulcers in relation to soluble salt exposure. Historically, workers in extraction also were described as having chemical nasopharyngitis, tracheobronchitis, and/or pneumonitis with subacute onset, which resolved with cessation of exposure to beryllium salts and always within 1 year of symptom onset. In contrast, the chronic disease may develop after workers have left the beryllium industry, sometimes with a latency of several decades from first exposure. With workforce screening, latencies as short as a few weeks from first employment have been recognized.

3. What is Salem sarcoid?

In the 1940s, beryllium oxide was used in making phosphors in the fluorescent light industry before its health hazards were recognized in the United States. With the entry of many women into the workforce during World War II, several cases of severe "sarcoidosis" occurred among young women in a light bulb plant in Salem, Massachusetts. This cluster of cases was suspected to have an occupational cause and led to the recognition of chronic beryllium disease for the first time. Beryllium has not been used in fluorescent light bulb manufacture since 1949.

4. How do cases of beryllium disease present?

The cardinal symptoms of clinical beryllium disease are chronic cough and exertional shortness of breath. In addition, patients may have wheezing, fevers, weight loss, and profound fatigue. Workforce screening programs may identify asymptomatic workers as well. The most

75

sensitive clinical test for abnormality is oxygen desaturation on exercise tolerance testing, which often long precedes abnormal pulmonary function tests (obstructive or restrictive), low diffusing capacity, interstitial changes on chest radiograph, or hilar adenopathy (in a minority of cases).

5. Why are only a small percentage of beryllium-exposed workers affected?

Beryllium disease arises only in workers who develop a cell-mediated immune response to beryllium. This T-helper cell response can be measured with the beryllium lymphocyte proliferation test, using mononuclear cells from peripheral blood or bronchoalveolar lavage. The sensitivity of the blood test varies from laboratory to laboratory and may be only 50%. In contrast, lavage cells nearly always respond to beryllium, although alveolar macrophages in smokers may inhibit the lymphocyte response and may need to be removed from the assay.

6. Describe the diagnostic criteria for beryllium disease.

The diagnosis of beryllium disease requires evidence of lymphocyte proliferation to beryllium in blood or lavage lymphocytes. This specific characteristic differentiates the disease from other granulomatous diseases, such as sarcoidosis and hypersensitivity pneumonitis. The diagnosis usually requires bronchoscopy for bronchoalveolar lavage and transbronchial lung biopsy in asymptomatic cases detected in screening programs. In clinically evident disease, a chest radiograph compatible with granulomatous disease may make tissue evidence of granulomas unnecessary in the setting of beryllium sensitivity.

7. Which screening tests are appropriate for beryllium-exposed workers?

Early diagnosis of beryllium sensitivity is now possible with the beryllium lymphocyte proliferation test on screening blood samples. Workers with abnormal blood tests may have sensitization only or subclinical beryllium disease, a diagnosis made on bronchoscopy. A small percentage of cases with abnormal lavage lymphocyte proliferation tests have normal blood tests; these cases can be identified with chest radiograph screening. Pulmonary function tests, diffusing capacity, and symptom questionnaires are too insensitive and nonspecific to be useful except in the extraction industry.

8. How do you judge whether a worker has had significant beryllium exposure?

Any beryllium exposure is significant. In nearly every plant studied, both historically and recently, cases of beryllium disease have occurred among persons without industrial job descriptions, including secretaries, accountants, security guards, and inspectors of final product. Thus, the physician evaluating a patient with granulomatous disease should inquire about the industry as well as the job description. Cases have occurred among workers in former beryllium plants who were hired long after beryllium production ceased. Similarly, cases have occurred among family members of beryllium workers and community residents living in proximity to beryllium plants.

9. Since idiosyncratic cases occur with brief or minimal exposures, what is the basis of the permissible exposure limits?

The permissible exposure limits of $2 \ \mu g/m^3$ for a time-weighted average, $5 \ \mu g/m^3$ for a short-term exposure limit, and $25 \ \mu g/m^3$ as a ceiling exposure limit were not based on empiric data. The standard is known as the "taxicab standard" because it was proposed on the basis of a conversation between experts in a cab who believed that the standard should be analogous to other toxic metals (proportional to atomic weight). Nevertheless, the occurrence of "chemical pneumonitis" in beryllium workers was thought to be eliminated by adherence to the taxicab standard. The incidence of chronic irreversible disease may not have changed with these standards. Nevertheless, cross-sectional studies of modern beryllium-exposed populations have uniformly found process-related risks, suggesting that exposure characteristics are critical to disease risk. In one plant with usable historical measurements, the machining jobs had highest risk and highest median exposures. In another plant, however, the process with the highest contemporary risk did not have the highest indices of gravimetric exposure. Reexamination of permissible exposure limits may take into account respirable beryllium exposures (or other characteristics apart from total mass of beryllium) that characterize high-risk processes.

10. Can susceptibility to disease be identified?

Approximately 80% of cases of beryllium disease are associated with a genetic marker, HLA-DP glu69, which is present in 30–40% of the general population as a normal variant. Accordingly, its predictive value for beryllium disease is very low. Even if it were to be used in preplacement evaluation (an ethically dubious practice), beryllium disease occurs among workers without the marker. Research continues on this and other markers with the hope that understanding of the molecular mechanism of beryllium disease may lead to secondary prevention.

The lymphocyte proliferation test is not a test of susceptibility to beryllium disease, although it identifies a postexposure group with the immunologic response necessary for disease, most of whom already have granulomatous disease. The remainder are at high risk of developing granulomatous disease.

11. Is there a role for determining beryllium concentrations in tissue, blood, or urine?

No relation has been shown between lung or urine concentrations of beryllium and risk or severity of disease. This finding may be predictable for a disease now known to be immunologically mediated. Beryllium remains in tissue and urine for decades after exposure to insoluble beryllium compounds, such as beryllium oxide in ceramics and metal industries. The only use of beryllium assays in biologic samples is in research. For example, demonstration of beryllium in lung granulomas by laser microprobe mass spectroscopy is of interest in current documentation of beryllium disease in a household contact of a beryllium worker. The presence of lymphocyte proliferation to beryllium indicates prior exposure, whether or not beryllium can be measured in biologic materials.

12. How should you pursue the diagnosis of beryllium disease in persons with known granulomatous lung disease?

Beryllium disease cannot be distinguished on pathologic grounds from sarcoidosis, hence the term "Salem sarcoid." The only way to ensure that a case of sarcoidosis is not due to beryllium is to test blood and lavage lymphocytes with the beryllium lymphocyte proliferation test. Bystander, household, and community cases make it difficult to rule out beryllium disease with personal work history alone. On the other hand, sarcoidosis does occur in beryllium workers.

13. Is beryllium disease curable?

The acute pneumonitis recognized in the 1940s was cured by exposure cessation if the patient survived the acute illness. In contrast, chronic beryllium disease is not usually improved by exposure cessation and indeed may develop decades after exposure has ceased. Although not curable, the disease is responsive to corticosteroids in most cases, particularly if the diagnosis is made before fibrosis is a dominant characteristic. Unfortunately, most patients with physiologic impairment require lifelong steroids for disease suppression. In asymptomatic cases identified in workplace screening programs, steroids are not commonly used until clinically indicated by objective deterioration.

14. A 26-year-old construction worker applies for a position in a beryllia ceramics plant as a plant facilities worker. On preplacement testing, he is found to have an abnormal beryllium lymphocyte proliferation test, a normal chest radiograph, normal pulmonary functions, and no chest symptoms. The plant physician learns that he was involved in demolition work at the Rocky Flats nuclear weapons plant after production ceased. What would you recommend for job placement and worker notification?

The applicant's abnormal lymphocyte proliferation test indicates that he is sensitized to beryllium as a result of prior exposure. In this case, the exposure was likely to have been in the former nuclear weapons plant. Most industrial facilities with beryllium production remain conta-minated despite clean-up efforts. In demolition work, settled dust in ventilation systems or on false ceilings leads to predictable but often unrecognized exposure. Although the applicant has no symptoms or signs of beryllium disease, he has not undergone bronchoscopy to rule out the diagnosis of granulomatous lung disease. With or without lung disease, it is medically prudent to restrict him from further beryllium exposure. In addition, he should be notified of the screening test result. He may want to consult his previous employer at Rocky Flats to participate in a worker surveillance program sponsored by the U.S. Department of Energy for former nuclear weapons workers. At a minimum, the applicant needs to bring his previous beryllium exposure and sensitization status to the attention of his physician if he develops chest symptoms.

CONTROVERSIES

15. Does beryllium cause cancer?

Beryllium causes lung cancer in several animal species. In addition, a small excess of lung cancer has been documented in an industry-wide cohort of beryllium workers and among persons with beryllium disease in the U.S. Beryllium Case Registry. On this basis, the International Agency for Research on Cancer designated beryllium as a probable human carcinogen. The beryllium industry disputes this designation, saying that the excess in lung cancer arose in only one or two plants among seven.

16. Is workplace screening warranted?

Although beryllium lymphocyte proliferation testing can identify sensitized persons, most of whom have beryllium disease in an asymptomatic stage, no investigators have studied whether early diagnosis changes prognosis, either by early treatment or by removal from beryllium expo-sure. Only in the beryllium extraction industry does evidence indicate that removal of sympto-matic workers can lead to resolution or improvement of symptoms. In the absence of data in the rest of the industry, some beryllium plants do not remove workers with sensitization or subclinical disease from beryllium exposure, although it seems prudent to do so from a medical point of view.

Because efficacy of screening in changing prognosis has not been studied, the rationale for screening is the identification of risk factors in the worker population that may lead to preventive measures. In contemporary screening, process-related risk factors have been demonstrated in every plant studied. These work factors can form the basis for preventing disease in the future and for understanding the qualitative and quantitative exposures that confer risk of beryllium disease. Screening is justified for surveillance, but the benefit for individual workers remains unclear.

17. Was acute beryllium disease a toxic pneumonitis?

Acute beryllium disease was not recognized in the United States after 1953, although expo-sures in excess of the standard have occurred in many plants. Has the disease really disappeared, or is it no longer diagnosed, even in the extraction industry where it occurred historically? In re-viewing the clinical descriptions of the disease from the 1940s, including pathologic reports for fatal cases, acute disease was accompanied by mononuclear cell alveolitis and interstitial infil-trate similar to what is seen in chronic disease. The radiographic abnormality lagged about 3 weeks after symptomatic presentation. Such features suggest that it was not a toxic pneumonitis with acute pulmonary edema as seen in phosgene poisoning. Symptomatic disease often recurred in workers who returned to beryllium work after resolution of acute pneumonitis. In light of cur-rent understanding of the cell-mediated immunologic nature of chronic beryllium disease, acute disease seems to be remarkably similar.

On the other hand, acute disease was clearly reversible with restriction from exposure, whereas the chronic disease recognized today is not. The time course of improvement of the acute disease was months. The explanation may lie in the biopersistence of different beryllium compounds. The acute disease arose in the setting of exposure to soluble salts. Persons sensitized to beryllium with such exposure are likely to improve as they clear the antigen over time. In contrast, beryllium metal or oxide is an insoluble antigen that may result in sensitization even years after workplace exposure has ceased. Once the worker is sensitized, the granulomatous reaction persists along with the antigen. Perhaps for this reason two distinct clinical courses of disease were described historically in different sectors of the industry. The possible identity of pathologic mechanism may explain why a high proportion of patients with acute beryllium disease eventually progressed to chronic beryllium disease in industrial sectors with exposure to both soluble and insoluble beryllium compounds.

BIBLIOGRAPHY

1. Eisenbud M, Lisson J: Epidemiologic aspects of beryllium-induced nonmalignant lung disease: A 30-year update. J Occup Med 25:196–202, 1983.
2. Kreiss K, Miller F, Newman LS, et al: Chronic beryllium disease—From the workplace to cellular immunology, molecular immunogenetics, and back. Clin Immunol Immunopath 71:123–129, 1994.
3. Kreiss K, Mroz MM, Newman LS, et al: Machining risk of beryllium disease and sensitization with median exposures below 2 μg/m³. Am J Indust Med 30:16–25, 1996.
4. Kreiss K, Mroz MM, Zhen B, et al: Epidemiology of beryllium sensitization and disease in nuclear workers. Am Rev Respir Dis 148:965–991, 1993.
5. Kreiss K, Mroz MM, Zhen B, et al: Risks of beryllium disease related to work processes at a metal, alloy, and oxide production plant. Occup Environ Med 54:605–612, 1997.
6. Kreiss K, Wasserman S, Mroz MM, Newman LS: Beryllium disease screening in the ceramics industry: Blood test performance and exposure-disease relations. J Occup Med 35:267–274, 1993.
7. Kriebel D, Brain JD, Sprince NL, Kazemi H: The pulmonary toxicity of beryllium. Am Rev Respir Dis 137:464–473, 1988.
8. McMahon B: The epidemiologic evidence on the carcinogenicity of beryllium in humans. J Occup Med 36:15–24, 1994.
9. Newman LS, Kreiss K: Non-occupational chronic beryllium disease masquerading as sarcoidosis: Identification by blood lymphocyte proliferative response to beryllium. Am J Respir Dis 145:1212–1214, 1992.
10. Pappas GP, Newman LS: Early pulmonary physiologic abnormalities in beryllium disease. Am Rev Respir Dis 148:661–666, 1993.
11. Richeldi L, Kreiss K, Mroz MM, et al: Interaction of genetic and environmental factors in the prevalence of berylliosis. Am J Indust Med 32:337–340, 1997.
12. Richeldi L, Sorrentino R, Saltini C: HLA-DPB1 glutamate 69: A genetic marker of beryllium disease. Science 262:242–244, 1993.
13. Steenland K, Ward E: Lung cancer incidence among patients with beryllium disease: A cohort mortality study. J Natl Cancer Inst 83:1380–1385, 1991.
14. Ward E, Okun A, Ruder A, et al: A mortality study of workers at seven beryllium processing plants. Am J Indust Med 22:885–904, 1992.

13. MANGANESE: ESSENTIAL ELEMENT AND NEUROTOXIN

H. Kenneth Hudnell, Ph.D., and Donna Mergler, Ph.D.

1. Why is manganese (Mn) an essential nutrient?

The trace element Mn makes up about 0.1% of the earth's crust in over 100 mineral forms and is an essential nutrient because of its involvement in enzymatic reactions. It also is a prominent cofactor in phosphorylation and the synthesis of cholesterol and fatty acids.

2. How much dietary Mn intake is recommended?

Due to the lack of data about daily Mn requirements and the uncertainty of the level at which toxicity begins, only provisional ranges of recommended intake are available.

Estimated Safe and Adequate Daily Dietary Intakes (ESADDI)

	AGE (Years)	MANGANESE REQUIREMENT (Mg/Day)
Infants	0–0.5	0.3–0.6
	0.5–1	0.6–1
Children	1–3	1–1.5
	4–6	1.5–2
Adolescents	7–10	2–3
	11+	2–5
Adults		2–5

Modified from Food and Nutrition Board: Recommended Dietary Allowances. Washington, DC, National Academy of Science–National Research Council, 1989.

The Environmental Protection Agency's (EPA) Integrated Risk Information System (IRIS) database lists a total oral Reference Dose (RfD) for Mn of 0.14 mg/kg/day (~ 10 mg/day for a 70 kg person) with a modifying factor of 3 if the source is other than food. The RfD is intended to represent a safe intake level, with higher levels posing a potential human health risk.

3. What are the sources of dietary Mn?

Foods rich in Mn include green and leafy vegetables, the germinal portion of grains, nuts, tea, and some fruits and spices. Some processed foods are enriched with Mn. Concern has been expressed that some processed foods may be overly enriched with Mn. The consumption of infant formulas (particularly soy-based), in which Mn levels may be up to 50–100 times higher than in breast milk, has been associated with elevated body Mn levels in infants and subsequent learning disabilities.

4. How does the body process dietary Mn?

Less than 5% of ingested Mn is absorbed through the gastrointestinal system. The principal route of excretion is in the feces. Most absorbed Mn is transported in plasma bound to a β1-globulin, probably transferrin. Mn concentrates in mitochondria, so organs with high mitochondria density such as the liver, pancreas, kidney, and intestines have high Mn concentrations. The biologic half-life of Mn in the body is about 37 days, but in the brain, which Mn readily accesses, the half-life is 2–3 times longer. Mn is sequestered in bile, so some is reabsorbed in the intestines. Homeostatic processes alter Mn absorption and elimination rates as intake varies.

5. Describe Mn neurotoxicity.

Occupational exposures to high concentrations of airborne Mn may cause a neurologic disease: manganism. Nonspecific symptoms, such as headache, weariness, sleep disturbance, and irritability, generally precede the frank manifestation of manganism, which often emerges with the psychotic condition *locura manganica* (manganese madness). Concomitant or subsequent Parkinson-like signs of extrapyramidal motor dysfunction are observed, including muscular rigidity, altered gait (cock walk), lack of facial expression, and fine tremor. Recovery is rare and dysfunction generally persists or progresses after cessation of exposure.

More recent occupational Mn exposure studies of active industrial and agricultural workers have associated increasingly lower exposure levels and shorter exposure durations with subclinical neurologic dysfunction, including motor slowing, increased tremor, olfactory suprasensitivity, and learning and memory decline. Severity of effects increase with exposure duration and concentration, and Mn may interact with the aging process, causing older individuals to be at increased risk for developing a Parkinson-like syndrome.

6. How does manganism differ from idiopathic Parkinson disease?

Calne et al. have reported several distinctions between manganism and idiopathic Parkinson disease:

1. Unlike idiopathic Parkinson disease, manganism may involve damage downstream of the nigrostriatal dopaminergic pathways. In addition, manganism has a low response rate to levodopa, and normal fluorodopa positron emission tomography (PET) scans indicate intact dopaminergic cells.

2. Primary damage may be in neurons with dopaminergic receptors. The reduced intensity in raclopride PET scans suggests a low density of dopaminergic receptors.

3. Mn damage is most prominent in the pallidal nuclei, whereas the pigmented, dopaminergic neurons of the *pars compacta* of the substantia nigra are the primary target in idiopathic Parkinson disease.

4. Some clinical signs help distinguish Parkinson disease and manganism. In manganism, for example, a propensity to fall backward is seen and tremor is less prevalent.

7. What clinical conditions have been associated with elevated Mn levels?

Several studies have described excessive Mn distribution in the central nervous system (CNS) in patients with liver damage and in patients receiving total parenteral feeding. Using high-field strength T-1 weighted magnetic resonance imaging (MRI), the presence of Mn in the blood of 11 cirrhosis patients correlated significantly with signal intensity, which showed high, bilateral signal intensity, primarily in the globus pallidus, putamen, and substantia nigra.

8. Are there other susceptibility factors for elevated Mn concentrations in the CNS?

Individual differences in susceptibility for excessive Mn concentrations in the CNS may involve coexposures or nutrient deficiencies. Exposures that compromised the integrity of the blood-brain-barrier are expected to facilitate Mn access to the interstitial fluid of the CNS. Enhanced CNS access also may involve deficiencies in magnesium, zinc, calcium, and iron. Mn^{+3} is thought to compete with iron for transport into the CNS via transferrin.

9. Can drinking water be a significant source of Mn exposure?

Some areas in the world have high, naturally occurring levels of Mn in drinking water (MnW). Until recently, the EPA's IRIS database listed a drinking water RfD of 200 mg/l, which was assumed to represent a safe Mn level for consumption of 2L of water/day. Evidence shows, however, that higher levels of Mn in drinking water are associated with higher levels of hair Mn and a greater prevalence of clinical signs of extrpyramidal motor dysfunction.

10. Can airborne Mn be a significant source of exposure?

The production of Mn ore, industrial use of Mn, and ambient air levels of Mn have increased during the 20th century. The production of Mn ore has risen from about one million tons to over

20 million tons per year since the beginning of the 20th century. Previous use of Mn was primarily limited to steel-alloy production, but new applications include the production of aluminum beverage cans, fungicides, fertilizers, dry-cell batteries, glass, ceramics, electronics, and gasoline.

Another important source of Mn in ambient air is fossil fuel combustion. Mean atmospheric concentrations of fine Mn (aerodynamic diameter < 2.5 μm) in recent years ranged from 0.001 mg/m^3 in rural areas to 0.003 mg/m^3 in primarily urban areas, to 0.007 mg/m^3 in Riverside, California (fall, 1990), to 0.012 mg/m^3 in Canada, where methylcyclopentadienyl manganese tricarbonyl (MMT) is used extensively in gasoline as a lead substitute. The potential for increased industrial and consumer release of Mn into the air as applications are discovered or expanded, such as the addition of MMT to all unleaded gasoline in the United States, suggests that a prudent course of action requires increased research on the possibility of adverse human-health effects from low-level, environmental exposure to Mn.

11. Is inhaled Mn processed differently than ingested Mn?

Inhaled Mn may be a critical route of Mn entry because it bypasses the liver and blood-brain barrier (CNS protective systems), thereby accessing the CNS directly. Only the fine Mn fraction was previously thought to pose a substantial human-health risk due to its ability to reach deep lung. The ciliary-mucosal cleansing system transports larger Mn compounds to the gut, where it is processed homeostatically as food. However, an evolving issue concerns a newly discovered route of Mn entry into the CNS. Recent rodent studies have demonstrated that $MnCl_2$ placed on the nasal mucosa is taken up by the olfactory nerve and transported to the olfactory bulb; unlike cadmium, Mn then readily crosses synapses to spread throughout the CNS, even into the spinal column. This evidence suggests that some of the course fraction of Mn that deposits in the nasal mucosa may have direct CNS access.

12. Can airborn environmental Mn exposure affect neurologic function?

Recent evidence suggests that environmental exposures to Mn may affect neurologic function. Results from a recent study in Québec, Canada indicate that blood Mn levels in a population with no occupational exposure to Mn were higher in areas with higher airborn levels, and were significantly associated with passive tremor and deficits in the functional domains of coordinated upper-limb movements, learning, and recall. Men with higher Mn blood levels manifested slower postural sway, and neuropsychiatric test results indicated that Mn affected men more than women.

13. What effects of environmental Mn exposure have been reported in children?

Two reports from China described a study of children who lived in an area with moderately high Mn levels in drinking water (241–346 μg/l) due to extensive field irrigation with sewage products (see reference 7). Relative to matched-control children from an area with much lower Mn levels, hair and blood levels were elevated and school performance was poorer. Neurobehavioral performance was significantly lower in the functional domains of coordinated upper-limb movement, learning, and recall. Significantly, negative correlations between Mn in hair and most of the endpoints were reported. These results are consistent with an earlier report of higher levels of Mn found in the hair of learning-disabled children than in children with normal Mn levels.

14. Has violent behavior been associated with excessive body burdens of Mn?

Gottschalk et al. measured significantly higher hair Mn levels in several cohorts of prisoners incarcerated for violent crimes than in nonviolent prisoners and other control populations. Hair Mn concentrations in the violent criminals were reported to be 2–6 times lower than levels seen in clinical manganism cases. Masters et al. examined an environmental pollutant-release database, the EPA Toxic Release Inventory, and a Federal Bureau of Investigation database on the incidence of violent crimes in each county of the United States to identify potential associations between metal releases and violence. After controlling for many socioeconomic and demographic variables, significant positive associations were seen between releases of Mn and lead (Pb) and increases in violent crimes. More research is needed in this area.

15. What are the relationships between air Mn concentrations, biologic levels, and neurobehavioral performance?

Several occupational Mn exposure studies have observed significantly higher blood and/or urine Mn levels in the exposed participants compared to unexposed control participants, as well as poorer performance on tests of cognitive and neuromotor functions. In some occupational studies, neurobehavioral performance was significantly related to cumulative airborne-Mn exposure estimates or to biologic Mn levels.

However, occupational studies have generally failed to find relationships between estimates of cumulative Mn exposure or measurements of current airborne exposure and biologic levels. It is thought that biologic levels may reflect past exposure integrated over the last few weeks better than very recent or cumulative exposure in currently exposed individuals. A review of studies on bioindicators of Mn suggests that biologic Mn levels measured during environmental exposure may reflect current exposure and predict neurobehavioral performance, whereas strong relationships with occupational Mn exposure may require the measurement of biologic levels following a short period of exposure cessation.

16. In addition to neurotoxicity, do excessive Mn concentrations have other health effects?

Like most particulate matter, inhaled Mn is a respiratory irritant that may induce an inflammatory response and bronchitis. Occupational exposure may lead to pneumonitis and act synergistically with cigarette smoke. Occupational exposure to airborne Mn often induces impotency in men, and high environmental exposures may increase the incidence of birth defects. No data on reproductive effects in women are available.

Disclaimer: This chapter has been reviewed by the National Health and Environmental Research Laboratory, U.S. Environmental Protection Agency, and has been approved for publication. Approval does not signify that the contents necessarily reflect the views and policies of the Agency.

BIBLIOGRAPHY

1. Collipp PJ, Chen SY, Maitinsky S: Manganese in infant formulas and learning disability. Ann Nutr Metab 27:488–494, 1983.
2. Huang C-C, Chu N-S, Lu C-S, et al: Long-term progression in chronic manganism: Ten years of follow-up. Neurology 50:698–700, 1998.
3. Mergler D, Baldwin M: Early manifestations of manganese neurotoxicity in humans: An update. Environ Res 73:92–100, 1997.
4. Calne DB, Chu N-S, Huang C-C, Lu C-S, Olanow W. Manganism and idiopathic Parkinsonism: Similarities and differences. Neurology 44:1583–1586, 1994.
5. Hauser RA, Zesiewicz TA, Martinez C, et al: Blood manganese correlates with brain magnetic imaging changes in patients with liver disease. Can J Neurol Sci 23:95–98, 1996.
6. Alessio L, Lucchini R: Manganese and manganese compounds. In Argentesi F, Roi R, Sevilla Marcos JM (eds): Data profiles for selected chemicals and pharmaceuticals: 3 2,4-dinitrophenol, 4 manganese and manganese compounds, 5 trichloroethylene. Joint Research Centre, Ispra (I), European Commission (S.P.I. 96.59), 1996, pp 75–162.
7. Hudnell HK: Effects from evironmental Mn exposures: A review of the evidence from non-occupational exposure studies. NeuroTox 20(2–3):223–241, 1999.
8. Mergler D, Baldwin M, Belanger S, et al: Manganese neurotoxicity: A continuum of dysfunction: Results from a community based study. NeuroTox 20(2–3):243–258, 1999.
9. Gottschalk LA, Rebello T, Buchsbaum MS, et al: Abnormalities in hair trace elements as indicators of aberrant behavior. Compr Psychiatry 32:229–237, 1991.
10. Masters RD, Hone B, Doshi A: Environmental pollution, neurotoxicity, and criminal violence. In Rose J (ed): Environmental Toxicology. London, Gordon and Breach, 1997.

14. RADON OCCURRENCE AND HEALTH RISK

R. William Field, Ph.D.

1. What are the chemical and radiologic characteristics of radon?

Radon is a colorless, odorless, tasteless, radioactive noble gas that generally lacks activity toward other chemical agents. However, radon occasionally forms clathrate compounds with some organic compounds and may form ionic or covalent bonds with highly reactive elements such as oxygen or fluorine. Radon is the heaviest noble gas and exhibits the highest boiling point, melting point, critical temperature, and critical pressure of all noble gases. Radon is highly soluble in non-polar solvents and moderately soluble in cold water. Radon's isotopes, all of which are radioactive, include mass numbers ranging from 200–226. Radon-222 (^{222}Rn), formed in the ^{238}U decay chain, is the most important isotope because of its relatively long half-life of 3.82 days, which is the longest half-life of the radon isotopes formed in the ^{238}U decay chain. The short half-life beta- and gamma-emitting decay products of ^{222}Rn achieve equilibrium with the parent isotope within several hours.

2. Draw the ^{226}Ra decay chain. Include the half-life and major emission type of each decay product.

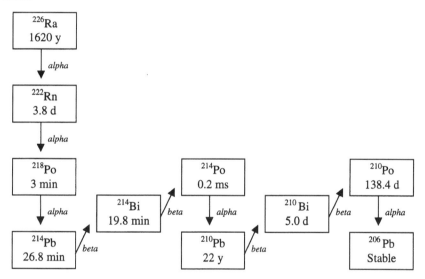

3. What are ^{222}Rn progeny? Why are they important?

Radon-222 progeny is another name for the ^{222}Rn decay products or ^{222}Rn daughters. Radon-222 progeny rather than ^{222}Rn gas deliver the actual radiation dose to lung tissues. The solid airborne ^{222}Rn progeny, particularly ^{218}Po, ^{214}Pb, and ^{214}Bi, are of health importance because they can be inspired and retained in the lung. The radiation released during the subsequent decay of the alpha-emitting decay products ^{218}Po and ^{214}Po delivers a radiologically significant dose to the respiratory epithelium. The ratio of progeny to ^{222}Rn gas ranges from 0.2–0.8 with a typical value of 0.4. The ratio between progeny and ^{222}Rn gas is called the equilibrium factor.

4. How does the behavior of ^{222}Rn progeny in air affect the dose delivered to lung tissues?

After decay of the ^{222}Rn gas, a high percentage of the decay products attaches to ambient aerosols. A small percentage of the decay products remains unattached; others increase their diameter through chemical and physical processes. The percent attachment depends on numerous factors, including the size and concentration of the airborne particles. The size and density of a particle determine its behavior in the respiratory tract. The unattached particle fraction with a 1-nm diameter is generally removed in the nose and mouth during breathing and has limited penetration of the bronchi. Maximal deposition occurs as the particles with diameters ranging from 3–10 nm increase their rate of penetration through the mouth and nose, ultimately depositing in the bronchial region. The deposition rate decreases for particles as their diameter increases toward 100 nm and larger because the particles are less able to diffuse to the airway surface. However, particle deposition into the respiratory tract through impaction starts to increase again for particles above 500 nm. Larger particles with a diameter exceeding 3.5 μm deposit predominantly in the nose and mouth during inhalation and do not reach the sensitive respiratory epithelium.

5. List the physical and biologic factors that affect the dose delivered by ^{222}Rn progeny to the target cells in the respiratory epithelium.
- Aerosol size distribution
- Equilibrium between ^{222}Rn gas and ^{222}Rn progeny
- Respiratory rate
- Lung tidal volume
- Oral vs. nasal inhalation route
- Bronchial morphometry
- Clearance rate from lung
- Thickness of mucus in respiratory tract

6. When was the link between ^{222}Rn exposure and lung cancer first postulated?
As early as 1556, Agricola described high mortality rates from respiratory diseases among underground metal miners at Schneeberg in the Erz Mountains of Eastern Europe. Harting and Hesse first linked the high mortality rates at Schneeberg to lung cancer in 1879 on the basis of autopsy findings. In 1921 Margaret Uhlig suggested that radium emanation, later known as ^{222}Rn, may be the cause of the lung cancers. In 1939 Peller wrote the first review of mining-related cancers, which described the occurrence of lung cancers in Schneeberg and Joachimsthal miners. Finally, in the mid 1950s ^{222}Rn progeny inhalation rather than ^{222}Rn gas was implicated as the causative agent in the excessive lung cancer deaths noted for miners in both the United States and Europe.

7. What is the evidence that ^{222}Rn progeny exposure causes lung cancer?
Laboratory animals exposed to high concentrations of ^{222}Rn progeny display lung carcinoma, emphysema, pulmonary fibrosis, and a shortened life span. However, the International Agency for Research on Cancer has classified ^{222}Rn as a human carcinogen primarily on the basis of findings in underground miners exposed to ^{222}Rn progeny. The lung cancer risk attributable to ^{222}Rn progeny exposure has been examined in over 20 different populations of underground miners, including uranium, fluorspar, shale, and metal miners from the United States, Canada, Australia, China, and Europe.

The findings from these studies overwhelmingly document that ^{222}Rn progeny exposure causes lung cancers in miners. An analysis of the pooled data from 11 major studies involving 68,000 miners found that lung cancer was linearly related to ^{222}Rn progeny concentrations in underground mines and that overall about 40% of miners' lung cancers were attributable to ^{222}Rn progeny exposure. A subset analysis of the miner data suggests a synergistic (submultiplicative) effect for combined exposure to ^{222}Rn progeny and cigarette smoke. Other factors possibly influencing the relationship between ^{222}Rn progeny exposure and lung cancer include age at exposure, age at risk, exposure rate, sex, other carcinogens, and nonspecific inflammation of the airways. No data are available to determine whether the risk estimates attributable to ^{222}Rn for male miners are applicable to nonmining women.

8. Does ^{222}Rn progeny exposure induce a specific subtype of lung cancer?

Lung cancer encompasses a clinically and histologically diverse group of carcinomas. The major histologic types of lung cancer include squamous cell carcinoma, small cell carcinoma, adenocarcinoma, and large cell carcinoma. Early findings from the miner epidemiologic studies noted a high frequency of small cell carcinoma in both smokers and nonsmokers. Recent findings from the miner data have indicated that all major subtypes have occurred in excess. Therefore, a specific histologic subtype of lung cancer has not been associated with ^{222}Rn progeny exposure.

9. What units are used to express ^{222}Rn gas concentrations and ^{222}Rn progeny exposure?

The activity (rate of decay) of ^{222}Rn is expressed in units called curies. The curie is based on the rate of decay of one gram of ^{226}Ra or 3.7×10^{10} disintegrations per second. The International System of Units (SI) measure of activity is becquerels per cubic meter (Bq/m^3). One Bq equals 1 disintegration per minute.

Historically, ^{222}Rn progeny exposure rates have been expressed as working levels (WLs); 1 WL equals any combination of short-lived ^{222}Rn progeny (^{218}Po, ^{214}Pb, ^{214}Bi, and ^{214}Po) in 1 liter of air that releases 1.3×10^5 MeV of potential alpha energy. The value of 1.3×10^5 MeV derives from the energy produced by complete decay of the short-lived ^{222}Rn progeny in radioactive equilibrium with 100 pCi/L of ^{222}Rn. A unit that incorporates both dose and time is the working level month (WLM). Exposure to 1 WL for 1 working month (170 hours) equals 1 WLM cumulative exposure. The SI unit of cumulative exposure is expressed in joule-hours per cubic meter (Jh/m^3). One WLM is equivalent to 3.5×10^{-3} Jh/m^3.

10. List common occupations that have the potential for high ^{222}Rn progeny exposure.
- Mine workers, including uranium, hard rock, and vanadium
- Workers remediating radioactive contaminated sites, including uranium mill sites and mill tailings
- Workers at underground nuclear waste repositories
- Radon mitigation contractors and testers
- Employees of natural caves
- Phosphate fertilizer plant workers
- Oil refinery workers
- Utility tunnel workers
- Subway tunnel workers
- Construction excavators
- Power plant workers, including geothermal power and coal
- Employees of radon health mines
- Employees of radon balneotherapy spas (waterborne ^{222}Rn source)
- Water plant operators (waterborne ^{222}Rn source)
- Fish hatchery attendants (waterborne ^{222}Rn source)
- Employees who come in contact with technologically enhanced sources of naturally occurring radioactive materials
- Incidental exposure in almost any occupation from local geologic ^{222}Rn sources

11. What is the occupational exposure limit for ^{222}Rn?

The exposure limit varies by regulating agency and type of worker. The Miners Safety and Health Act (MSHA) covers underground miners, whereas the Occupational Safety and Health Act (OSHA) regulates exposure to ^{222}Rn gas and ^{222}Rn progeny for workers other than miners. The MSHA sets limits so that no employee can be exposed to air containing ^{222}Rn progeny in excess of 1.0 WL (100 pCi/L) in active work areas. The MSHA also limits annual exposure to ^{222}Rn progeny to less than 4 WLM per year. OSHA limits exposure to either 30 pCi/L or 0.33 WL based on continuous workplace exposure for 40 hours per week, 52 weeks per year.

The Nuclear Regulatory Commission (NRC) and Department of Energy (DOE) generally exclude ^{222}Rn from their occupational exposure regulations. However, when the materials generating the ^{222}Rn are or were under the control of a licensee (e.g., uranium mill, in situ leach facility), dose limits are enforced. When ^{222}Rn progeny are present in equilibrium with ^{222}Rn gas, the derived air concentration (DAC) is 30 pCi/L or 0.33 WL and the annual limit on intake (ALI) is 4 WLM.

12. What is the principal site of ^{222}Rn exposure for most people?

The primary site of ^{222}Rn exposure for most people is the home. The average person in the United States receives over one-half their annual average radiation dose equivalent from ^{222}Rn progeny exposure. The ^{222}Rn progeny exposure imparts a greater effective dose equivalent to the average person than all other natural and man-made sources combined. The high percentage of radiation dose contributed by ^{222}Rn progeny is attributable to both the extended time spent in the home and the frequent occurrence of ^{222}Rn within the home. In some cases, long-term residents of homes with high ^{222}Rn concentrations exceed the cumulative ^{222}Rn progeny exposure noted for some underground miner cohorts.

13. What is the source of ^{222}Rn in homes?

Radon-222 is present in the natural environment because of the spontaneous fission of ^{238}U. Four intermediate decay products follow the decay of ^{238}U and precede ^{226}Ra, the direct source of ^{222}Rn. Because ^{222}Rn is a gas, it readily travels through several meters of permeable soils before decaying. The major sources of ^{222}Rn in indoor air are (1) soil gas emanations from soils and rocks, (2) off-gassing of waterborne ^{222}Rn into indoor air, (3) building materials, and (4) outdoor air. Of these four sources, soil gas represents the predominant source of indoor ^{222}Rn gas. The primary limiting factor for ^{222}Rn gas migration in the soil is its half-life of 3.8 days. Radon-222 gas enters the home from the soil through cracks in the home, including cracks in the home's foundation, loose-fitting pipe penetrations, sump openings, crawl spaces, and open top of block walls.

In the United States waterborne ^{222}Rn accounts for approximately 5% of the total indoor air ^{222}Rn concentrations for homes utilizing ground-water sources. Waterborne ^{222}Rn may account for a higher percentage of total indoor ^{222}Rn concentrations in some areas of the United States, such as Maine and New Hampshire, where waterborne ^{222}Rn concentrations occasionally exceed 1,000,000 pCi/L. The inhalation exposure from waterborne ^{222}Rn occurs when it off-gasses from the water supply during activities such as showering, washing clothes, and washing dishes. Researchers estimate that 10,000 pCi/L of ^{222}Rn in water contributes about 1 pCi/L of ^{222}Rn to the indoor air of a home.

Building materials generally contribute only a small percentage of the indoor air ^{222}Rn concentrations. However, building materials may impart a greater ^{222}Rn contribution when waste products from uranium mining were used to make concrete, concrete blocks, or wallboard. In some areas with a high geologic ^{222}Rn source, outdoor ^{222}Rn gas concentrations exceed several pCi/L for short periods, depending on meteorologic conditions.

14. Which areas of the United States have the greatest potential for elevated ^{222}Rn gas concentrations?

The United States Geological Survey Bureau assessed the potential for geologic ^{222}Rn using five main types of data: (1) geologic (litholithic); (2) aerial radiometric; (3) soil characteristics, including soil moisture and permeability; (4) indoor ^{222}Rn gas data from ^{222}Rn surveys; and (5) building architecture. The areas of the United States with high geologic ^{222}Rn potential are shown on the map on the following page.

From a limited national survey, the EPA has estimated an average outdoor ^{222}Rn concentration of 0.4 pCi/L for the United States. An average indoor ^{222}Rn concentration of 1.5 pCi/L has been estimated for single family homes from summary data from numerous state residential ^{222}Rn surveys. However, some yearly average outdoor ^{222}Rn concentrations in areas of high geologic radon potential exceed the national indoor average.

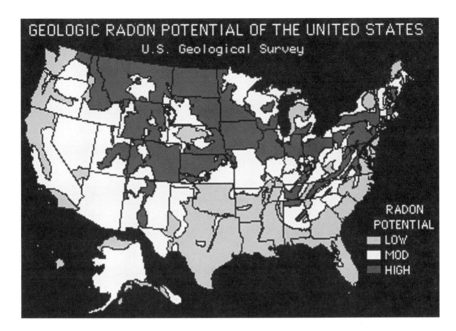

GEOLOGIC RADON POTENTIAL OF THE UNITED STATES
U.S. Geological Survey

RADON
POTENTIAL
■ LOW
■ MOD
■ HIGH

15. What has served as the basis for risk estimates for residential ^{222}Rn progeny exposure?

In 1998 the National Academy of Sciences (NAS) used data compiled from studies of underground miners exposed to ^{222}Rn progeny to project that 18,600 (range: 3,000–32,000) lung cancer deaths each year in the United States are attributable to residential ^{222}Rn progeny exposure. Therefore, numerous public health agencies rank residential ^{222}Rn exposure as the second leading cause of lung cancer after cigarette smoking. The authors of the NAS report cautioned that their approach to assessing risks posed by indoor ^{222}Rn exposure was subject to considerable uncertainty because of gaps in knowledge about the effects of low levels of exposure. Risk estimates derived from miners for the general population must be interpreted cautiously because of inherent differences between the two populations as well as differences between mine and home environments.

16. What differences between mine and residential environments may limit the generalizability of risk estimates based on miner data?

- Relatively higher ^{222}Rn gas concentrations in mines than in homes
- Greater concentrations of airborne dust in mines than in homes
- Particle diameter higher in mines than in homes
- Different activity size distributions of radon progeny and rates of attachment for the two environments
- Presence of other toxic pollutants in mine air, which may act as confounders
- Age and sex differences between miners and the general population
- Higher level of physical activity among miners, which affects respiration rates
- Greater extent of oral vs. nasal breathing in the miners, which leads to increased deposition of larger particles into the lung
- Different exposure patterns and rates for miners vs. the general population (miners have shorter-term high exposure compared with the lifelong lower concentration exposure for the general population)
- Most miners were smokers compared with a minority of the general population

Even with these physical and biologic differences, the NAS estimated that the dose per unit ^{222}Rn concentration was essentially the same for mine and residential environments.

17. What studies have assessed directly the risk posed by residential ^{222}Rn exposure?

Residential epidemiologic case-control studies examining the relationship between contemporary ^{222}Rn gas concentrations and lung cancer have been performed in Canada, China, Finland, Germany, Sweden, the United Kingdom, and the United States. A meta-analysis of eight studies using weighted linear regression found a summary excessive risk of 14% at an average indoor ^{222}Rn gas concentration of 4 pCi/L. The excess risk at 4 pCi/L in recent studies in Germany and the United Kingdom was in close agreement with risk estimates obtained from the meta-analysis. The meta-analysis risk estimate was also consistent with the risk estimate extrapolated from miner studies. Additional residential case-control studies currently in progress in the United States (Missouri and Iowa) and Europe incorporate improved estimates of retrospective exposure to ^{222}Rn progeny. In addition, the pooling of data from published and ongoing case-control studies is currently in progress.

18. How can a homeowner test for ^{222}Rn gas?

Short-term ^{222}Rn test gas kits, which use charcoal detectors, or longer-term test kits, which use an alpha track detector to provide a year-long average ^{222}Rn concentration, are available at most hardware or discount stores.

19. What are the recommended residential ^{222}Rn exposure limits? Where can I get more information about ^{222}Rn?

The EPA recommends that ^{222}Rn gas concentrations not exceed a year-long average concentration of 4 pCi/L in any livable area of the home. Instructions for testing and interpreting residential ^{222}Rn concentrations are available from the EPA in " A Citizen's Guide to Radon" (2nd edition), "Guide to Protecting Yourself and Your Family from Radon," and "Radon, The Health Threat with a Simple Solution: A Physician's Guide." These booklets also list state radon contacts who can provide information about testing and reducing the radon concentrations in the home.

20. Where do elevated waterborne ^{222}Rn concentrations occur?

The highest concentrations of waterborne ^{222}Rn are found in groundwater sources. Surface water sources have much lower concentrations. In addition, water distribution systems with historically high ^{226}Ra concentrations are a source of waterborne ^{222}Rn. Radium-226 adsorbed onto pipe scale within the water distribution system produces ^{222}Rn gas, which significantly increases waterborne ^{222}Rn concentrations by the time the water reaches the point of use.

21. Does ingestion of waterborne ^{222}Rn present a hazard?

The NAS estimates that 160 lung cancer deaths occur each year in the United States as a result of inhaling ^{222}Rn progeny produced by the decay of ^{222}Rn gas emanated from a waterborne source within the home. In comparison, the NAS estimates that 700 lung cancer deaths each year in the United States are attributable to natural outdoor exposure to ^{222}Rn progeny. The NAS also predicted that ingested radon causes about 20 deaths annually in the United States from stomach cancer. The EPA has previously proposed a waterborne ^{222}Rn standard of 300 pCi/L for public water supplies in the United States. The EPA is considering an alternative waterborne ^{222}Rn standard of 4,000 pCi/L for communities that make a concerted effort to reduce indoor ^{222}Rn gas concentrations.

BIBLIOGRAPHY

1. Alavanja MCR, Lubin JH, Mahaffey J, et al: Cumulative residential radon exposure and risk of lung cancer in Missouri: A population-based case-control study. Am J Public Health [in press].
2. Cothern CR, Smith JE (eds): Environmental Radon. New York, Plenum Press, 1987.
3. Darby S, Whitley E, Silcocks P, et al: Risk of lung cancer associated with residential radon exposure in South-West England: A case-control study. Br J Cancer 78:394–408, 1998.
4. Field RW, Steck DJ, Smith BJ, et al: Residential radon gas exposure and lung cancer: The Iowa radon lung cancer study. Radiat Res 151:101–103, 1999.

5. Field RW, Fisher E, Valentine R, Kross BC: Radium-bearing pipe scale deposits: Implications for national waterborne radon sampling methods. Am J Public Health 85:567–570, 1995.
6. Lubin JH, Boice JD Jr: Lung cancer risk from residential radon: Meta-analysis of eight epidemiologic studies, J Natl Cancer Inst 89(1): 49-57, 1997.
7. Lubin JH, Boice JD, Edling C, et al: Radon and Lung Cancer Risk: A Joint Analysis of 11 Underground Miner Studies, Rockville, MD, National Institutes of Health, NIH Publication No. 94-3644, 1994.
8. Lubin JH: Invited commentary: Lung cancer and exposure to residential radon. Am J Epidemiol 140:323–332, 1994.
9. National Research Council: Risk Assessment of Radon in Drinking Water, Committee on the Assessment of Exposures to Radon in Drinking Water, Board on Radiation Effects Research, Commission on Life Sciences, Washington, DC, National Academy Press, 1998.
10. National Research Council: Health Effects of Exposure to Radon, BEIR VI, Committee on Health Risks of Exposure to Radon (BEIR VI), Board on Radiation Effects Research, Commission on Life Sciences, Washington, DC, National Academy Press, 1998.
11. National Research Council: Comparative Dosimetry of Radon in Mines and Homes, Board on Radiation Effects Research, Commission on Life Sciences, Panel on Dosimetric Assumptions Affecting the Applications of Radon Risk Estimates, Washington, DC, National Academy Press, 1991.
12. National Research Council: Report of the Committee on the Biological Effects of Ionizing Radiation: Health Effects of Radon and Other Internally Deposited Alpha Emitters, BEIR IV. Washington, DC, National Academy Press, 1988.
13. Nazaroff WW, Nero AV (eds): Radon and Its Decay Products in Indoor Air. New York, John Wiley & Sons, 1988.
14. Nero AV, Schwehr MB, Nazaroff WW, Revzan KL: Distribution of airborne radon-222 concentrations in U.S. homes. Science 234: 992–997, 1986.
15. Neuberger JS: Residential radon exposure and lung cancer: An overview of published studies. Cancer Detect Prevent 15(6):435–441, 1991.
16. Samet JM: Radon and lung cancer. J Natl Cancer Inst 81:745–757, 1989.
17. Steck DJ, Field RW: Exposure to atmospheric radon. Environ Health Perspect 107(2):123–127, 1999.

15. ASBESTOS

E. Brigitte Gottschall, M.D.

1. What is asbestos?

The word *asbestos* is derived from the Greek word for *noncombustible*. It refers to a family of naturally occurring fibrous, hydrated silicates present everywhere in the soil. The six distinct types of asbestos—chrysotile, crocidolite, amosite, anthophyllite, actinolite, and tremolite—are divided into two major fiber types: serpentine (curly and long) and amphibole (rodlike and straight) fibers. Chrysotile, the only serpentine asbestos fiber, accounts for 95% of all asbestos used commercially worldwide. Of the amphibole fibers, crocidolite and amosite were most often used commercially in the United States. The six mineral types share physical properties that have led to more than 3,000 commercial uses of asbestos-containing products: resistance to heat, insulation against cold and noise, great tensile strength, flexibility and weavability, and resistance to corrosion by alkalis and most acids.

2. What occupations are associated with asbestos exposure?

Asbestos miners/millers	Insulators
Asbestos removal workers	Laborers
Automobile repair workers	Maintenance and custodial workers
Asbestos paper makers and users	Petroleum refinery workers
Brake lining makers/repair workers	Pipefitters
Boilermakers	Plumbers
Construction workers	Railroad workers
Demolition workers	Roofers
Electricians	Sheet metal workers
Gasket makers	Shipyard workers
Glass workers	Textile workers

A listing of all occupations associated with asbestos exposure is not feasible. Because of its widespread use and resistance to degradation, asbestos remains virtually ubiquitous.

3. Are people still exposed to asbestos?

Yes. From the beginning of the 20th century until 1973 asbestos was used extensively in a large number of construction materials because of its heat resistance, flexibility, acid/alkali resistance, and tensile strength. In 1973 the U.S. Environmental Protection Agency banned its use in many but not all applications; however, large numbers of schools, public and commercial buildings, and even private homes continue to house asbestos-containing materials (acoustic ceiling tiles, vinyl floor tiles, paints, walls, plasters, and insulation materials on pipes, boilers, and structural beams). Currently exposure to asbestos may occur largely during the degradation of asbestos-containing materials in existing buildings. The airborne concentrations of asbestos fibers in most buildings studied have been low (0.0002–0.002 fibers/ml) compared with the occupational permissible exposure limit (PEL) of 0.1 fiber/ml mandated by the U.S. Occupational Safety and Health Administration (OSHA). However, assuming a nonthreshold relationship between exposure to asbestos and occurrence of malignancies, a small risk for lung cancer and mesothelioma may exist with these low exposures. Occupational exposure to asbestos is still of concern. Asbestos removal workers, brake and clutch repair workers, construction workers involved in remodeling, and many others are still exposed to asbestos on their jobs.

4. What is paraoccupational exposure to asbestos?

Paraoccupational exposure refers to exposure to a hazardous agent that is not directly associated with an individual's job or activity. Many construction workers who did not handle asbestos directly may have experienced significant exposure due to use of asbestos by coworkers in their vicinity. For example, electricians and laborers were exposed as bystanders when insulators prepared asbestos mixtures to insulate steam pipes in shared working areas. Inadvertent domestic exposures occurred when asbestos workers carried large fiber burdens into the home on work clothing and hair. This "fowling of the nest" led to an increased incidence of mesothelioma and lung cancer in the families (including children) of asbestos workers.

5. With which diseases is asbestos exposure associated?

Inhalation of asbestos fibers into the lungs is by far the most important route of exposure. Both nonmalignant and malignant asbestos-related respiratory diseases may result. The nonmalignant manifestations are asbestosis, pleural plaques, benign pleural effusions, diffuse pleural thickening, rounded atelectasis, and benign lung nodules. Lung cancer (bronchogenic carcinoma) and mesothelioma are the two malignancies associated with asbestos inhalation.

Laryngeal, gastrointestinal tract, and kidney cancers as well as lymphoma and leukemia have been associated with asbestos exposure, but the risk is much less than that for lung cancer and mesothelioma and the data suggesting these associations are controversial.

6. What is a latency period?

A latency period is the time between first exposure and clinical manifestations of disease. The latency period varies for the different manifestations of asbestos-related lung disease. Pleural plaques have the shortest latency at 10–20 years. Asbestosis develops over 20–30 years. Lung cancer has a latency of 20–40 years, and mesotheliomas often occur 30–40 years after exposure. These ranges are averages and may vary, depending on exposure intensity and other factors. A manifestation of asbestos inhalation that develops outside these ranges may still be related to asbestos exposure.

7. What is asbestosis?

Asbestosis is sometimes used colloquially for any thoracic manifestations due to asbestos exposure. Strictly speaking it describes *only* the bilateral interstitial fibrosis of the lung parenchyma caused by inhalation of asbestos fibers.

8. Describe the symptoms of asbestosis.

The symptoms of asbestosis are similar to those of other interstitial lung fibroses and include slowly progressive dyspnea on exertion and dry cough. Chest pain, weight loss, and hemoptysis are not common and should raise the suspicion of asbestos-related malignancy.

9. How is asbestosis diagnosed?

The diagnosis of asbestosis usually can be based on clinical findings without histologic proof. A history of significant exposure (asbestosis has a well-established dose-response relationship), an appropriate interval between exposure and disease detection (20–30 year latency), and radiographic evidence of interstitial fibrosis on chest radiograph or chest CT scan are the primary means to establish the diagnosis. Confirmatory but nonessential findings include other radiographic evidence of asbestos exposure, such as pleural thickening or pleural calcification; pulmonary function tests with a restrictive pattern and decreased diffusing capacity (DLCO); and fixed bilateral end-expiratory crackles on physical exam. Digital clubbing, cyanosis, and signs of cor pulmonale are seen in late, severe stages of asbestosis. The main differential diagnoses are the other pneumoconioses and other causes of pulmonary fibrosis, such as metal or organic dusts, drugs, infectious agents, collagen vascular disorders, and idiopathic pulmonary fibrosis.

Although clinical assessment is usually sufficient to make a probabilistic determination of asbestosis for medical and legal purposes, a more sensitive and specific method is the histologic and mineralogic evaluation of lung tissue. Lung tissue, however, can be obtained only through an invasive biopsy procedure with all of its associated risks. Transbronchial lung biopsy is generally inadequate to diagnose asbestosis. Biopsy should be obtained only if a thorough history and non-invasive testing yield no clues to the causes of pulmonary fibrosis. Even then, the risk-benefit ratio for biopsy must be weighed carefully.

10. What is a chest radiograph B-reading?

During the past 50 years the International Labor Organization (ILO) has assisted in designing a system of classifying chest radiographs of persons with pneumoconiosis to achieve better standardization for epidemiologic use. The strength of the ILO system lies in its systematic and more reproducible manner of assessing pneumoconiosis chest radiographs. The ILO classification, which is based on the posteroanterior chest radiograph, is a descriptive system consisting of a glossary of terms and a set of 22 standard radiographs illustrative of the pleural and parenchymal changes of the pneumoconioses. The classification grades the parenchymal, typically reticulonodular pattern of the pneumoconioses based on size, shape, extent, and profusion (severity). Pleural abnormalities are also categorized and quantified. The National Institute of Occupational Safety and Health (NIOSH) in conjunction with the American College of Radiology (ACR) offers courses on the ILO classification. A physician who attends the course and passes a subsequent test is a NIOSH-certified B-reader. The interpretation of a chest radiograph by a certified B-reader is considered authoritative in regard to whether the radiograph shows evidence of pneumoconiosis. The implications for patients may be important because the B-reader's interpretation is often pivotal in court cases. Of interest, 10–20% of symptomatic patients with asbestosis and gas exchange abnormalities have a normal chest radiograph. In such patients high-resolution CT scan (HRCT) often shows early interstitial changes. HRCT has therefore become an important tool in the diagnosis of asbestosis.

11. How does asbestosis appear microscopically?

Lung tissue taken from the lower lobes adjacent to the pleura is most likely to show histologic evidence of asbestosis. The development of end-stage asbestosis with severe lung fibrosis and honeycombing is a process that takes many years. The evolution of asbestosis lesions from the early appearance of fibrosis surrounding only the respiratory bronchiole to honeycombing with destruction of alveoli has been divided into four grades of severity by a panel from the College of American Pathologists:

Grade 1: discrete foci of fibrosis limited to the walls of first-order respiratory bronchioles
Grade 2: fibrosis extends into some adjacent alveolar ducts and septae
Grade 3: grade 2 fibrosis with more diffuse coalescent involvement of the respiratory bronchioles and surrounding alveoli
Grade 4: obliteration of the parenchyma with fibrous tissue, honeycombing

12. What is an asbestos body?

Characteristically two different types of asbestos are found in the lungs: the uncoated, bare fiber and the coated fiber, also called **asbestos body**. The bare fiber is an inhaled particle that may have undergone change due to fracture or digestion; however, it has not accumulated a coating. The asbestos body is an asbestos fiber coated with proteins and iron compounds. It is a histologic marker of asbestos exposure, associated more with amphibole than with chrysotile fibers. Occasionally the term **ferruginous body** is used in this context. Strictly speaking, a ferruginous body is any fiber coated by protein and iron compounds. Thus the asbestos body is a specific kind of ferruginous body: a coated asbestos fiber.

13. Is asbestosis treatable?

There is no specific treatment for asbestosis. Corticosteroids and immunosuppressive agents have been tried without success and generally are not indicated. Treatment is supportive. Intercurrent respiratory infections may occur frequently and should be treated aggressively. Oxygen therapy is necessary for patients with hypoxemia at rest or with exercise. In the late stages of asbestosis right heart failure (cor pulmonale) may develop; treatment consists of oxygen and diuretics. Influenza and pneumococcal vaccinations are warranted. Patients should be counseled to abstain from smoking to decrease the risk of developing lung cancer as well as to minimize the risks of other smoking-related diseases. The lack of viable treatment options for asbestosis emphasizes the critical need for primary prevention—reduction or elimination of asbestos exposure by using asbestos substitutes, engineering controls, or administrative controls.

14. What is the pathogenesis of asbestosis?

Much of our knowledge about the pathogenesis of asbestosis is derived from experimental animal and cellular studies. After a 1-hour inhalation of asbestos fibers, animals develop evidence of lung injury within 48 hours. Asbestos fibers deposit at the bifurcations of the terminal bronchioles. Type I alveolar epithelial cells take up some fibers, whereas others pierce the alveolar wall. Both lead to cell injury and cell death. Increased numbers of alveolar macrophages gather at the alveolar duct bifurcations. Macrophages are activated by asbestos and release reactive oxygen species, which damage surrounding lung tissue through peroxidation and direct cytotoxicity. Asbestos also induces toxicity by interaction with macromolecules in target cells, which leads to genetic alterations that activate oncogenes, inactivate tumor suppressor genes, and modify the expression of genes coding for proinflammatory proteins. This complex series of events, which is only partially understood, eventually leads to the release of a number of substances, including interleukin-8, gamma-interferon, platelet-derived growth factor (PDGF), insulinlike growth factor (IGF-1), fibroblast growth factor (FGF), and tumor necrosis factor-alpha (TNF-α). The result is promotion of fibroblast proliferation and eventual formation of scar tissue.

15. Does everyone exposed to asbestos develop asbestosis?

No. The most important factor in the development of asbestosis is the cumulative fiber dose to which a person is exposed. When exposure levels were very high in the early part of the century, the time from first asbestos exposure to clinical manifestations of asbestosis (latency period) was reported to be around 5 years. With the introduction and implementation of exposure limits, latency periods have increased. Latency is inversely proportional to cumulative fiber dose. Some data suggest that the threshold fiber dose, below which asbestosis is not seen, is 25–100 fibers/ml/year. Although cumulative fiber dose remains the strongest predictor of asbestosis, recent research suggests a possible component of individual susceptibility. What renders one person potentially susceptible at a lower cumulative dose than another is under intense investigation. Susceptibility probably is influenced by many factors, including genetics, gender, ethnic origin, immune function, and fiber clearance.

16. What is the significance of pleural plaques?

Pleural plaques are focal, irregular fibrous tissue collections on the parietal pleura, diaphragm, or mediastinum. They are the most frequent manifestation of asbestos exposure and typically develop bilaterally with a latency of 10–20 years. Often they are noticed incidentally on a chest radiograph taken for a different reason. Pleural plaques alone rarely if ever lead to symptoms. A standard chest radiograph can identify 50–80% of pleural plaques actually present on chest CT scan. Over time, pleural plaques may calcify, making them more easily visible on plain chest radiograph. The greatest significance of pleural plaques lies in their recognition as markers of asbestos exposure.

Although the most common cause of pleural plaques is asbestos exposure, other diagnoses should be considered. Previous hemothorax, empyema, or repeated pneumothorax associated with tuberculosis may be implicated, especially if the pleural thickening or calcification is unilateral. Mesothelioma, lymphoma, multiple myeloma, and pleural metastasis may lead to localized pleural thickening. Occasionally the callus of an old rib fracture may give the appearance of pleural thickening. Other exposures connected with pleural plaques are talc, mica, tin, barite, and silica; however, concomitant exposure to asbestos cannot be excluded.

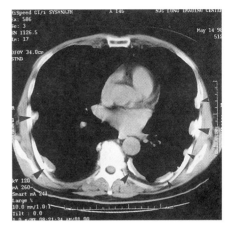

Conventional CT scan of a retired pipefitter shows multiple, focal areas of pleural thickening (*arrows*) with partial calcification.

17. What is rounded atelectasis?

Rounded atelectasis is a form of partial collapse in the peripheral part of the lung. Synonyms include folded lung syndrome, Blesovsky's syndrome, shrinking pleuritis with atelectasis, atelectatic pseudotumor, and pleuroma. The pathogenesis is controversial. The most accepted theory postulates that a pleural inflammatory reaction is followed by pleural shrinkage, which causes atelectasis in the immediately adjacent lung parenchyma that assumes a rounded configuration. The principal cause is believed to be asbestos exposure; however, conditions such as parapneumonic effusions, congestive heart failure, Dressler's syndrome, pulmonary infarcts, chest trauma, and therapeutic pneumothoraces have been associated with rounded atelectasis. Its clinical significance lies in its presentation as a pulmonary mass that must be distinguished from a malignancy. It is often an incidental finding on chest radiograph, ranging from 2.5–7 cm in size. The angle between the pleura and the mass is usually sharp. Rounded atelectasis occurs predominantly in the lower lobes. The classic radiographic feature is a "comet tail" extending from the hilum toward the base of the lung, then sweeping into the inferior pole of the lesion. In the past the diagnosis often was made only at decortication, but CT of the chest permits recognition of this benign condition noninvasively. No specific treatment is needed.

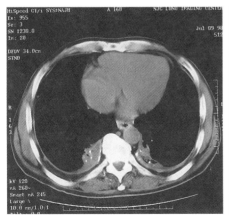 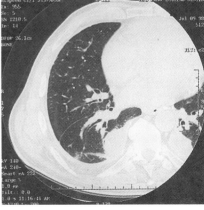

Left, Conventional CT scan (mediastinal window) of a retired pipefitter shows bilateral lower lobe mass-like opacities typical of rounded atelectasis. The right lower lobe mass contains air bronchograms. Both masses contain punctate areas of calcification. *Right,* High-resolution CT scan of the same pipefitter demonstrates a "comet tail." Bronchi and blood vessels swirl into the lateral aspect of the mass on the right.

18. How do you diagnose an asbestos-related benign pleural effusion?

Benign asbestos-related effusion is a diagnosis of exclusion. In patients with a significant history of asbestos exposure and an appropriate latency interval, in whom other causes (including bronchogenic carcinoma, mesothelioma, tuberculosis, pulmonary embolism) have been considered, exudative, serosanguineous pleural effusions are probably due to asbestos exposure. These benign effusions may have white blood cell (WBC) counts up to 28,000/mm^3, and polymorphonuclear or mononuclear cells may predominate in the WBC differential. Some series have shown pleural fluid eosinophilia. Asbestos-related benign pleural effusions produce few symptoms and may be discovered incidentally on serial chest radiographs. The effusion on average lasts several months and eventually clears without residual.

19. What is mesothelioma?

Mesothelioma is an uncommon but increasingly recognized malignant neoplasm, typically of the pleura (80%), rarely of other mesothelial surfaces (e.g., peritoneum, pericardium, or tunica vaginalis testis). It is one of the few malignant tumors for which the specific etiologic agent has been identified. Eighty to 85% of patients diagnosed with malignant mesothelioma have had occupational, paraoccupational, or environmental exposure to asbestos. The latent period between first exposure and clinical detection of the neoplasm is 30–40 years. All of the major commercial forms of asbestos have been reported to induce mesotheliomas. Fiber size appears to be important in terms of tumor risk. Fibers smaller than 0.2 μm in diameter and at least 8 μm long are believed to have the greatest potential for inducing mesothelioma (Stanton theory). Unlike bronchogenic carcinoma, cigarette smoking does not confer an increased risk of developing mesothelioma.

Dull, aching chest pain combined with slowly progressive dyspnea and weight loss are often the presenting symptoms. Pleural effusions occur in approximately 60% of patients. A biopsy obtained at open thoracotomy or video-assisted thoracoscopy is usually needed to establish the diagnosis; only one-third of blind, closed pleural biopsies yield a diagnosis. Treatment of mesotheliomas, either by surgery or chemotherapy, has extended survival by only a few months, if at all. Typically treatment is supportive, including pain management, nutritional support, treatment of infections and counseling of patient and family. Death usually occurs 8 months to 2 years after diagnosis as a result of extensive spread, infection, or respiratory failure.

20. How do you counsel a patient with asbestos-related disease?

The care of a patient with a work-related disorder does not stop with medical treatment and psychological support. Each patient should be counseled that the diagnosis of an asbestos-related disorder may raise legal issues, which can be further explored with a knowledgeable lawyer. Either written or verbal communication of a diagnosis of work-related disease may trigger the legal statute of limitations (the time frame in which the patient must file a legal claim for benefits). Thus patients should be counseled to seek appropriate legal support.

21. What hazards are associated with work in the asbestos removal industry?

Because of the known hazard of asbestos, asbestos abatement is heavily regulated. The asbestos-containing work area has to be strictly isolated, often by erection of physical barriers and maintenance of an air pressure differential. Abatement workers undergo extensive training and must wear protective equipment, including a full-face respirator and impermeable protective clothing. Abatement sites may be hot. The use of water spray to minimize airborne dust levels increases the humidity. Such conditions may lead to significant heat stress as well as psychological stress. If the work area cannot be cooled to comfortable temperatures, a cool rest area must be provided and working time between rest periods must be limited. Many respirators are made of rubber. Because of the increasing incidence of latex allergy, it is prudent for clinicians to ask workers about skin and respiratory reactions to latex or rubber products.

22. How are asbestos fibers measured?

To enforce the Occupational Safety and Health Administration's (OSHA) standard of 0.1 asbestos fibers/cc^3 of workplace air, concentrations of airborne asbestos fibers must be measured.

Air samples are pulled through a filter over time so that suspended dust settles onto the filter. The collected dust is then precipitated for examination under the light microscope. With magnification up to 500×, fibers with a length ≥ 5 μm and a diameter ≥ 0.1 μm can be detected. This means that many of the smaller fibers, mostly chrysotile fibers, will be missed. Transmission electron microscopy (TEM) allows magnification up to 100,000×. This technique, however, may miss some of the larger fibers. Thus light microscopy combined with TEM gives a more representative picture of asbestos fiber air contamination.

BIBLIOGRAPHY

 1. Aberle DR, Balmes JR: Computed tomography of asbestos-related pulmonary parenchymal and pleural diseases. Clin Chest Med 12:115–131, 1991.
 2. Bates DV: Environmental Health Risks and Public Policy: Decision Making in Free Societies. Seattle, University of Washington Press, 1994, pp 27–35.
 3. Begin R, Samet JM, Shaikh RA: Asbestos. In Harber P, Schenker MB, Balmes JR (eds): Occupational and Environmental Respiratory Disease. St. Louis, Mosby, 1996, pp 293–329.
 4. Burgess WA: Asbestos products. In Burgess WA: Recognition of Health Hazards in Industry. New York, John Wiley & Sons, 1995, pp 443–451.
 5. Craighead JE, Abraham JL, Churg A, et al: The pathology of asbestos-associated diseases of the lungs and pleural cavities: Diagnostic criteria and proposed grading schema. Arch Pathol Lab Invest 106:544–595, 1982.
 6. Epler GR, McLoud TC, Gaensler EA: Prevalence and incidence of benign asbestos pleural effusions in a working population. JAMA 247:617–622, 1982.
 7. Light RW: Malignant and benign mesotheliomas. In Light RW: Pleural Diseases. Baltimore, Williams & Wilkins, 1995, pp 117–128.
 8. Mossman BT, Churg A: Mechanisms in the pathogenesis of asbestosis and silicosis. Am J Respir Crit Care Med 157:1666–1680, 1998.
 9. Schwartz DA, Galvin JR, Speakman SB, et al: Restrictive lung function and asbestos-induced pleural fibrosis. J Clin Invest 91:2685–2692, 1993.
10. Wagner GR: Mineral dusts. In Rosenstock L, Cullen MR (eds): Textbook of Clinical Occupational and Environmental Medicine. Philadelphia, W.B. Saunders, 1994, pp 825–837.

16. SILICOSIS, COAL WORKERS' PNEUMOCONIOSIS, AND BYSSINOSIS

William G. Hughson, M.D., D.Phil.

SILICOSIS

1. What is silicosis?

Silicosis is a fibrotic lung disease caused by inhalation of crystalline silicon dioxide (SiO_2), which is the major constituent of minerals. The main forms of SiO_2 are quartz, cristobalite, and tridymite. Occupations at risk include miners, foundry workers, sandblasters, and manufacturers of products such as glass and ceramics.

2. How does SiO_2 cause silicosis?

Particles of SiO_2 are trapped in the alveoli, where they provoke an inflammatory response. Pulmonary alveolar macrophages phagocytose the particles and are subsequently killed by the cytotoxicity of SiO_2. Lysis of the macrophages releases their proteolytic enzymes, causing a cascade of parenchymal destruction and inflammation. This process occurs repeatedly, as successive generations of macrophages are destroyed during the futile attempt to ingest SiO_2 particles. Release of inflammatory mediators causes recruitment of neutrophils and plasma cells to the lung. Over time, repeated injury results in pulmonary fibrosis. Many patients with silicosis have circulating antinuclear antibodies and polyclonal hypergammaglobulinemia, although their role in the pathogenesis of silicosis is uncertain.

3. What is the pathologic appearance of silicosis?

The basic lesion of **chronic and accelerated silicosis** is the silicotic nodule, which begins as a collection of dust-laden macrophages and reticulin fibers in the interstitium. As the nodule develops, hyalinized collagen fibers accumulate in the center. Examination by polarized light microscopy reveals birefringent SiO_2 crystals. The central zone expands gradually, and adjacent nodules may coalesce. The term **simple silicosis** is used when the nodules are smaller than 1 cm. The term **progressive massive fibrosis** (PMF) is used when nodules larger than 1 cm are present.

The pathology of **acute silicosis** is quite different. The air spaces are filled with lipoproteinaceous material similar to that seen in idiopathic pulmonary alveolar proteinosis. Macrophages are filled with SiO_2. Nodules are not a major feature, possibly because the fulminant course of acute silicosis kills the patient before fibrosis can occur.

4. How long does it take to develop silicosis?

The clinical presentations of silicosis are described as chronic, accelerated, and acute. Chronic silicosis is the most common and becomes evident more than 20 years after exposure to SiO_2. Accelerated silicosis develops in 5–15 years. Acute silicosis occurs within 2 years. The accelerated and acute forms are associated with higher levels of exposure. The acute form is rapidly fatal and has occurred in groups of workers with intense exposures, such as tunneling through granite. The incidence of silicosis has declined sharply with better dust control.

5. How is silicosis diagnosed?

The occupational history is crucial. Detailed questions about the patient's entire working life are necessary, since exposures as a young adult can cause disease many years later. Failure to ask the right questions prevents accurate diagnosis. Patients with simple silicosis are often asymptomatic, whereas patients with more advanced disease report dyspnea and cough. The physical examination is usually not helpful. Pulmonary function tests are often normal, and abnormalities are not specific. The chest radiograph is the key. Silicotic nodules are located predominantly in the upper lobes. They cause round nodular densities that are small in simple silicosis. PMF is used to describe masses > 1 cm. Cavitation of larger masses is usually due to tuberculosis. Hilar and mediastinal lymph nodes are often enlarged and may become calcified in an egg-shell pattern. Pleural thickening adjacent to pulmonary masses is common.

6. What are the complications of silicosis?

Silicotics have a threefold risk of tuberculosis compared with silica-exposed people of similar age without silicosis. Included are infections with *Mycobacterium tuberculosis* and atypical strains such as *M. avium-intracellulare* and *M. kansasii*. There is also an increased incidence of fungal infections, such as nocardiosis, cryptococcosis, and those due to *Aspergillus* species.

After years of controversy, silicosis is now an accepted risk factor for lung cancer. In 1996 the International Agency for Research on Cancer (IARC) reclassified silica as a group 1 carcinogen in humans. As with asbestosis, the risk appears confined to patients with silicosis and is not due simply to silica exposure. The degree of risk varies from study to study, and confounding problems result from the greater prevalence of smoking among blue collar workers and radon exposure during mining operations.

Patients with silicosis have a greater incidence of collagen vascular disease, particularly scleroderma. Patients with rheumatoid arthritis or circulating rheumatoid factor without arthritis may develop nodules that are somewhat larger than those in simple silicosis. Pulmonary hypertension and cor pulmonale are features of PMF. Renal disease characterized by glomerular injury has been described in patients with heavy exposure.

7. How is silicosis treated?

Removal from further exposure is essential, as is smoking cessation. In patients with advanced disease, supportive measures such as supplemental oxygen and treatment of heart failure may be needed. Careful observation is necessary for early detection and treatment of tuberculosis and other infections. Bronchoalveolar lavage has been recommended for treatment of acute silicosis, although its efficacy is unproved.

8. What is the prognosis?

Patients with simple silicosis usually have a good prognosis, although the disease may progress even after exposure ceases. Patients with PMF and other complications do not fare as well.

COAL WORKERS' PNEUMOCONIOSIS

9. What is coal workers' pneumoconiosis?

Coal workers' pneumoconiosis (CWP) is a fibrotic lung disease caused by inhalation of coal dust and other carbonaceous materials such as graphite and carbon black. Occupations at risk include coal miners and trimmers, graphite miners and millers, and workers manufacturing carbon electrodes.

10. How does coal dust cause CWP?

There is no such thing as "pure" coal. Coal is predominantly elemental carbon, with varying amounts of minerals, metals, and organic compounds. It is much less cytotoxic than silica. Until the 1940s CWP was thought to be caused by silica present as a byproduct of mining operations. It is now known that CWP is related to the total mass of dust in the lungs. The risk of CWP increases with the degree of hardness (rank) of the coal being mined. Anthracite is the highest rank, followed by bituminous and lignite coal. The higher ranks have lower silica content, which is inconsistent with the theory that silica causes CWP. However, the role of silica and other mineral dusts in the pathogenesis of CWP is still a subject of discussion, and patients with CWP also may have features of silicosis. As in silicosis, the pulmonary alveolar macrophage is believed to play a central role in CWP by releasing inflammatory mediators, recruiting neutrophils into the lung, and stimulating fibroblast production of collagen. A number of immunologic abnormalities have been found in miners with CWP, including elevated levels of IgA, IgG, complement, antinuclear antibodies, and rheumatoid factor. Their role in the pathogenesis of CWP is uncertain.

11. What is the pathologic appearance of CWP?

The basic pathologic lesion is the coal macule, a collection of coal dust-laden macrophages, reticulin, and collagen located in the walls of respiratory bronchioles and adjacent alveoli. A zone of emphysema surrounds the macules, caused by traction on adjacent parenchyma or destruction of alveolar walls by proteolytic enzymes released by inflammatory cells. With time, macules can expand and coalesce. PMF is diagnosed when lesions > 1 cm in diameter are present.

12. How long does it take to develop CWP?

The time course for CWP is similar to that of silicosis and the other pneumoconioses; presentation is typically 20 years or more after onset of exposure. The incidence of CWP has declined with better dust control.

13. How is CWP diagnosed?

As with silicosis, a detailed occupational history is necessary. Patients with simple CWP are often asymptomatic. Dyspnea is present with advanced simple CWP and PMF. Cough and sputum are usually attributable to smoking. The physical examination is usually not helpful. Pulmonary function tests are often normal, and abnormalities are not specific. The chest radiograph in simple CWP reveals round nodules located predominantly in the mid and upper lung zones. PMF is used to describe masses > 1 cm. Cavitation of larger masses may be seen, usually due to necrosis rather than infection, although tuberculosis must be excluded.

Rheumatoid coal pneumoconiosis, also known as Caplan's syndrome, deserves special mention. Radiographs show rapidly enlarging nodules evenly distributed in the lungs. Microscopically, they are similar to rheumatoid nodules. Arthritis may precede or follow the lung nodules by years and in some cases never develops.

14. What are the complications of CWP?

The major complication of CWP is obstructive lung disease. Smoking plays a major role, but bronchitis and emphysema are increased in nonsmoking miners. Tuberculosis and other infections are common, particularly when PMF is present. Lung cancer is not increased in CWP.

15. How is CWP treated?

There is no specific treatment. Avoidance of further pulmonary injury, particularly smoking, is important. Otherwise the approach is similar to that for silicosis (see above).

16. What is the prognosis of CWP?

The life expectancy of a coal miner is similar to that of the general public. Patients with simple CWP have a good prognosis. Patients with PMF are at risk for cardiorespiratory failure and infection.

BYSSINOSIS

17. What is byssinosis?

Byssinosis describes a spectrum of respiratory symptoms and functional impairment in workers exposed to dust from cotton, flax, soft hemp, and sisal. It has many features of asthma. A unique aspect of byssinosis is "the Monday feeling"; affected workers have more problems on the first day of the week. Symptoms then improve after successive work shifts, only to recur following weekends and holidays. Occupations at risk include cotton mill workers, weavers, mattress makers, and makers of yarn and rope.

18. How do plant materials cause byssinosis?

The mechanisms by which cotton and other plant fiber dusts cause byssinosis are not clearly understood. The most important theories are (1) nonimmunologic release of histamine, (2) antigen-antibody reaction, (3) bacterial endotoxins, (4) fungal enzymes, and (5) nonspecific pharmacologic mediator release. Cotton is the most important cause of byssinosis in terms of both number of workers exposed and potency. It is believed that bract, the leaf-like structure that enfolds the cotton boll, causes byssinosis in cotton workers. The bioactivity of cotton is greatly reduced by washing and steaming before processing. Therefore, the active agent is probably water-soluble. Inhalation of cotton dust aerosols provokes symptoms and respiratory function decrements in previously unexposed volunteers. This finding is consistent with nonimmunologic release of histamine or other mediators. Precipitating IgG antibodies against an antigen in cotton are present in exposed workers, but current evidence suggests that they do not play a direct role in byssinosis. Cotton dust contains bacteria and fungi, but they are also found in other industries that are not associated with a byssinosis-like syndrome. In summary, we do not know the exact mechanisms for byssinosis; several mechanisms may occur simultaneously.

19. What is the pathologic appearance of byssinosis?

No specific pathologic abnormalities are associated with byssinosis. Airway inflammation and mucous gland hyperplasia are found in patients with chronic disease.

20. How long does it take to develop byssinosis?

It usually takes more than 10 years of exposure before byssinosis develops. This latent period distinguishes byssinosis from occupational asthma, making specific sensitization a less likely mechanism. A self-selection process is probably involved, because patients with asthma and allergies leave the industry at an early stage. Smokers have a higher incidence and more severe ventilatory impairment. The frequency of byssinosis has decreased with better dust control, but up to one-half of workers in developing countries are still affected.

21. How is byssinosis diagnosed?

The diagnosis requires an appropriate exposure history. Symptoms include chest tightness and dyspnea. Physical signs are cough and sputum production. Wheezing is not a regular feature but may be present in more severe cases. Pulmonary function testing before, during, and after a work shift demonstrates airway obstruction. Classically, the greatest decline occurs on the first day following a weekend or vacation. In more severe cases fixed expiratory obstruction may make it difficult to demonstrate cross-shift changes. Chest radiographs are often normal but may show hyperinflation. The World Health Organization (WHO) has proposed a new grading system based on symptoms, evidence of respiratory tract irritation, and acute or chronic changes in lung function.

22. What are the complications of byssinosis?

Chronic obstructive lung disease is the major problem. Studies have shown increased morbidity and mortality due to respiratory diseases.

23. How is byssinosis treated?

Avoidance of further exposure is recommended for patients with more than mild symptoms or with evidence of significant pulmonary function impairment. However, this goal is difficult to achieve because of the negative economic and social consequences for the worker, particularly in developing countries. Inhaled bronchodilators, steroids, and sodium cromoglycate can ameliorate symptoms but may not prevent chronic obstructive lung disease if exposure continues. Smoking cessation is essential.

24. What is the prognosis of byssinosis?

The prognosis is uncertain. Once established, airways hyperreactivity may persist even after exposure ceases. Patients with more advanced disease have airway obstruction that may be permanent.

BIBLIOGRAPHY

Silicosis
 1. Brown LM, Gridley G, Olsen JH, et al: Cancer risk and mortality patterns among silicotic men in Sweden and Denmark. J Occup Environ Med 39:633–638, 1997.
 2. Beckett W, Abraham J, Becklake M, et al: Adverse effects of crystalline silica exposure. Am J Respir Crit Care Med 155:761–765, 1997.
 3. Mossman BT, Churg A: Mechanisms in the pathogenesis of asbestosis and silicosis. Am J Respir Crit Care Med 157:1666–1680, 1998.
 4. Steenland K, Stayner L: Silica, asbestos, man-made mineral fibers and cancer. Cancer Causes Control 8:491–503, 1997.
 5. Wagner GR: Asbestosis and silicosis. Lancet 349:1311–1315, 1997.

Coal workers' pneumoconiosis
 6. Henneberger PK, Attfield MD: Respiratory symptoms and spirometry in experienced coal miners: Effects of both distant and recent coal mine dust exposures. Am J Indust Med 32:268–274, 1997.
 7. Heppleston AG: Coal workers' pneumoconiosis: A historical perspective on its pathogenesis. Am J Indust Med 22:905–923, 1992.
 8. Hughson WG: Coal workers' pneumoconiosis. In Bordow RA, Moser KM (eds): Manual of Clinical Problems in Pulmonary Medicine, 4th ed. Boston, Little, Brown, 1996, pp 367–370.
 9. Lapp NL, Parker JE: Coal workers' pneumoconiosis. Clin Chest Med 13:243–252, 1992.
10. Wang X, Yano E, Nonaka K, et al: Respiratory impairments due to dust exposure: A comparative study among workers exposed to silica, asbestos, and coalmine dust. Am J Indust Med 31:495–502, 1997.

Byssinosis
11. Beckett WS, Pope CA, Xu XP, Christiani DC: Women's respiratory health in the cotton textile industry: An analysis of respiratory symptoms in 973 non-smoking female workers. Occup Environ Med 51:14–18, 1994.
12. Hodgson JT, Jones RD: Mortality of workers in the British cotton industry in 1968–84. Scand J Environ Health 16:113–120, 1990.
13. McL Niven R, Fletcher AM, Pickering CAC, et al: Chronic bronchitis in textile workers. Thorax 52:22–27, 1997.
14. McL Niven R, Pickering CAC: Byssinosis: A review. Thorax 51:632–637, 1996.
15. Newman-Taylor AJ, Pickering CAC: Occupational asthma and byssinosis. In Parkes WR (ed): Occupational Lung Disorders, 3rd ed. Oxford, Butterworth-Heinemann, 1994, pp 729–754.

17. MAN-MADE VITREOUS FIBERS

Stuart M. Brooks, M.D., and Wasif M. Alam, M.D., M.S.P.H.

1. What are man-made vitreous fibers (MMVFs)? What is their exposure prevalence?

MMVFs are a variety of manufactured materials with excellent insulating properties. They are used with increasing frequency as asbestos substitutes and have thousands of applications in industrial and nonindustrial settings. They are used for reinforcement in buildings, ships, and automobiles, as well as home appliances, industrial kilns, and furnaces. Exposure to MMVFs occurs during production, fabrication, and application of materials. According to the National Occupational Exposure Survey, approximately 500,000 American workers are potentially exposed to MMVFs.

2. Differentiate MMVFs from man-made mineral fibers (MMMFs).

MMVFs and MMMFs are essentially the same. MMVFs are not true minerals; they are amorphous silicates manufactured into a fibrous form. They are grouped, according to origin, into glass fiber (from glass; also called fiberglass), ceramic fiber (from kaolin clay), and mineral wool (from rock or slag).

3. Why are MMVFs considered superior to asbestos?

MMVFs have generally replaced asbestos as insulating agents in recent years, even though data continue to support the 1988 judgment by the International Association for Research on Cancer (IARC) that mineral fibers are a possible human carcinogen (group 2B). Recent epidemiologic studies provide little evidence of lung carcinogenicity for either glass wool or rock/slag wool. Ceramic fibers, a much less common source of exposure than glass wool and rock/slag wool, are of concern because of positive animal studies, but human data are insufficient. The carcinogenicity of asbestos for the lung and mesothelium is well established.

4. Name the fibrous minerals most commonly used in industry.

MMVFs include glass wool, rock wool, slag wool, glass filaments and microglass fibers, and refractory ceramic fibers (RCFs). RCFs are manufactured for high-temperature applications.

5. What physical characteristics of fibers determine their toxicity and carcinogenicity?

The carcinogenic potential of any fiber is related to its dimension and biopersistence. According to experimental evidence, only fibers longer than 5 microns, thinner than 3 microns, and with a length-to-diameter ratio more than 3 are able to reach the periphery of the lung. In addition to the traditionally considered variables of particle size and shape, mineralogic characteristics such as dissolution behavior, ion exchange, sorptive properties, and the nature of the mineral surface (e.g., surface reactivity) play important roles in determining toxicity and carcinogenicity. The biologic activity of MMVFs made of glass, rock, slag, or other minerals does not depend only on their respirability but also on their chemical durability and persistency. In the use of MMVFs, the goal is to decrease their harmful effects by increasing their dissolution and removal from the lungs.

6. Discuss the pathophysiology of disease caused by MMVFs.

How fibers cause diseases and what specific determinants are critical to fiber-induced toxicity and carcinogenicity are still not completely understood. Further research in fiber toxicology and additional toxicity and exposure data are needed to characterize more accurately the health risks of inhaled fibers. Scanning electron micrographs, however, show that MMVFs are readily phagocytized by rat alveolar macrophages (AMs) in culture. The phagocytosis begins within

30 minutes after the onset of the exposure and continues for a 96-hour observation period. Short fibers (< 20 microns in length) are readily phagocytized by AMs, whereas longer fibers are attacked with a large number of AMs. In all studies, ceramic fibers phagocytized by AMs were characterized by moderate fibrotic activity. A statistically significant increase in the incidence of tumor (mesothelioma) was observed in RCFs, which show a carcinogenic potential similar to that of natural asbestos (crocidolite or chrysotile).

7. How is the risk of fiber exposures measured?

Naturally occurring and man-made fibers of respirable sizes have been identified by the U.S. Environmental Protection Agency (EPA) as priority substances for risk reduction and pollution prevention under the Toxic Substances Control Act (TSCA). The health concern for respirable fibers is based on the association of occupational asbestos exposure and environmental erionite exposure with the development of chronic respiratory diseases in humans, including interstitial lung fibrosis, lung cancer, and mesothelioma. Considerable laboratory evidence also indicates that fibers of varying physical and chemical characteristics may elicit fibrogenic and carcinogenic effects in animals under certain exposure conditions. To assess the potential risk associated with production and use of certain man-made materials for which human data are either unavailable or inadequate, it has been necessary to use data from studies conducted in laboratory animals and with cells or tissues. During the past several decades, it has been suggested that data about the mechanisms by which particles cause disease may be used to reduce the uncertainty in estimates of human risks.

8. What are the occupational exposure limits (OELs) for MMVFs?

To set OELs for aerosol particles, dusts, or chemicals, one must evaluate whether mechanistic factors permit identification of a no-observed-effect level (NOEL). In the case of carcinogenic effects, an NOEL can be assumed if no genotoxicity is involved, and exposure is considered safe if it does not exceed the NOEL. If tumor induction is associated with genotoxicity, any exposure is considered to be a risk, although an NOEL may be identified in the animal or human exposure studies. The same assumption is made when no information about the carcinogenic mechanism is available. Because carcinogenic effects have been associated with long-thin fiber geometry and high durability in vivo, all fibers meeting such criteria are considered to be unsafe. Investigations of fiber tumorigenicity/genotoxicity should include information about dose-response relationship, pathobiochemistry, particle clearance, and persistence of the material in the target organ. Such information introduces quantitative aspects into the qualitative approach that has so far been used to classify fibrous dusts as carcinogens.

9. How serious are the health effects of MMVFs?

Increasing knowledge about the carcinogenic properties of asbestos has given rise to extensive research into possible adverse health effects of alternative materials. MMVFs turned out to be of unique interest, because they have already been used for several decades for isolation purposes. Except for RCFs, studies show that inhalation does not provoke tumors in rodents, whereas intratracheal, intrapleural, and intraperitoneal instillation induces a carcinogenic effect for most kinds of MMVFs. Compared with asbestos, MMVFs clear much faster from lung tissue. No consistent epidemiologic evidence indicates an increased standardized mortality ratio due to malignant tumors of the airways and malignant mesotheliomas in people formerly exposed to MMVFs. An itchy skin problem (glass-fiber dermatitis) appears appears to be far more common than the rather theoretic tumor risk in workers who handle thicker and therefore more stinging fibers without protection. Based on these facts and the actual exposure situation, handling of glass fibers and wool poses no clear-cut cancer risk; however, the potential risk of exposure to RCFs has to be evaluated with more caution. In 1988 the IARC classified such mineral fibers as glass wool, rock wool, and slag wool as probably carcinogenic in humans. MMVFs break transversely, but do not split longitudinally in the manner of asbestos to produce thinner fibers. Thus airborne dust inhaled by workers does not penetrate beyond the longer bronchi.

10. MMVFs are classified as "probably carcinogenic." What is the likely mechanism of their carcinogenicity?

The mechanism of MMVF carcinogenicity remains unclear. It is assumed that their involvement in the production of free oxygen radicals is one of the most important factors contributing to the initiation of carcinogenesis. When free oxygen radicals are produced at a fast rate, the cell is exposed to oxidative stress. DNA damage is an important consequence of oxidative stress. New oxygen radicals may modify DNA and lead to mutation; finally, they may contribute to the occurrence of neoplastic cells. MMVFs also may contribute to the increase of the number and activity of neutrophilic granulocytes and macrophages. The appearance of MMVF fractions in granulocytes results in increased production of free oxygen radicals, which may damage the DNA of epithelial cells.

11. Does smoking affect MMVF exposure?

Experimental studies indicate that the production of free oxygen radicals by neutrophilic granulocytes and macrophages activated by MMVFs increases under the influence of chemicals in tobacco smoke. The combination of fibers with tobacco smoke may amplify DNA damage and contribute to the occurrence of neoplastic cells.

12. In a workers' compensation case, when can you say that ill health effects are most likely due to MMVFs?

Before jumping into a diagnosis, one should ask the following important decision-making questions:

History. A thorough history of workers' past and present employment together with their leisure activities (e.g., hobbies) should be taken. A detailed history is often enough to make a diagnosis. MMVFs have thousands of applications in nonindustrial settings.

Risk assessment. Determine whether the person is at all exposed to MMVF and, if so, to what degree and for how long. It is essential to understand dose-response relationships. Workers newly exposed to MMVFs may develop acute respiratory and skin irritation. Pneumoconiosis, chronic bronchitis, pleural plaques and pleural thickening, and asbestos-like effects—particularly lung cancer—should be related to long-term exposure. It is important to know the fiber's physical characteristics, biodurability and type (e.g., RCFs rather than glass wool may result in lung cancer). Therefore, biomonitoring is needed.

Biomonitoring. Biomonitoring may be divided into two general categories. Bulk sample analysis, which determines whether MMVFs are present in bulk material (usually some sort of building product) and estimates the amount, may be done by polarized light microscopy or electron microscopy. Air sampling and analysis estimate the number of fibers present per volume of air. Light microscopy with phase-contrast enhancement is commonly used. Direct reading meters, as used for asbestos, are also available for estimating concentrations of airborne fiber.

Physical examination. Glass-fiber dermatitis is commonly associated with exposure to thicker and therefore more stinging fibers. Mechanical irritation of the skin may result from fibers more than 5 µm in diameter. Punctate erythema and itching may be produced when the exposure is recent, whereas long-term exposure leads to hardening of the skin, usually without itching discomfort. Glass-fiber dermatitis is one of the most common forms of occupational dermatitis resulting from mechanical irritation. Intense itching accompanied by erythematous macules, papules, and folliculitis with excoriation over arms, neck, face, and upper chest has been reported after the first 2 weeks of employment. Paronychia and warts may result from implanted splinters of glass fibers. When glass fibers contaminate an indoor environment (as detected by indoor air sampling), the direct trauma of inhalation may cause cough, epistaxis, and sore throat. Glass blowers have a significantly higher prevalence of chronic bronchitis, nasal catarrh, chronic sinusitis, and nasal bleeding than control workers. Therefore, measurement of lung function among glass blowers may show chronic respiratory findings.

Determination of the relationship of MMVFs to the health complaints of a worker is sometimes complex. An interdisciplinary approach must focus on the occupation medicine specialist, industrial hygienist, employee, employer, and workplace. However, decision making is the responsibility of the occupational medicine specialist with the required knowledge and training.

BIBLIOGRAPHY

1. Alam WM: Manufactured mineral fibers. In Harbison R (ed): Hamilton & Hardy's Industrial Toxicology 5th ed. St. Louis, Mosby, 1998.
2. Brooks S, Gochfeld M, Herzstein J, et al (eds): Environmental Medicine. St. Louis, Mosby, 1994.
3. Greim HA, Ziegler-Skylakakis K: Strategies for setting occupational exposure limits for particles. Environ Health Perspect 105(Suppl 5):1357–1361, 1997.
4. Guthrie GD Jr: Mineral properties and their contributions to particle toxicity. Environ Health Perspect 105(Suppl 5):1003–1011, 1997.
5. Lutz W, Krajewska B: Oxidative stress as a basic mechanism of the carcinogenic effect of man made mineral fibers on the human body. Med Pr 46:275–284, 1995.
6. McClellan RO: Use of mechanistic data in assessing human risks from exposure to particles. Environ Health Perspect 105(Suppl 5):1363–1372, 1997.
7. Morimoto Y, Tsuda T, Nakamura H, et al: Expression of metalloproteinases, tissue inhibitors of metalloproteinases, and extracellular matrix mRNA following exposure to mineral fibers and cigarette smoke in vivo. Environ Health Perspect 105(Suppl 5):1247–1251, 1997.
8. Muhle H, Bellmann B: Significance of the biodurability of man-made vitreous fibers to risk assessment. Environ Health Perspect 105(Suppl 5):1045–1047, 1997.
9. Plato N, Westerholm P, Gustavsson P, et al: Cancer incidence, mortality and exposure response among Swedish man-made vitreous fiber production workers. Scand J Work Environ Health 21:353–361, 1995.
10. Steenland K, Stayner L: Silica, asbestos, man-made mineral fibers, and cancer. Cancer Causes Control 8:491–503, 1997.
11. Vu VT, Lai DY: Approaches to characterizing human health risks of exposure to fibers. Environ Health Perspect 105(Suppl 5):1329–1336, 1997.
12. Wagner GR: Mineral dusts. In Rosenstock L, Cullen MR (eds): Textbook of Clinical Occupational and Environmental Medicine. Philadelphia, W.B. Saunders, 1994.

18. CARBON MONOXIDE AND OTHER COMBUSTION PRODUCTS

Elizabeth A. Katz, M.P.H., C.I.H., and James E. Cone, M.D., M.P.H.

1. What substance is the leading cause of fatal poisonings in the United States?

Carbon monoxide (CO) causes over 800 unintended fatalities each year. Lost work days due to acute CO illness exceed 10,000 nationally. CO is an odorless and colorless gas that is a natural byproduct of combustion.

2. What are the symptoms of acute CO poisoning?

Symptoms of acute CO poisoning include headache, nausea, dizziness, muscle weakness, chest pain, visual disturbances, decreased muscle coordination, and persistent fatigue. Mental stupor may progress to unconsciousness. Onset may be acute, insidious, or delayed.

3. Why does mild-to-moderate CO intoxication often go unrecognized?

The nonspecific symptoms, which mimic those of influenza and other common illnesses, result in widespread undiagnosed morbidity due to CO. Similar concurrent symptoms in coworkers or household members may be misinterpreted as evidence of contagious illness. An elevated alcohol level, which has been noted in many nonoccupational poisonings, may be an additional complicating factor, because signs and symptoms of alcohol intoxication may mask CO symptoms. CO is odorless and colorless and can be detected only if appropriate tests are performed on air or biologic samples.

4. What are the immediate sequelae of severe CO poisoning?

Severe, acute intoxication leads to loss of consciousness and insufficient oxygen supply to the heart and may cause death. A short period of apparent recovery may mask permanent neurologic and neuropsychological damage.

5. Besides CO, what other products of combustion may be hazardous?

Depending on the material undergoing combustion, temperature, and oxygen availability, other toxic materials may be formed. In addition, some of the unburned material can be expected to vaporize.

Toxic Products of Combustion

TOXIC PRODUCT	POTENTIAL PYROLYSIS SOURCE(S)
Cyanide gas	Urethane or polyurethane foams/rubbers
Dioxin	Municipal waste incineration
Hydrogen chloride	Chlorinated solvents
Respirable particulates	Diesel exhaust, fires
Sulfur dioxide	High-sulfur coal or crude oil
Nitrogen oxides (NO, NO_2)	Paint, solvents, motor vehicles
Formaldehyde	Diesel exhaust, polyvinyl chloride
Phosgene	Chlorinated solvents in presence of arc welding
Phthalic anhydride	Cutting polyvinyl chloride meat-wrapping film with a thermal film cutter

6. What are the most common occupations involving CO exposure?

Workers exposed in poorly ventilated areas to fires, furnaces, internal combustion engines, or diesel engines are at risk for CO poisoning. Auto mechanics, parking garage and gas station attendants, warehouse workers (particularly large refrigerated warehouses), firefighters, cooks, maintenance workers, and construction workers are commonly affected. Many poisonings result from improper use or inadequate maintenance of gasoline-powered equipment, such as concrete-cutting saws, compressors, power trowels, welding gear, pressure washers, and floor buffers. Even propane-powered equipment, formerly assumed to be CO-safe, is now recognized as an indoor hazard (propane-powered forklifts, ice-rink smoothing equipment). Other fuels generating CO include wood, kerosene, coal, and natural gas. In addition, most urban drivers (occupational and commuter) are exposed to CO levels exceeding 9 ppm (the Environmental Protection Agency's [EPA] ambient air quality standard) inside their vehicles. In addition, CO may be used as a calibration gas, in metallurgy, and in organic chemistry.

7. What is warehouse workers' headache?

Headache and other general gastrointestinal and central nervous system symptoms result from CO poisoning in warehouse workers exposed to forklift exhaust.

8. During what season does most CO intoxication occur?

In winter, in part because garage and warehouse doors are more often kept closed, decreasing natural ventilation. Increased use of furnaces and portable space heaters is also a factor. However, many cases occur year-round wherever ventilation is inadequate, even though windows and doors may be open and some forced-air ventilation may be provided. One investigator estimated that 3–5% of winter headaches are due to CO.

9. What about classic signs of CO poisoning such as cherry-red cyanosis?

Cherry-red mucous membranes are rarely seen. Carboxyhemoglobin (COHb) is indeed red, but most poisonings do not cause altered skin color. Nor is retinal hemorrhage commonly seen in CO poisoning.

10. What is the half-life of CO in humans?

After cessation of exposure, the half-life of CO in blood (COHb) is 5 hours; factors that influence the half-life include age, activity level, and therapeutic oxygen administration.

11. What is the classic toxic mechanism of CO?

Formation of COHb with resultant hypoxia. CO has an affinity for hemoglobin 242 times higher than oxygen. The hypoxia primarily affects the central nervous system and the heart (especially in people with existing atherosclerotic coronary artery disease).

12. What are the other toxic mechanisms and target organs for CO?

Direct tissue effects have been observed. CO affects the cytochrome oxidase system, mitochondrial processes, and myoglobin (found mainly in heart and skeletal muscles). The clinical importance of the alternate toxic mechanisms is not well understood. CO may accumulate in tissue and plasma preferentially over hemoglobin, particularly over long periods of lower-level exposure; thus, direct tissue toxicity can result from poisoning with relatively low COHb levels. Although no clinical techniques are available for evaluation of intracellular CO binding, practitioners should consider the possibility of intracellular toxic effects when interpreting COHb and exhaled air CO tests. It is probably because of these alternative mechanisms that COHb levels may not correlate well with symptoms and signs of poisoning in individual cases.

13. What are the long-term sequelae of CO poisoning?

Neurologic and neuropsychiatric sequelae sometimes appear 2 days to 6 weeks after an acute intoxication. The likelihood of such sequelae seems to be greatest for older people with preexisting health problems and people with greater intensity or duration of exposure. (Also see reproductive and coronary effects below.) Signs and symptoms of such neuropsychological sequelae include language difficulties, attention and memory disturbance, slowed information processing, disorientation, gait and balance deficits, and hallucinations. Occasionally, peripheral neuropathy has been reported.

14. What steps do you recommend in evaluating a case of suspected occupational or environmental CO poisoning? What laboratory tests are most useful?

Check electrolytes in comatose patients because acidosis may occur. Assess the blood level of COHb (usually in the same arterial blood sample used for blood gas analysis). Check for hydrogen cyanide (HCN) poisoning; particularly in fire-exposed victims, CO and HCN poisoning may occur simultaneously.

History-taking should include symptoms in coworkers and household members; occupation, hobbies, and fuel-powered tool use; time pattern of symptoms (especially duration of likely exposure, time elapsed since removal from exposure); exposure to methylene chloride; and history of ischemic heart disease or anemia.

Laboratory testing should include a chest radiograph if the patient has been exposed to fire. Patients with neurologic or neuropsychologic damage should undergo neuropsychological testing, dynamic posturography, and gait assessment.

In cases of acute exposure (within 1 hour of exposure), exhaled breath samples should be obtained with maximal inspiration, followed by 20-second breath hold and exhalation into a monitor or 1-liter plastic sample bags. Analysis should be prompt.

15. To what extent should clinicians be concerned about CO exposure in cigarettes? What about passive smoking?

Cigarette smokers have mean COHb levels of approximately 4%, although the range can be 2–10% or even higher. Passive smoking usually results in a COHb increase of only a few percent above baseline levels that result from metabolism in the body. Cigar smoke may contain more CO than cigarette smoke.

16. What are the reproductive effects of CO?

Some investigators believe that CO from cigarette smoking accounts for some of the excessive rates of low birthweight among infants of smokers. However, low birthweight has not been shown to be associated with workplace exposure to CO. Severe CO poisoning during pregnancy may lead to neurologic malformations in the fetus or even fetal death. The maximal CO exposure level or COHb during pregnancy has not been well defined.

17. Does workers' compensation cover harm to a fetus carried by an employed mother?

No. The fetus is not covered. Therefore, the employer may be subject to third-party liability; some lawsuits against employers on behalf of infants damaged by CO have been successful.

18. A 50-year-old construction worker presents with complaints of chest pain consistent with angina. Questioning reveals that he uses tools powered by a gasoline-powered compressor. Can the angina be due to CO?

For persons with preexisting coronary heart disease, increased levels of COHb may precipitate angina or myocardial infarction because of the inability of the heart to increase blood flow to the myocardium in response to hypoxia.

19. What treatment regimens are useful for CO poisoning? What are the indications for hyperbaric oxygen (HBO) after CO poisoning?

Aggressive administration of hyperbaric oxygen, if available, is indicated for all levels of CO intoxication. HBO also treats concomitant HCN poisoning, if present. If neuropsychological deficits are found, cognitive retraining may assist in recovery.

20. Should a CO-poisoned pregnant woman be treated with HBO?

Yes. Because of the short duration of HBO treatment, it is believed to be well tolerated by the fetus in all stages of development. HBO treatment reduces risk of death or brain damage to the mother and fetus.

21. What are the most common sources of CO in the home?

Common sources include furnaces, water heaters, and stoves fueled by natural gas, oil, or propane; kerosene space heaters; charcoal-burning grills and hibachis; and wood-burning stoves and fireplaces. Vehicle exhaust often contains large amounts of CO; vehicles should not be warmed up in a garage, even with the door open.

Energy-efficient construction has tended to decrease natural ventilation in homes; thus the importance of proper venting and maintenance of combustion appliances is increased. Mobile homes and recreational vehicles also may be tightly constructed. They have been associated with a disproportionate number of poisoning incidents. Backdrafting of exhaust gases from flues and chimneys commonly occurs when the house air pressure drops during operation of powered exhaust fans (for example, in bathrooms and kitchen range hoods).

22. What are the maximal acceptable exposure standards for CO?

Maximal Acceptable Exposure Standards

AIR CONCENTRATION	EXPOSURE PERIOD	AGENCY
35 ppm	8 hr	National Institute of Occupational Safety and Health
35 ppm	8 hr	Occupational Safety and Health Administration
25 ppm	8 hr	American Conference of Governmental Industrial Hygienists
9 ppm	Continuous (ambient air)	Environmental Protection Agency

23. What prevention methods have been effective?

1. Each incident of CO poisoning should be considered an index case. Surveillance of CO poisonings by the Colorado Department of Public Health and Environment has been effective in the prevention of additional poisonings.

2. Regularly scheduled inspection and preventive maintenance of combustion appliances and their vents is recommended in residences and workplaces. Equipping propane forklifts with catalytic converters typically reduces CO output by more than 95%. Vehicle tune-ups also reduce CO output somewhat by increasing efficiency. Natural gas appliances adjusted for blue-flame operation emit much less CO than those with yellow-tipped flame.

3. Toll-booth workers can be protected by forced-air ventilation. Observation booths in tunnels can be replaced with remote video cameras.

4. Education is extremely important, particularly for immigrants unaccustomed to tightly constructed buildings. Charcoal grills and hibachis should not be used indoors or in tents. Cooking stoves should not be used for space heating.

5. Gasoline-powered machinery should not be used indoors, even in large spaces. Substitution with electrical or hydraulic equipment may be appropriate. For brief use in defined areas (vehicles during tune-up, fire stations) negative-pressure exhaust ductwork is often an effective control. A flexible duct must be slipped directly over the exhaust pipe and vented to the outdoors.

6. Investigation of complaints of poor indoor air quality sometimes uncovers elevated CO exposures. Typical causes of elevated CO in nonindustrial settings include building air intakes located near parked vehicles and loading docks, backdrafting of exhaust gases, blocked flues, and propane-powered floor buffers.

7. Installation of CO alarms has prevented poisonings; see below.

24. How useful are CO alarm monitors in workplaces?

CO monitors have long been used in industry and are extremely useful if properly selected and maintained. They should be considered wherever ventilation failure, worker error, or other variables may result in a dangerous CO level. According to a recent National Institute for Occupational Safety and Health (NIOSH) Health Alert, portable gasoline-powered equipment should be equipped with CO monitors. NIOSH can assist in selection of workplace CO monitors.

25. What field instruments are available for monitoring CO exposure levels?

Real-time monitors and grab-sampling detector tubes are useful for industrial hygiene investigations. The real-time monitors are generally used for short-term observations (because of their expense, they are impractical for shift-long monitoring of numerous employees).

For time-weighted average measurement, the most accurate results are obtained by integrating bag sampling. Passive lapel-worn, length-of-stain indicator tubes are available for time-weighted average measurements, but their accuracy may vary significantly. No validated passive time-weighted average dosimeters are currently available. Lawrence Berkeley National Laboratory is currently developing such a monitor with an 8-hour occupational version and a 1-week nonoccupational version.

CONTROVERSY

26. Should CO alarm monitors be used in the home?

CO monitors are now mass-marketed for home installation. Some authorities do not recommend them, primarily because of numerous "false alarms" that occur during local temperature inversions. However, if a model with a full-range digital readout is selected and the user becomes familiar with usual exposure levels, undue episodes of alarm can be avoided and the source of elevated CO can be located. Many home CO monitors, priced between $30 and $95, were rated "acceptable" by *Consumer Reports*, which states that the quality of home CO monitors has improved since they first appeared on the market. The first CO monitor in a home should be installed in the sleeping area. The expense of universal home use of CO monitors would be high; mandatory or universal use may not be justifiable in terms of societal cost-benefit. In cases where CO intoxication is suspected, however, home CO monitors can certainly be useful.

BIBLIOGRAPHY

1. Apte M: An Inexpensive CO Sensor. Center for Building Science News, Lawrence Berkeley National Laboratory, Berkeley, CA, 1995.
2. Carbon-monoxide detectors. Consumer Rep 16(11)58–59, 1996.
3. Kelefant GA: Encephalopathy and peripheral neuropathy following carbon monoxide poisoning from a propane-fueled vehicle. Am J Indust Med 30:765–768, 1996.
4. Lee K, Yanagisawa Y: Sampler for measurement of alveolar carbon monoxide. Environ Sci Technol 29:104–107, 1995.
5. National Institute of Occupational Safety and Health, Colorado Department of Public Health and Environment, U.S. Consumer Product Safety Commission, Occupational Safety and Health Administration, U.S. Environmental Protection Agency: ALERT: Preventing Carbon Monoxide Poisoning from Small Gasoline-Powered Engines and Tools. NIOSH Publication No. 96-118, 1996.
6. U.S. Environmental Protection Agency: Air Quality Criteria for Carbon Monoxide, EPA/600/8-90/045F 1991.
7. Van Hoesen KB, Camporesi EM, Moon RE, et al: Should hyperbaric oxygen be used to treat the pregnant patient for acute carbon monoxide poisoning? JAMA 261:1039–1043, 1989.

19. TUBERCULOSIS

Neil W. Schluger, M.D.

1. What causes tuberculosis? How is it spread?

Tuberculosis (TB) is a disease caused by *Mycobacterium tuberculosis*, a slow-growing bacterium that is found throughout the world. The disease is most commonly spread by the airborne route when respiratory droplet nuclei less than 5 microns in diameter are inhaled by persons in close contact with a person who has active disease. TB also may be spread by inhalation of aerosolized contents of abscesses or tissue (for example, at autopsy), although this route of exposure is less common now than in the past. The chance that someone will become infected with *M. tuberculosis* is difficult to quantify. Older studies suggest that only 50% of people sharing living space with a person with active TB become infected if exposed for as long as 6 months, but many recent studies suggest that infection occurs with apparently trivial exposures.

2. What is the difference between TB infection and TB disease?

After a person inhales tubercle bacteria, the immune system may be able to control the growth of the organism, which may remain dormant in the lungs. This stage of dormancy in a host with no signs or symptoms of respiratory illness is **TB infection**. Most infected patients do not develop actual **TB disease**. However, in 10% of cases of infection (often when the immune system of the infected host has become depressed by malnutrition, advanced malignancy, use of immunosuppressive drugs, end-stage renal disease, diabetes mellitus, underlying silicosis, or acquired immunodeficiency syndrome), the host develops active disease, as manifest by the development of symptoms such as fever, sweat, cough, and weight loss. Thus, most persons exposed to an active case do not develop TB. In fact, the World Health Organization estimates that one-third of the world's population is infected with TB, although there are "only" 8–12 million cases of active disease each year. Three million persons with active TB will die, making TB the world's leading infectious cause of death in adults. The rationale for use of chemoprophylaxis such as isoniazid is that the risk of developing active TB is highest in the first 2 years after initial infection, although the risk probably increases with advanced age.

3. Can multidrug-resistant TB be prevented?

The increase in cases of multidrug-resistant tuberculosis (MDR-TB) has been a particularly worrisome feature of the recent TB epidemic in the United States. As opposed to drug-susceptible TB, for which cure rates are essentially 100%, MDR-TB is associated with substantial morbidity (from both the disease itself and the prolonged 18–24-month drug regimens used for treatment) and mortality. By far the best way to reduce morbidity and mortality from MDR-TB is prevention, which depends primarily on proper prescription and administration of medication (programs of directly observed therapy reduce the incidence and spread of MDR-TB) and maintenance of proper infection control practices for hospitals and other facilities where patients with MDR-TB reside.

4. How should occupational exposure to MDR-TB be treated?

Occupational exposure to MDR-TB is probably inevitable from time to time. It is impossible to know with certainty the drug susceptibility pattern of an isolate causing latent infection, although in an occupational setting one should try to determine the likely source case. If a worker probably was exposed to a case of MDR-TB, a preventive regimen should be based on the susceptibility pattern of the source case. In cases of exposure to strains of TB resistant to isoniazid and rifampin, some authorities have recommended pyrazinamide and a quinolone, but no data prove the efficacy of this regimen. Alternatively, if a worker is in a situation where exposure to

MDR-TB is inevitable and infection has not yet occurred, the bacille Calmette-Guérin (BCG) vaccine may be a reasonable alternative.

5. Can an asymptomatic person with TB infection spread TB to others?

No. Asymptomatic people with TB infection, with normal chest radiographs and negative sputum for acid-fast bacillus (AFB) usually cannot spread TB to others. The only manifestation of infection is a positive tuberculin skin test, demonstrating delayed-type hypersensitivity against the purified protein derivative (PPD) of *M. tuberculosis*.

6. What occupations place workers at increased risk of TB infection?

Certain workers are obviously at increased risk for TB infection, including physicians, nurses, respiratory therapists involved in the care of patients with active TB, workers in correctional institutions, dentists, workers in homeless shelters, microbiology laboratory workers, pathologists, and morticians. The risk of infection is not equal among all types of health care workers caring for patients with TB. One study examined the occupational risk of TB infection for fellows in infectious diseases compared with fellows training in pulmonary medicine and found that pulmonary fellows had a substantially increased risk of TB infection. The most likely reason is the elevated risk of infection associated with invasive procedures performed on patients with TB, such as bronchoscopy, although other explanations are possible.

In addition to health care workers, other occupations have been associated with an increased risk of TB infection. Workers with silicosis have a much higher rate of developing TB than the general population. Morgue workers and undertakers also have a higher risk of developing TB than persons in other jobs. The higher risk is probably due to exposure to previously undiagnosed cases of TB during the performance of autopsy. Finally, TB cases are overrepresented among migrant farm workers, restaurant workers, and factory workers. Such cases are probably related less to specific environmental or occupational risks than to socioeconomic status and demographic characteristics associated with significant risk of TB (residence in areas with high rates of TB, low income, poor nutritional status).

7. Can a person get TB from riding the subway or bus?

As stated above, TB is transmitted by respiratory droplet nuclei that are 5 microns in diameter or less. Because droplets of this size cannot travel far when expelled by coughing, the chance of becoming infected in a brief bus or subway ride is very small. The chance is made even smaller by the fact that in the United States the overall incidence of active TB is less than 9 cases per 100,000 persons. Thus the chance of finding oneself on a bus or subway car with a person with active TB is extremely low. However, in situations in which air is shared, it is theoretically possible to become infected by a ventilation system into which an infectious patient has coughed tubercle bacilli. Recently, for example, several cases of TB infection were believed to have occurred in airplane passengers seated several rows from the source case. When a patient known to have TB travels by plane, at a minimum he or she should wear a mask. However, to the extent possible, no person with infectious TB should travel in a setting with a recirculating air supply shared by others.

8. What diagnostic methods are available for people at risk for occupational or environmental exposure to tuberculosis?

Monitoring people at high risk for TB infection is an essential component of any program in occupational medicine. Monitoring is done with the tuberculin skin test, in which 5 tuberculin units (TU) of PPD are injected intradermally, usually in a location such as the volar forearm. The test is read 48–72 hours after placement. A positive result is 10 mm (or 5 mm in close contacts of an active case) of induration (not erythema) at the site of injection. The test should be performed in all new employees to screen for prior infection and repeated yearly (or every 6 months for higher-risk workers). Any person with a positive test should have a chest radiograph to exclude active disease. In persons with a previously negative skin test, a newly positive test indicates recent infection and is an indication for preventive drug therapy.

For people in whom the initial skin test is positive or who later develop a positive test result, subsequent skin testing is useless because the result will remain positive. In such cases, surveillance is probably best done by careful history-taking on a regular basis to elicit symptoms of active TB. Yearly chest radiographic examination of asymptomatic tuberculin-positive patients is not warranted because of the extremely low yield and the needless radiation exposure.

Although no other test can reliably detect TB infection, the PPD skin test has a significant false-negative rate (10–15%), due in part to anergy. Sputum cultures are negative in patients with TB infection, but culture and sensitivity testing should be the main guides to treatment of active disease.

9. What is the booster effect?

In some people who have been previously infected with TB, the delayed-type hypersensitivity skin test response wanes with time but is "boosted" when a second tuberculin skin test is done shortly after the initial, apparently negative one. Thus, an important component of skin test monitoring for TB exposure is initial two-step testing to account for the booster effect. If at the time of initial screening the tuberculin skin test is negative, it should be repeated within 2 weeks. If the test is positive at that time, the *initial* skin test result should be recorded as positive. The importance of checking for boosted responses is obvious if one considers that a second test, performed 6 months after the first test as a part of routine employee screening, will be falsely interpreted as representing a new infection rather than prior immunity.

10. What safeguards can be used to reduce occupational transmission of TB?

In recent years the concept of reducing the risk of occupational TB in institutions has evolved into a three-pronged strategy of administrative, environmental, and personal protection. The most important element is administrative control, which must maintain a high index of suspicion for TB in patients (particularly those with HIV infection) admitted with respiratory symptoms and an abnormal chest radiograph. Such patients should be rapidly isolated and their sputum examined for AFB; patients with AFB-positive sputum are the most infectious. A hospital laboratory capable of rapid turnaround (< 24 hours) for AFB examinations is thus an important part of good infection control.

The second prong of reducing occupational and environmental risk of TB exposure is use of environmental or engineering controls. Examples include negative-pressure isolation rooms with greater than 12 air exchanges per hour to remove potentially infected air from the environment, use of high-efficiency particulate air (HEPA) filters to eliminate small particles from the air, and ultraviolet germicidal irradiation to kill infectious particles.

The final component of occupational protection is personal and includes the use of particulate respirator masks. Standard surgical masks are designed to protect patients from becoming infected by surgeons and provide no protection to the wearer from inhalation of airborne tubercle bacilli. Specially designed masks, termed N95 particulate respirators (95% filter efficiency in a non-oilmist environment), are capable of filtering small particles and theoretically provide protection against environmental TB transmission. However, such masks must be individually fitted and are often uncomfortable. Higher levels of respiratory protection are needed, such as powered air-purifying respirators, for cough-inducing procedures, such as bronchoscopy.

11. Should health care workers and others at risk for occupational tuberculosis receive BCG vaccine?

A truly effective vaccine against tuberculosis would be one of the greatest achievements of medical science. The currently available BCG vaccine, which is a live vaccine using an attenuated strain of *Mycobacterium bovis* to provide immunity, has been estimated to be roughly 40–80% protective in preventing cases of TB. Although it is the most widely used vaccine in the world, it has not been used in the United States as a routine preventive health measure, because TB is not considered a sufficient threat to public health to warrant vaccination of the entire population. Control efforts in the U.S. have focused on identifying and treating all cases of active TB and then identifying and treating people with latent infection. The second goal can be accomplished quite well with isoniazid preventive therapy; if there is a high likelihood of infection with an isoniazid-resistant strain of *M. tuberculosis*, rifampin may be substituted—provided that the patient does not have rifampin-resistant TB.

The best protection against occupational TB infection is the series of administrative, environmental, and personal measures detailed above. However, if these measures are not successful **and** the possibility of occupational exposure to strains of *M. tuberculosis* resistant to isoniazid and rifampin is substantial, vaccination of health care workers with BCG may be an appropriate strategy. The Centers for Disease Control and Prevention and the Occupational Safety and Health Administration recommend vaccination only as a last line of defense. For years after BCG is given, the PPD test may be mildly positive, but it usually reverts to negative (< 10-mm induration) over time. Thus, adults with a remote history of BCG inoculation—for example, in childhood—should be followed with serial PPDs and treated for new infection if a conversion from < 10-mm induration to > 10-mm induration occurs.

12. What is the appropriate evaluation for a person with suspected exposure to TB?

Persons exposed to a case of active TB should have a tuberculin skin test, using 5 TU of PPD. The test should be interpreted in 48–72 hours after placement. Some studies of specific occupational groups, such as firefighters who have been adequately trained and motivated, have shown that self-reading of negative PPD results may be reliable. In general, however, the best practice is to require all PPD tests to be read by experienced personnel. If the skin test is negative, no further investigation need be taken, and preventive therapy is not indicated unless a condition causing potential immune deficiency is suspected. If the skin test is positive and represents a new conversion, careful symptom screening should be done and a chest radiograph should be obtained. If the radiograph is normal and the health care worker is asymptomatic, TB infection is present and the health care worker should receive preventive isoniazid therapy. If there is a strong likelihood of exposure to isoniazid-resistant TB, rifampin should be substituted. In cases of exposure to MDR-TB, preventive therapy should be instituted under the guidance of an expert in its management. If the radiograph is abnormal and suggestive of active TB, sputum should be collected for microscopy and culture, and multiagent chemotherapy for active disease should be started until culture results are available.

13. How can molecular biology be used to investigate environmental spread of TB?

Restriction fragment-length polymorphism (RFLP) analysis has become a powerful tool to investigate the relatedness among strains of *M. tuberculosis* isolated from different patients. RFLP can create a "DNA fingerprint" of individual *M. tuberculosis* strains by comparing the frequency and location in the genome of a segment of DNA called IS6110, a unique nucleotide sequence found only among the *M. tuberculosis* complex of organisms. When IS6110-based DNA fingerprints are obtained from isolates from different patients, one expects that if the two (or more) patients have no epidemiologic link, the DNA fingerprints will be different. If, on the other hand, DNA fingerprints from *M. tuberculosis* isolates from several different patients are identical, a chain of transmission is strongly implied. Thus, the use of RFLP analysis to investigate outbreaks of TB helps to identify a significant environmental risk of TB and may lead to corrective action to reduce such risk. RFLP has been used to identify numerous hospital-based outbreaks of TB. It also identified a number of TB cases spread by a single patron of a bar in Minneapolis.

14. How should patients with TB be transported through the hospital to reduce the risk of spreading infection to other patients or health care workers?

The best way to reduce the risk of spreading TB during transport of patients through the hospital, of course, is to order only tests that are absolutely necessary. However, when a test is truly necessary, certain precautions may help to reduce the spread of TB. The patient should wear a surgical mask during transport, and the transporters should wear N95 or better particulate respirators. Whenever possible, tests in patients with TB should be done at a time when few other patients are likely to be in the same area. For example, an ultrasound examination should be scheduled as the last test of the day to minimize exposure to other patients both during and after the test. The same strategy should be used for tuberculosis patients going to the operating room for resectional surgery for MDR-TB.

15. Is fresh air good for patients with TB?

In the preantibiotic era, it was believed that fresh air (particularly cold, fresh air) was an important part of treatment for TB. A number of TB sanitoria were established in elegant resort settings so that patients could "take the cure." Such sanitoria were immortalized in many literary works, including *The Magic Mountain*, by the Nobel-prize winner Thomas Mann. Poorer patients often slept on rooftops in cold weather to achieve the desired effect. However, with the advent of antibiotics, it became apparent that no amount of "fresh air" can cure TB in the absence of effective chemotherapy. A vacation in the mountains may have a salutary effect on the psyche, but it cannot be recommended as a medical prescription.

16. How should a contact investigation for TB be carried out?

When a case of TB is diagnosed, close contacts of the source case should be examined, and those with evidence of TB infection should be offered preventive therapy with isoniazid (or other appropriate therapy). Consult the local TB controller and the current Centers for Disease Control and Prevention guidelines for prevention of the spread of TB before embarking on a case contact investigation. Determining who should be included in the contact investigation is often the difficult part of the process, because contact investigations consume significant resources and time. In general, contact tracing follows the concentric circle model, based on the assumption that people most closely sharing the environment of the source case are most likely to be infected. If the closest contacts are free of infection, more casual contacts are unlikely to be infected and therefore need not be investigated. The contact investigation can stop. If people in the first circle of contacts demonstrate infection, the next ring of investigation generally focuses on people with somewhat less, but regular contact, such as coworkers. The investigation expands until a circle of contacts is reached that shows no infection. The contact tracing can stop at that point.

CONTROVERSY

17. Are health care workers or other persons with positive tuberculin skin tests immune to reinfection with TB?

The link between a positive tuberculin skin test, representing a delayed-type hypersensitivity type of immune reaction, and true cell-mediated immunity is complex. Certainly, after receiving BCG vaccine, many persons manifest a positive tuberculin skin test, and many seem to be protected against developing TB in the future. An analogous situation may occur in patients who are diagnosed with latent TB infection by a PPD skin test and take a course of isoniazid preventive therapy, thereby killing the small number of dormant *M. tuberculosis* bacilli in the body. After such a course of therapy, the tuberculin skin test invariably remains positive, implying that the body retains T-cell memory for TB antigens that may represent immunity against reinfection.

William Stead of the Arkansas Department of Health found that despite heavy exposure to environmental TB, active TB developed in only 2.4% of persons with previously positive tuberculin skin test compared with 19% of new converters with similar exposure. The 19% developed TB within 3 months of exposure before isoniazid preventive therapy could be given. Stead interpreted these data to indicate that "a previous infection with *M. tuberculosis*, as shown by a skin test result of greater than 10 mm induration, affords excellent protection of a healthy person against reinfection and that preventive therapy is not indicated." He concludes that workers in urban medical centers or other high-risk environments fare better with cellular immunity resulting from "previous natural infection."

Opposing this view is the observation that many persons who are skin-test converters in fact develop active TB; the correlation between delayed-type hypersensitivity reaction and true cellular immunity is less than perfect. Furthermore, as Stead is careful to point out, persons with impaired immune systems are certainly susceptible to reinfection. This fact has been convincingly demonstrated in studies using RFLP analysis to demonstrate recovery of different strains of *M. tuberculosis* from the same AIDS patient at different times.

Although the data presented by Stead are provocative, health care workers and others in high-risk environments with previously positive skin tests should not be cavalier about future TB exposure.

BIBLIOGRAPHY

1. Blumberg HM, Watkins DL, Berschling JD, et al: Preventing the nosocomial transmission of tuberculosis. Ann Intern Med 122:58–63, 1995.
2. Bowden KM, McDiarmid MA: Occupationally acquired tuberculosis: What's known. J Occup Med 36:320–325, 1994.
3. Centers for Disease Control and Prevention: Guidelines for preventing the transmission of *Mycobacterium tuberculosis* in health-care facilities, 1994. MMWR 43:1–132, 1994.
4. Centers for Disease Control and Prevention: Proportionate mortality from pulmonary tuberculosis associated with occupations—28 states, 1979–1990. MMWR 44:14–9, 1995.
5. Centers for Disease Control and Prevention: The role of BCG vaccine in the prevention and control of tuberculosis in the United States. A joint statement by the Advisory Council for the Elimination of Tuberculosis and the Advisory Committee on Immunization Practices. MMWR 45:1–18, 1996.
6. Jarvis WR, Boylard EA, Bozzi CJ, et al: Respirators, recommendations, and regulations: The controversy surrounding protection of health care workers from tuberculosis. Ann Intern Med 122:142–146, 1995.
7. Maloney SA, Pearson ML, Gordon MT, et al: Efficacy of control measures in preventing nosocomial transmission of multidrug-resistant tuberculosis to patients and health care workers. Ann Intern Med 122:90–95, 1995.
8. McGowan JE: Nosocomial tuberculosis: New progress in control and prevention. Clin Infect Dis 21:489–505, 1995.
9. Nettleman MD, Fredrickson M, Good NL, Hunter SA: Tuberculosis control strategies: The cost of particulate respirators. Ann Intern Med 121:37–40, 1994.
10. Pearson ML, Jereb JA, Frieden TR, et al: Nosocomial transmission of multidrug-resistant *Mycobacterium tuberculosis:* A risk to patients and health care workers. Ann Intern Med 117:191–196, 1992.
11. Sepkowitz KA: Tuberculosis and the health care worker: A historical perspective. Ann Intern Med 120:71–79, 1994.
12. Stead WW: Management of health care workers after inadvertent exposure to tuberculosis: A guide for the use of preventive therapy. Ann Intern Med 122:906–912, 1995.
13. Templeton GL, Illing LA, Young L, et al: The risk for transmission of *Mycobacterium tuberculosis* at the bedside and during autopsy. Ann Intern Med 122:922–925, 1995.

20. OCCUPATIONAL LYME DISEASE

Brian S. Schwartz, M.D., M.S.

1. What is Lyme disease?

Lyme disease is the most common vector-borne disease in the United States. It is caused by the spirochetal bacterium *Borrelia burgdorferi*, and it is transmitted to humans by the bites of certain kinds of ticks. The infection can involve multiple organ systems and has myriad manifestations.

2. How do people get Lyme disease?

Lyme disease is transmitted to people by ticks of the *Ixodes ricinus* complex: *I. scapularis* in the eastern United States, *I. pacificus* in the western United States, *I. ricinus* in Europe, and *I. persulcatus* in Asia. There is some controversy about the tick species in the northeastern United States. In the 1980s, some investigators asserted that the vector of Lyme disease in the Northeast was a new tick species, which they called *I. dammini*. Recent data suggest that the tick is probably the same species that has been known in the southeastern United States for around a hundred years, *I. scapularis*. Most scientists accept that the two species are the same, although a minority maintains that they are, in fact, different.

B. burgdorferi has been identified in other ticks, including *Dermacentor variabilis* and *Amblyomma americanum*, but little convincing epidemiologic evidence suggests that they are important vectors of Lyme disease. Ticks generally also have common names, which are used most often by patients. There have also been case reports of Lyme disease after bites of certain kinds of flies.

Tick Species and Common Names

TICK SPECIES	COMMON NAME	COMMENT
Amblyomma americanum	Lone star tick	Probably uncommon vector
Dermacentor variabilis	Dog tick	Probably uncommon vector
Ixodes scapularis	Black-legged tick	Vector species
Ixodes pacificus	Western black-legged tick	Vector species
Ixodes dammini	Northern deer tick	Common name applied to ticks in the northeastern United States, but many scientists do not believe that this species is distinct from *I. scapularis*

Ticks seek blood meals from a variety of mammal, reptile, and bird species. The animal that provides the blood meal is termed the **host**. An animal in which *B. burgdorferi* can live and from which a feeding tick can acquire the bacteria for subsequent transmission to the next host is termed a **reservoir** of infection. Data suggest that *I. scapularis* must feed for 24–48 hours before *B. burgdorferi* is transmitted to the host. This important point in the prevention of Lyme disease is discussed below.

I. scapularis has a two-year life cycle in three stages. Larvae, the first stage, appear in the late summer and fall. The larva feeds once, then molts to the next stage (nymph), which appears in the spring of the second year of the two-year life cycle. The nymph feeds once, then molts to the adult form, which appears in the fall of the second year. Male and female adults then mate. The female overwinters, then lays eggs that produce larvae within a few months. Subadult forms (larvae, nymphs) feed on a wide variety of small mammals, birds, and reptiles but prefer to feed on white-footed mice *(Peromyscus leukopus)*, which are the important reservoir of infection. Adults prefer to feed and mate on white-tailed deer *(Odocoileus virginianus)*.

3. What are the high-risk areas for Lyme disease in the United States?

Over 95% of cases of Lyme disease come from from three distinct geographic regions of the U.S.: the Northeast from Maryland to Maine, parts of the upper Midwest in Wisconsin and Minnesota, and parts of northern California and southern Oregon. Several important points must be emphasized. First, adequate tick habitats are highly localized. Even within endemic areas, vector ticks are not homogeneously dispersed throughout the area. Second, cases of Lyme disease have been reported from almost every state in the U.S., including some states where vector ticks, infected reservoirs, or infected human tissues have not been identified. This fact illustrates difficulties in diagnosis of the disease. The vast majority of cases have been reported from a handful of states—New York, Connecticut, New Jersey, and Pennsylvania—and from several specific counties within each state.

Approximately 8,000–16,000 cases of Lyme disease have been reported in the U.S. annually from 1990–1997. In 1997 approximately 23% of cases were reported from New York, 19% from Connecticut, 18% and 14% from Pennsylvania and New Jersey respectively, and 14% each from Wisconsin, Rhode Island, Massachusetts, and Maryland. In 1994 the national incidence rate was 5.2 per 100,000, and incidence rates were highest in Connecticut (62.2 per 100,000), followed by Rhode Island (47.2), New York (29.2), New Jersey (19.6), Delaware (15.5), Pennsylvania (11.9), Wisconsin (8.4), and Maryland (8.3). Some authors estimate that the actual incidence may be 10-fold higher.

4. Are workers at increased risk of Lyme disease? If so, which workers?

Several epidemiologic studies—some based in the general population, some confined to groups of workers—have documented that outdoor workers have an increased risk of Lyme disease. Seroprevalences of Lyme disease antibody, as measured by enzyme-linked immunosorbent assay (ELISA) or indirect fluorescent antibody, have ranged from 5.6–35% in populations with varying degrees of risk in several areas of the U.S. and Europe. In these cross-sectional studies, outdoor workers have been reported to have a 4–6-fold increase in risk of clinical Lyme disease or seropositivity for antibodies to *B. burgdorferi*. Seroprevalence in populations of normal, healthy volunteers from low-to-moderate risk areas have been as high as 5–10%.

Annual or seasonal risk of seroconversion in several longitudinal studies of *B. burgdorferi* infection have ranged from 0.4–10% in populations at high risk by virtue of area of residence or outdoor employment. Seroconversion was associated with an asymptomatic infection in 26–98% of cases. The average annual risk of clinical Lyme disease in several high-risk populations has ranged from 0–3.3%.

5. What is the clinical presentation of early Lyme disease?

The classic presentation of early Lyme disease is the appearance of a characteristic rash, termed erythema migrans (previously named erythema chronicum migrans). The rash begins as a small red papule at the site of a tick bite, generally 3–30 days after a tick bite of sufficient duration to transmit the bacteria. Most patients (66-86%), however, do not recall a tick bite at the site. Over several days to weeks, the papule grows in size, with red expanding borders and often a clearing center. Several concentric rings of redness may appear, resembling a target. The rash may grow to over 20 cm in diameter, and its specificity for the diagnosis of Lyme disease probably improves with increasing diameter (a minimal diameter of 5 cm is suggested by the Centers for Disease Control and Prevention for diagnosis). *B. burgdorferi* can be detected (by culture or polymerase chain reaction) at the leading edge of the rash.

Although most patients (60–80%) develop a rash, the classic target shape is not the most common appearance. Central clearing occurs in less than 40% of cases, and solid red rashes are probably most common. Vesicular eruptions have been uncommonly reported; scaling lesions are not likely to be Lyme disease. Multiple lesions occur in approximately 20% of cases. Up to 80% of patients have associated symptoms, including fatigue (54%), myalgia (44%), arthralgia (44%), headaches (42%), fever and/or chills (39%), and stiff neck (35%). Specific respiratory or gastrointestinal complaints (other than anorexia) are rare, and the presence of such symptoms argues against a diagnosis of Lyme disease.

6. Are all target-shaped rashes due to Lyme disease?

It was previously thought that all target-shaped rashes (i.e., circular with red border and clearing center) were erythema migrans and that the appearance of this rash was pathognomonic for Lyme disease. Increasing clinical suspicion, however, indicates that many rashes reported by patients as resembling erythema migrans are not Lyme disease. Furthermore, most Lyme disease skin rashes are not target-shaped. It appears increasingly likely that immune responses to tick salivary gland antigens and reactions to spider bites can result in rashes that may be mistaken for erythema migrans by the patient or the physician.

7. What are the later manifestations of Lyme disease?

Within weeks to months of becoming infected, **early disseminated Lyme disease** may develop (formerly termed stage 2). Approximately 4–10% of patients in the U.S. develop cardiac manifestations, including conduction defects (e.g., atrioventricular block, complete heart block, bundle-branch block, fascicular block), tachyarrhythmias (e.g., atrial tachyarrhythmia due to pericarditis or, uncommonly, ventricular tachyarrhythmia as an escape rhythm), myopericarditis, and mild myocardial dysfunction. The central or peripheral nervous system may be involved in 10–20% of cases, as manifested by headache, fatigue, stiff neck, and malaise. Possible diagnoses include Lyme meningitis, neuroborreliosis, cranial neuropathies (especially facial nerve palsy, which may be bilateral), peripheral neuropathy, radiculitis, myelopathy, or brachial plexopathy. Lyme disease also may involve the eye (e.g., follicular conjunctivitis, keratitis, and, rarely, uveitis or vitritis). Musculoskleletal manifestations of Lyme disease are quite common. During early infection, most patients report migratory arthralgias and pain in bursae, tendon, muscle, or bone. Weeks to months later, frank arthritis may develop—most commonly mono- or oligoarticular arthritis involving large joints (usually knees, but also shoulders, ankles, elbows, and other sites). Lyme arthritis is one manifestation of **persistent** or **late Lyme disease** (previously termed stage 3).

8. How is Lyme disease diagnosed?

The diagnosis of Lyme disease is clinical, and the diagnostician must consider many types of evidence. The history is important to the diagnosis of the disease (e.g, opportunity for tick exposure, residence or employment in endemic area, recent tick bites). The temporality and pattern of the development of symptoms are critical to the diagnosis. Many patients have access to scientific and lay publications about Lyme disease and use a "checklist" to self-diagnosis by circling the several symptoms that they have experienced from the list of 50 symptoms attributed by some authors to Lyme disease. The description of the rash is important if it is not present at the time of the examination. A history of expansion over several days, eventually beyond 5 cm in diameter, is a useful clue.

Classic later presentations, such as unilateral facial palsy, heart block, or frank monoarticular arthritis of the knee, should motivate the physician to obtain appropriate diagnostic tests for Lyme disease and to exclude other causes. Diagnosis of Lyme disease is aided by serologic testing, which should include antibody testing by ELISA and, if positive, follow-up with Western blot testing for both immunoglobulin G and M antibodies. By 6–8 weeks of infection, most patients have an appropriate antibody response. The sensitivity of serologic testing is approximately 50% at the erythema migrans stage but increases to over 90% by the later stages of the disease. Serologic testing is thus not very helpful in a patient with classic erythema migrans, who will be treated for Lyme disease regardless of the result. The specificity of serologic testing is approximately 90–95% for all stages of the disease.

A positive ELISA result must be followed by Western blot testing. The usual criterion for positive Western blot for IgM is at least two bands corresponding to proteins of specific molecular weights (two of the following three: 24, 39, or 41 kDa). For Western blot testing for IgG, the usual criterion is five bands corresponding to proteins of specific molecular weights (five of the following ten: 18, 21, 28, 30, 39, 41, 45, 58, 66, or 93 kDa). Most laboratory reports of Western blot results include the molecular weights of the important proteins, both of the criterion proteins and the proteins to which the patient has produced antibodies.

In the patient with numerous nonspecific symptoms that may or may not be compatible with Lyme disease, the clinician must understand that if the pretest probability of Lyme disease is low, a positive serologic test result is more likely to be false than true. Lyme disease serologic testing should be used with caution in patients complaining solely of nonspecific symptoms—for example, chronic fatigue, headaches, or diffuse musculoskeletal pain.

9. How is Lyme disease treated?

Lyme disease is treatable at all stages with either oral or intravenous antibiotics. Treatment decisions are often complex and differ somewhat for children and adults. Because there have been few randomized clinical trials, optimal choice of antibiotic and optimal duration of treatment are not known. In general, early Lyme disease in adults is treated with doxycycline, 100 mg orally twice daily, or amoxicillin, 500 mg orally 3 times/day, for 10–30 days. Doxycycline should not be used in children under age 9 years or pregnant women. Other antibiotic choices include phenoxymethyl penicillin, tetracycline, and cefuroxime axetil; erythromycin and azithromycin are second-line choices. Doxycycline for 30 days has been used to treat certain cardiac, nervous system, and joint manifestations of Lyme disease. Other specific manifestations of Lyme disease, including Lyme meningitis, neuroborrelliosis, arthritis not responsive to doxycycline, and severe cardiac manifestations, are generally treated with intravenous antibiotics, most often ceftriaxone, 2 gm twice daily for 14–30 days.

Symptomatic relief after treatment should be evaluated not on a day-to-day basis but rather over several months. Patients should progress slowly but steadily to their premorbid state. Patients who have lingering symptoms after treatment should not be routinely retreated with antibiotics without clear evidence of antibiotic failure. Nonsteroidal antiinflammatory medications, antidepressants, exercise, and physical therapy have been used for symptomatic relief after an adequate trial of antibiotic therapy.

10. What proportion of all adult cases of Lyme disease are occupational in origin?

This number is not known. Data from the northeastern U.S. suggest that in the most endemic areas most patients probably acquire Lyme disease around the residence or during recreational activities. Far more persons are at increased risk of Lyme disease by virtue of residence or recreational activities than by virtue of work activities. Despite this fact, work can clearly place people at increased risk for the disease.

11. What aspects of work have been shown to be risk factors for Lyme disease?

The obvious risk factor for occupational Lyme disease is exposure to tick-infested habitats during work. At-risk workers are often quite knowledgeable about ticks and know what species are present in their work areas. Habitats that support deer often have been shown to be tick-infested. Habitats with wooded areas abutting grassy areas also may be tick-infested. Work in such areas can increase the risk for tick exposure and Lyme disease. However, work activities also must be considered. For example, workers in toxic waste sites with extensive personal protection from chemical exposures are generally protected from tick bites.

Studies designed to identify risk factors for prevalent or incident *B. burgdorferi* infection in outdoor workers have been inconclusive. Self-reported tick exposure, age, outdoor recreational activities, pet ownership, residential area, and other factors have not been consistently identified as conferring risk. One cross-sectional study of outdoor workers in New Jersey identified occupational tick exposure, hunting, and male sex as risk factors for anti-*B. burgdorferi* antibody seropositivity; antibiotic use and insect repellent use were identified as protective factors.

12. What environmental factors favor increased tick abundance?

Some studies have shown that certain soil types, elevations, watersheds, and ground cover are associated with tick abundance, but these factors are of little clinical relevance. The most important questions to ask patients are whether they are bitten by ticks at work and whether they work in areas where deer are common.

13. How should the clinical evaluation differ for outdoor workers and other patients with suspected Lyme disease?

The clinical evaluation for suspected Lyme disease is the same, regardless of where the disease was acquired. The fact that the patient acquired the disease at work may have legal implications, but it is not likely to have medical implications.

14. What workers with Lyme disease should apply for workers' compensation? How does the clinician decide whether Lyme disease is work-related?

Some states consider infectious diseases to be "ordinary diseases of life" under workers' compensation systems. In other states, however, physicians can offer an opinion, based on the patient's medical and occupational histories, about where the disease was likely to be acquired; in such states workers have received compensation coverage for Lyme disease. The clinician should consider aspects of the patient's work; outdoor activities and tasks; tick bite history; history of other cases of Lyme disease at work; epidemiologic data about Lyme disease risk for the patient's specific job, if available; recreational activities; and area of residence and activities around the home. After careful consideration of these factors, the physician can offer an opinion whether it is "more likely than not" (the legal standard under workers' compensation law) that the disease was acquired at work. The workers' compensation system will consider the physician's opinion and reasoning in determining whether the Lyme disease is eligible for coverage.

15. What medical surveillance activities are recommended for workers at risk for Lyme disease?

Routine serologic testing is not recommended because the predictive value of a positive test (the proportion of all positive tests that are positive in people who have active Lyme disease) is low. Medical surveillance activities that involve a questionnaire to elicit information about the development of new rashes, new central or peripheral nervous system symptoms, new joint pain, or new flulike illness without upper respiratory system symptoms may be reasonable. Positive responses should be followed by appropriate medical evaluation. Worker training and education also can be included at the time of questionnaire administration and are important to the prevention of Lyme disease.

16. How can workers protect themselves from Lyme disease?

Workers should be educated to check themselves carefully at the end of each work day for ticks on their skin. Any ticks should be removed and discarded. Because *I. scapularis* must feed for 24–48 hours to transmit the disease, this strategy will probably prevent most, if not all, Lyme disease. Other behaviors such as use of DEET (an insect repellent) on skin or premethrin (an insecticide derived from flowers approved for this use) on clothing, tucking pants into socks, wearing long sleeves and long pants, and wearing light-colored clothing for easier spotting of ticks, also may be used. In 1998, two published studies documented the safety and effectiveness of the different recombinant protein vaccines (outer-surface protein A) for prevention of Lyme disease. Patients who receive the vaccine will have a positive serologic test by ELISA for Lyme disease.

Several unanswered questions remain: the duration of protection and the need for boosters, alternative dosing schedules, use of the vaccines in children, and the possibility of immunopathogenicity resulting in rare or late adverse reactions all require further attention. As of late 1998, the vaccines had yet to receive FDA approval, but were expected to do so. Vaccination may be appropriate for some workers at risk for the disease.

CONTROVERSIES

17. A worker is worried about Lyme disease because of a recent tick bite. He is asymptomatic. Should he be offered prophylactic treatment with antibiotics?

There are two schools of thought. Many academic researchers in Lyme disease note that the overall average risk of infection with *B. burgdorferi* after a single tick bite is low (probably around 1–3%); that people in endemic areas can have numerous tick bites each season; and that no randomized trials have shown that prophylactic antibiotics definitely prevent Lyme disease when given shortly after a tick bite. Other physicians note that the risk of Lyme disease is higher when the tick fed to engorgement and that certain subgroups (e.g, pregnant women) may suffer severe morbidity (especially to the fetus) if they become infected. The first group strongly advises against prophylactic administration of antibiotics and instead suggests that patients should be educated to look for the development of a rash and treated if a rash appears. The second group argues that because some patients are very worried about the development of Lyme disease and the side effects and cost of doxycycline or amoxicillin are low, prophylactic administration is warranted in selected cases. Strategies advising that all or no such patients should receive prophylactic antibiotics seem unwarranted. An individualized approach that considers likely tick-feeding duration, associated medical problems, degree of patient anxiety, and probable morbidity if Lyme disease develops is preferable; it may be reasonable to offer a small subset of patients prophylactic antibiotics after an *I. scapularis* bite. Needless to say, prophylaxis for Lyme disease should not be given for bites from other ticks or insects.

18. A patient presents with erythema migrans and left-sided facial palsy. A Lyme disease serologic test is positive. The cerebrospinal fluid (CSF) reveals lymphocytic pleocytosis and slightly elevated protein, but CSF Lyme antibody testing is negative. A diagnosis of Lyme disease is made, and the patient receives 3 weeks of intravenous ceftriaxone with good response. One month after completion of antibiotics, the patient returns, complaining of joint pain and fatigue. The physical examination is normal. What should be done next?

Some physicians believe that such patients represent failure of antibiotic treatment and recommend long-duration (months to years) oral or intravenous antibiotic therapy. Some physicians recommend unusual dosing protocols, such as two doses per week followed by weeks without treatment. No data suggest that such long-term or unusual regimens are necessary or better than standard regimens. Other physicians diagnose such patients as having post-Lyme disease fibromyalgia and treat them with antidepressants, physical therapy, and exercise programs. Increasing evidence indicates that such patients do not get better with continued antibiotic therapy and thus may not represent treatment failures. An increasing literature discusses post-Lyme disease symptom persistence, possible explanations for persistent symptoms, and options for therapy. Unfortunately, the literature also suggests that some such patients have received years of antibiotic therapy without clear objective benefit.

BIBLIOGRAPHY

1. Centers for Disease Control and Prevention: Lyme disease—United States, 1994. MMWR 44:459–462, 1995.
2. Gardner P: Lyme disease vaccines. Ann Intern Med 129:583–585, 1998.
3. Magid DJ, Schwartz BS, Craft J, Schwartz JS: Prevention of Lyme disease after tick bite: A cost-effectiveness analysis. N Engl J Med 327:534–542, 1992.
4. Nadelman RB, Wormser GP: Erythema migrans and early Lyme disease. Am J Med 98(Suppl 4A):15S–25S, 1995.
5. Pachner AR: Early disseminated Lyme disease: Lyme meningitis. Am J Med 98(Suppl 4A):30S–43S, 1995.
6. Schwartz BS, Goldstein MD: Lyme disease: A review for the occupational physician. J Occup Med 31:735–742, 1989.
7. Schwartz BS, Goldstein MD: Lyme disease in outdoor workers: Risk factors, preventive measures, and tick removal methods. Am J Epidemiol 131:877–885, 1990.
8. Schwartz BS, Goldstein MD, Childs JE: A longitudinal study of *Borrelia burgdorferi* infection in New Jersey outdoor workers, 1988–1991. Am J Epidemiol 139:504–512, 1994.
9. Sigal LH, Zahradnik JM, Lavin P, et al: A vaccine consisting of recombinant *Borerelia burgdorferi* outer-surface protein A to prevent Lyme disease. N Engl J Med 339:216–222, 1998.
10. Steere AC: Lyme disease. N Engl J Med 321:586–596, 1989.
11. Steere AC: Musculoskeletal manifestations of Lyme disease. Am J Med 98(Suppl 4A):44S–51S, 1995.
12. Steere AC, Sikand VK, Meuria F, et al: Vaccination against Lyme disease with recombinant *Borrelia burgdorferi* outer-surface lipoprotein A with adjuvant. N Engl J Med 339:209–215, 1998.

21. BRUCELLOSIS

Sharmeen S. Gettner, M.S., Ph.D.

1. What is brucellosis? Is it contagious?

Brucellosis is a systemic infection caused by gram-negative coccobacilli of the genus *Brucella*. Brucellosis is an important zoonotic disease but is not contagious in humans. *Brucella* spp. have been cultured from human milk, urine, and sperm, but the disease has not been known to spread to secondary contacts. Of the six recognized species of *Brucella*, the most pathogenic for humans are associated with different animal reservoirs: *B. melitensis* (goats), *B. suis* (swine), *B. abortus* (cattle), and *B. canis* (dogs). *B. melitensis* and *B. suis* are more virulent for humans than *B. abortus* or *B. canis*.

2. How common is human brucellosis? What is its public health importance?

In the United States, fewer than 300 cases of human brucellosis have been reported each year since 1965. Although brucellosis is a reportable disease in all states except Nevada, because of the variability in clinical manifestations and the infrequency with which physicians diagnose cases of brucellosis, only an estimated 50% of the cases are recognized and reported. The public health importance of brucellosis in many countries is significant because of economic losses from abortions in domestic animals and declining milk and meat products. Although human brucellosis is an uncommon diagnosis in Western countries, it remains an important zoonotic disease elsewhere, particularly in Mediterranean countries, north and east Africa, India, Central Asia, Mexico, and Central and South America. The disease in humans causes considerable debility and loss of active work days; it is potentially life threatening. Death due to brucellosis is rare; a case fatality rate of 0.9% has been reported. Endocarditis is the most common cause of death.

3. What is the epidemiology of brucellosis? How has it changed in recent years?

Persons of all ages are susceptible to brucellosis, but most cases are reported in patients between 20 and 60 years old, compatible with the age of the work force. In fact, human brucellosis (especially infection with *B. abortus* or *B. suis*) has long been recognized as an occupation-associated disease. Although most reported cases in the U.S. have occurred among abattoir workers and have been typed as *B. suis*, sporadic outbreaks involving a few cases have been associated with other species (*B. melitensis* and *B. abortus*). In the U.S., the largest number of cases reported to the Centers for Disease Control and Prevention in recent years have occurred in Texas, California, Florida, and North Carolina. The highest seasonal incidence of human brucellosis is in the spring and early summer (March to July). The epidemiology of the disease has undergone some changes over the past 20 years. Increasing evidence suggests that, with the advent of vaccination of cattle and stricter control of infected animals, brucellosis is slowly shifting from an occupational disease to a food-borne disease, especially among travelers to countries where brucellosis is endemic.

4. What industries and occupations are at risk of exposure to *Brucella* spp.?

Human brucellosis is predominantly an occupational disease associated with close contact with infected animals or their tissues or secretions. Occupational sources of infection include blood, urine, vaginal discharges, milk secretions, placenta, and other tissue from infected cattle, swine, sheep, goats, caribou, and dogs. Occupations with increased risk of exposure include slaughterhouse workers, farm workers, veterinarians, livestock producers, laboratory technicians, breeders, dairy workers, wildlife workers, hide and wool handlers, ranchers, pet shop workers, taxidermists, zoo attendants, butchers, and hunters.

The persons at greatest risk of exposure are slaughterhouse workers engaged in killing and processing pigs infected with *B. suis*. Attack rates have been calculated to be higher for hog-kill employees, who have high frequencies of skin cuts, exposure to fresh animal blood and lymph, ingestion of potentially contaminated animal products, and conjunctival contact with animal tissue and infection. Among slaughter and packinghouse workers, the differential risk of exposure to the microorganism appears to be proportional to the amount of time spent in contact with infected animal tissues. The process of beheading, eviscerating, and handling meats and organ products places the worker at highest risk of exposure, whereas activities involving the actual packaging, smoking, or curing pose relatively lower risk.

Brucellosis also may affect workers in other occupational settings, including meat inspectors and butchers. Veterinarians and farm families have an increased risk, especially if they work with aborting animals, remove retained placenta from infected animals, or vaccinate animals with live brucella vaccines.

Among laboratory workers, brucellosis is one of the 10 most frequently reported laboratory-acquired bacterial infections. Infections are known to occur among laboratory technicians who handle *Brucella* isolates through direct contact of mucosal membranes with infected tissues or urine. *Brucella* spp. are biosafety level three (BSL3) organisms; they are highly infectious and can easily be transmitted via aerosols. It is believed that less than 20% of laboratory-acquired infections are related to recognized accidents; most are thought to be associated with inhalation of infective aerosols produced by numerous microbiologic techniques, including subculturing from blood broth to solid media, staining for identification, and dividing samples for multiple assays.

5. What are the known transmission routes of infection?

Common routes of transmission are through the skin via minor cuts and abrasions, by inhalation of aerosols, through splashing of blood or lymph into conjunctival sac, or by accidental inoculation with live *Brucella* vaccines. The mucosa of the gastrointestinal tract is another portal of entry; gastric achlorhydria with antacids or histamine blocking drugs, such as cimetidine, appears to increase susceptibility. Person-to-person transmission of brucellosis is extremely rare, if it occurs at all. Unusual cases have been traced to transfusions of blood or bone marrow cells and through intravenous drug use. Although *Brucella* spp. have been found in mosquitoes and hematophagous ticks feeding on bacteremic animals, transmission to other animals or humans through their bites has not been reported.

6. What is the incubation period?

The incubation period is highly variable and difficult to ascertain, ranging from 1–6 weeks and rarely even several months. Almost one-half of patients with brucellosis experience an insidious onset of symptoms. The wide range of incubation times probably reflects differences in the size of inoculum, the virulence of *Brucella* species, and different routes of infection.

7. How do cases of brucellosis present?

Human brucellosis presents as a spectrum of nonspecific symptoms. In fact, many common illnesses, such as infectious mononucleosis, toxoplasmosis, tuberculosis, hepatitis, systemic lupus erythematosus, lymphoma, tularemia, malaria, influenza, and typhoid fever, may mimic the most frequent presentation (i.e., fever without localizing symptoms or physical findings). Furthermore, because the disease is relatively rare, recognition and diagnosis are often challenging.

The fever pattern in brucellosis is intermittent and, if monitored over time without the use of antibiotics or antipyretics, can be shown to be undulant. Brucellosis is a systemic infection and may result in gastric, intestinal, neurologic, hepatic, or musculoskeletal involvement. Clinical manifestations include lymphadenopathy, splenomegaly, and/or hepatomegaly. Occasionally, the infection may become localized and produce orchitis, meningitis, pneumonitis, endocarditis, osteomyelitis, or prepatellar bursitis. In localized brucellosis, the organisms are usually not present in the blood but are found in specific tissues such as the bones, joints, liver, kidney, spleen, or skin. Localization may be the principal manifestation (or complication) of systemic (bacteremic) infection.

Brucellosis during human pregnancy is not common, but it is of special interest because abortions are common in animals infected with *Brucella* spp. *Brucella* spp. tend to localize to the placenta in pregnant ungulates because of the presence of erythritol, which is a growth factor for *Brucella* spp. However, erythritol is not found in significant concentrations in humans, and it is thought that abortions do not occur any more frequently in brucellosis than in other bacteremias. The degree of virulence varies among the species; *B. melitensis* is the most invasive and produces the most severe illness and toxic effects; *B. suis* and *B. canis* are also quite invasive; and *B. abortus* is the least invasive.

8. When is the infection considered chronic?

Chronic brucellosis is often used to define a history of symptoms extending over 1 year after a positive serology or culture for *Brucella* spp. However, the diagnosis of chronic brucellosis per se is difficult and somewhat controversial. Because the onset of symptoms of brucellosis can be insidious, it is often difficult to distinguish acute from chronic forms of the disease. Furthermore, the clinical and laboratory findings in relapsed patients appear to be milder than during the initial disease, which makes the diagnosis sometimes difficult. Historically, a subset of patients with "chronic brucellosis" lacks objective signs of infection and is believed to suffer from psychoneurosis, which presents a challenge for disease management. Common reasons for the relapse of illness include localization of infection and inadequate treatment of initial infection.

9. Discuss the pathogenesis and pathology of brucellosis.

After invading the body, *Brucella* spp. are phagocytized by polymorphonuclear leukocytes and macrophages early in the course of infection (within 3–4 days). *Brucella* spp. are able to survive inside phagocytes, where they are protected against antibody and many antibiotics. Organisms are thought to spread via lymphatics to regional lymph nodes and, if not contained, to the blood stream.

Differences in host response to various *Brucella* spp. are suggested by experimental animal studies. *B. abortus* induces hepatic granulomas, associated with limitation of the spread of infection (persisting for more than 30 days), whereas *B. melitensis* and *B. suis* produce tissue abscesses (which normally resolve before 30 days). The liver is almost always involved in brucellosis. Hepatic involvement in brucellosis may include granulomas (infection with *B. abortus*), diffuse hepatitis with hepatic necrosis and absence of granulomas (infection with *B. melitensis*), or occasional clusters of mononucleated cells with histiocytes that form loose granulomas (infection with *B. suis*). Hepatic lesions resolve with antibiotic therapy, and, in absence of other toxins, cirrhosis does not occur. The histologic appearance of *Brucella* spp. in hepatic granuloma tends to be indistinguishable from sarcoidosis. The analysis of synovial fluid from peripheral joint effusions usually shows a predominance of mononuclear cells.

10. What diagnostic tests may be used to evaluate *Brucella* infection?

The diagnosis of brucellosis is based on history of exposure, compatible signs and symptoms, high antibody titer, and/or positive culture of the clinical specimen. Although anemia, leukopenia, and thrombocytopenia are common, routine laboratory tests such as erythrocyte sedimentation rate (ESR) and white blood cell count (WBC) are of little diagnostic value. Microbiologic isolation and identification are the most reliable methods of diagnosing brucellosis. These procedures, however, are not always successful and therefore should be done in conjunction with serologic testing.

Various serologic techniques can be used for diagnosis; among the most commonly performed is the standard tube agglutination test (STA), which is usually done in combination with the 2-mercaptoethanol test (2-ME) or complement fixation test. However, STA methods tend to have imperfect sensitivity and specificity (especially in cases of localization of infection or in the presence of cross-reacting antibodies), as discussed below, and warrant concurrent microbiologic isolation and identification. A serologic diagnosis of brucellosis is made by a fourfold rise in convalescent titer or by a single titer of 160 or greater and the presence of IgG antibodies with the STA method. Usually antibodies to *Brucella* spp. appear in the serum 1–2 weeks after infection. IgM antibody titers rise early in brucellosis, peak at 3 months, and then fall; they can be measured using both the STA and 2-ME methods. IgG antibodies peak at about 8 weeks after infection and remain high as long as the infection is active. A decline of IgG antibodies over time is prognostic of a good response to antibiotic therapy, whereas a persistently high IgG or a second rise in IgG indicates bacteriologic relapse. IgG antibody is considered a marker for active infection, and residual low titers of IgM are indicative of previous exposure to brucella.

The brucellosis skin test, a measure of past infection, is not advisable because it may cause a rise in antibody titers, confusing the interpretation of serology. Finally, the source and epidemiologic circumstances involved in the acquisition of infection should be defined by careful investigation of each case, because additional infections or secondary cases may be detected or prevented.

11. Discuss the challenges of making a positive diagnosis of brucellosis.

There are multiple challenges at every stage of diagnosis. In the clinical setting, some of the complications of brucellosis (prostatitis, cystitis, pyelonephritis) can easily be mistaken for tuberculosis.

With less than perfect sensitivity and specificity, serologic tests sometimes give false-positive or false-negative results. In the presence of cross-reacting bacterial antibodies, one may observe low titers of *Brucella* antibodies in persons infected with or immunized with *Francisella tularensis, Yersinia enterocolitica, Salmonella,* or *Vibrio cholerae.* Likewise, the presence of blocking antibodies or prozones (specifically IgA antibodies) may result in a false-negative tube agglutination test. Furthermore, very early treatment with antimicrobial drugs may suppress the production of antibodies. In some cases of localized brucellosis, agglutinating antibodies may not be detected in the serum, and diagnosis depends on culture of organisms from the involved organ.

Blood cultures are positive in up to 70% of acute cases, but *Brucella* bacteria are slow-growing in vitro; cultures must be incubated for at least 4 weeks before they can be declared negative. Because of the long delay in culture growth, a clinician may choose to start treatment or prophylactic therapy before culture results are available. The administration of antibiotics early in the course of the disease, before diagnostic studies have been obtained, may contribute to poor sensitivity of laboratory diagnostic tests (suppressed antibody response, especially with convalescent titers, and negative culture growth).

12. What treatments are usually recommended?

The treatment of brucellosis requires a combination of two antimicrobial agents: doxycycline (200 mg/day orally for 6 weeks) and streptomycin (1 gm/day intramuscularly for 3 weeks). This regimen is preferred because it is associated with a high cure rate and a low rate of relapse. However, because of the adverse side effects and the inconvenience of administration of streptomycin, clinicians often prefer the combination of doxycycline (200 mg/day orally for 6 weeks) and rifampin (600–900 mg/day orally for 6 weeks). Cotrimoxazole is effective but relapses are common. In severely ill patients, steroids may be administered to decrease systemic toxicity.

Tetracycline therapy should be avoided in pregnant women. Trimethoprim-sulfamethoxazole should be considered for women between 13 and 36 weeks of pregnancy (before 13 weeks teratogenic effects are possible, and after 36 weeks kernicterus is a concern). Rifampin is not contraindicated in pregnancy. Most patients respond to antibiotic treatment, although relapse rates of 12–17% have been reported. Relapsing illness is not due to development of resistant organisms and should be treated with the original regimen.

13. What occupational preventive measures help to reduce the risk of brucellosis?

Several useful preventive measures can be undertaken in occupational settings where the risk of exposure is determined to be high. Some are commonsense measures applicable to all settings, whereas others are occupation-specific. Examples include employee education, use of appropriate personal protective equipment (PPE), proper personal hygiene, familiarity with facility operations, and participation in ongoing medical surveillance. In addition, regulations of the Occupational Safety and Health Administration (OSHA) require employers to provide frequent safety programs addressing these issues.

The employee's understanding of the nature of the disease, risks involved in handling infected materials, and method of transmission is perhaps the most important step in promoting preventive measures. In practice, the risk of brucellosis can be reduced in workers at risk of exposure through the availability and use of effective PPE (including gowns or lab coats, disposable gloves, face shields or goggles, or splatter shields, masks, and respirators). Personal hygiene and protective precautions should be observed in handling potentially infected animal or human tissue or secretions, particularly those resulting from abortions. Furthermore, the workplace should enforce prohibitions against eating, smoking, and cosmetic application in areas where contaminated materials are handled and provide appropriate waste management practices (e.g., routine disinfection of all contaminated areas with chloramine, use of closed top waste bins, and proper labeling of infectious waste material). Waste management is especially important for workers at risk of inadvertent exposure (e.g., janitors).

Medical surveillance to monitor health of employees is a further preventive measure that all workplaces should practice. Ideally, all workers should have preemployment medical examinations to identify prior exposure to infectious agents and underlying conditions that require special employment placement. It is highly recommended that the facility collect and store a baseline serum sample from all at-risk employees. Banked sera are especially helpful for diagnosis in the event of infection.

The laboratory setting presents a unique situation because infections occur even among workers who are most knowledgeable of the microorganism. Unfortunately, "unknown" specimens often are sent to the laboratory for identification, and the most stringent precautions are not followed. In such cases, it is highly recommended that specimens be labeled as "suspected brucellosis"; in the event of a truly unknown specimen, absolute precautions should be taken by the laboratory technician. Because *Brucella* species are BSL3 organisms (potential transmission by aerosols), all work on *Brucella* or possible *Brucella* organisms should take place in biosafety cabinets operating under negative pressure (or taking air away from the worker). In addition, high-efficiency particulate air (HEPA) filters should be used and their efficiency monitored on a weekly basis. In general, laboratories that handle and manipulate infectious agents should be equipped with a ventilation system that operates under a negative pressure system with respect to outside corridors (i.e., air flows from corridors into the lab) and should have approximately 10–15 air changes per hour.

14. What are the OSHA standards for brucellosis?

In 1993 OSHA issued "Occupational Exposure to Blood-borne Pathogens: Final Rule," which requires health care institutions to protect employees from all occupational exposure to blood-borne pathogens. This standard is designed to protect all vulnerable personnel, from clinical engineers who service contaminated equipment to staff in clinical laboratories, patient care of treatment areas, and housekeeping and laundry services—any location where the nature of the work poses the risk of exposure to blood-borne pathogens. Compliance is mandatory, and failure to comply results in fines and other penalties.

15. What controversies surround human vaccinations and use of prophylaxis?

In several countries where brucellosis is endemic (including China, Greece, and Russia), live attenuated *Brucella* vaccines have been developed for use among high-risk personnel. Attenuated strains of *B. abortus* (strain 19) and *B. melitensis* (Rev-1) have been used or considered for immunization of humans; however, because these strains are also pathogenic, they have *caused* illness. Inoculation produces a rise in serum titer above the baseline value and is often accompanied by the onset of systemic symptoms, which mimic the manifestations of acute brucellosis. In people with prior exposure to *Brucella* spp., the symptoms generally resolve spontaneously in a matter of days, with or without treatment. This reaction is believed to be a hypersensitivity reaction to *Brucella* antigens. In people with no prior exposure, however, inoculation with the attenuated vaccine produces an active infection, sometimes accompanied with milder clinical manifestations than exposure to more virulent strains. Some patients may require hospitalization.

In France, a phenol-insoluble fraction obtained from *Brucella* spp. has been used to vaccinate high-risk personnel, but the efficacy of the vaccine has not been well established. In the U.S., both killed and attenuated live vaccines have been tried. Killed or antigenic *Brucella* fractions have not proved effective, whereas live attenuated vaccines have produced systemic reactions and bacteremia and have not been approved for human use.

Another controversial issue is the use of antibiotic prophylaxis. Although tetracycline prophylaxis is sometimes prescribed for cases of accidental exposure to *Brucella* spp., its benefit has not been demonstrated.

16. Discuss recent advances in *Brucella* research.

Recent advances in research have included the development of more sensitive and specific methods of detection. A single step polymerase chain reaction test for the detection of *Brucella* spp. in body fluids of infected livestock and humans has recently been developed. This method appears to be reliable and highly sensitive and specific; however, its high cost may prohibit widespread use. Various enzyme-antibody immunoassays (ELISAs) for detecting low concentrations of antibodies against *Brucella* spp. in bovine milk and serum as well as human serum are also under development. Although ELISA tests promise to be more sensitive, specific, and economic than the widely used STA, more work needs to be done to determine their validity and reliability.

17. What problems remain unresolved?

The largest unsolved problem in the U.S. involves the development of porcine vaccine. Although *B. abortus* strain 19 and *B. melitensis* strain Rev-1 vaccines are currently used for the control of infection in cattle, sheep, and goats, no safe effective vaccine has been approved for swine. In China, the recently developed *B. suis* strain 2 oral vaccine has been shown to be effective.

BIBLIOGRAPHY

 1. Ariza J, Guidiol F, Pallares R, Viladrich PF, et al: Treatment of human brucellosis with doxycycline plus rifampin or doxycycline plus streptomycin. Ann Intern Med 117:25–30, 1992.
 2. Benenson AS (ed): Control of Communicable Diseases Manual 1995, 16th ed. Washington, D.C., American Public Health Association, 1995.
 3. Chomel BB, DeBess EE, Mangiamele DM, Reilly KF, et al: Changing trends in the epidemiology of human brucellosis in California from 1973 to 1992: A shift toward foodborne transmission. J Infect Dis 170:1216–1223, 1994.
 4. Evans AS, Brachman PS (eds): Bacterial Infections of Humans: Epidemiology and Control, 3rd ed. New York, Plenum, 1998.
 5. Frank J (ed): Networking in Brucellosis Research. Report of the United Nations University. New York, United Nations Press, 1991.
 6. Human exposure to *Brucella abortus* strain rB51—Kansas, 1997. MMWR 47:172–175, 1998.
 7. LaDou J (ed): Occupational and Environmental Medicine, 2nd ed. Norwalk, CT, Appleton & Lange, 1997.
 8. Miller MA, Paige JC: Other food borne infections. Vet Clin North Am Food Anim Pract 14:71–89, 1998.
 9. Pike RN: Laboratory associated infections: Incidence, fatalities, causes and prevention. Annu Rev Microbiol 33:41–66, 1979.
 9. Remington J, Swartz M (eds): Current Clinical Topics in Infectious Diseases. Oxford, Blackwell Scientific Publications, 1993.
10. Remington JS, Swartz MN (eds): Current Clinical Topics in Infectious Diseases, 18th ed. Malden, MA, Blackwell Science, 1998.
11. Rosenstock L, Cullen MR (eds): Textbook of Clinical Occupational and Environmental Medicine. Philadelphia, W.B. Saunders, 1994.
12. Solera J, Rodriguez-Zapata M, Geijo P, et al: Doxycycline-rifampin versus doxycycline-streptomycin in treatment of human brucellosis due to *Brucella melitensis*. Antimicrob Agents Chemother 39:2061–2067, 1995.
13. U.S. Department of Labor, Occupational Safety and Health Administration: Occupational Exposure to Bloodborne Pathogens. OSHA Reprint 3127, 1993.
14. Woods G, Gutierrez Y (eds): Diagnostic Pathology of Infectious Diseases. Philadelphia, Lea & Febiger, 1993.
15. Young E, Corbel M (eds): Brucellosis: Clinical and Laboratory Aspects. Boca Raton, FL, CRC Press, 1989.
16. Young EJ: An overview of human brucellosis. Clin Infect Dis 2:283–290, 1995.

22. FUNGAL AND RELATED EXPOSURES

Eckardt Johanning, M.D., M.Sc.

1. How does biologic exposure contribute to occupational and environmental health?

In occupational and environmental medicine health risks are related principally to chemical, physical, or biologic exposure factors. Among the important biologic agents are animal components, bacteria, viruses, insects and parasites, vegetable and plant materials, and naturally produced toxins. The exposure route may be ingestion, but the most relevant routes are skin contact and inhalation. Biologic exposures are found in indoor and outdoor environments and in many occupations or industries. Health risks and adverse health effects depend on the various types or intensities of exposure.

2. What occupations and environmental settings are associated with biologic exposure?
Occupations
- Animal handlers
- Agricultural workers and farmers, greenhouse workers
- Wood and paper workers
- Waste management and composting workers
- Food production and transport workers (grain, hay, crops, vegetables, flour)
- Animal laboratory personnel
- Biotechnology personnel
- Textile production workers

Environmental settings
- Offices, schools, and hospital buildings
- Private residences
- Buildings with contaminated ventilation systems
- Swimming pools, spas

3. What are organic dusts and bioaerosols?

Organic dusts and bioaerosols are important exposure sources in the assessment of occupational and environmental diseases. Organic dusts are defined by the Committee on Organic Dust as consisting of vegetable and animal materials and microbes such as bacteria and fungi. Bioaerosols are microscopic organisms and biologically significant materials that are transported through the atmosphere and deposited in areas where they may have consequences for life. Many specialties are involved in research and practical applications related to organic dusts and bioaerosols: industrial hygienists, microbiologists, mycologists, veterinarians and physicians, aerosol physicists, botanists, and environmental health scientists. Microorganisms and components in dust are made of various substances, including fungal spores and hyphae, bacterial cell walls, *Actinomyces* spores, endotoxin, mycotoxins, (1-3) β-D-glucan, and microbial volatile organic compounds (MVOCs). Organic dusts contain causative agents for airway disease (sinusitis, asthma), allergy, and toxic health reactions. Individual health reactions may vary with conditions of short- or long-term exposure and low- or high-level concentrations. Individual susceptibility (atopy) and environmental factors (e.g., temperature, humidity, water content, wind, ventilation rate) are additional modifiers.

4. What are fungi? With what medically important health risks are they associated?

Fungi are eukaryote organisms with cell walls; they lack chlorophyll and reproduce sexually or asexually (by means of spores). Examples include yeast, molds (filamentous fungi), rusts, and mushrooms. There are more than 100,000 species of fungi, but only a few hundred are of medical importance because of their potential for infection, allergy, and toxicity. Many fungal spores are in the respirable range of 2–20 μm; they vary in shape and color. Maximal dispersal occurs under dry conditions. Spores germinate and grow if organic materials are present and species-specific moisture conditions are met. Nutrient sources may be hay, crops, plant and food material, animal droppings, wood, paper, paint, mineral oil, and various building materials. Together with bacteria, fungi contribute to degradation of biologic materials. Fungi are named by genus and species according to the International Code of Botanical Nomenclature (e.g., *Aspergillus fumigatus*). Classification of fungi is ongoing.

5. Which fungi are found most commonly in damp buildings?

Fungal species	Materials and location
Alternaria alternata	Moist window-sills, walls
Aspergillus versicolor	Damp wood
Aureobasidium pullulans	Outlets from bathroom, kitchen
Cladosporium herbarum	Moist window-sills, wood
Penicillium brevicompactum	Wood chip boards
P. chrysogenum	Damp wall paper
Stachybotrys chartarum (atra)	Damp/wet wallpaper, gypsum board, paper insulation
Trichoderma viride	Damp wood materials

6. What are the medically important indoor pollutant sources?

Medically important indoor air pollution generally is divided into exposures from the following sources:

- Environmental tobacco smoke
- Combustion products
- Volatile organic compounds and pesticides
- Heavy metals
- Mineral fibers (asbestos and man-made fibers)
- Biologic agents

7. What are the signs and symptoms of exposure to indoor biologic pollutants?

Important diagnostic clues with an overview of signs and symptoms of health reactions related to various environmental exposures were prepared for health professionals by the Environmental Protection Agency (EPA) in 1994. Health problems from biologic pollutants (aerosols) may be related to animal dander, fungi, dust mites, bacteria, viruses, *Legionella* species, and protozoa. In susceptible individuals such exposure or contact may result in infection, hypersensitivity or allergic reactions, toxicosis, and irritation or inflammatory reactions. Signs and symptoms include cough, chest tightness, dyspnea, malaise, fever, skin and mucous membrane reactions, cognitive abnormalities (due to conditions such as infectious disease or toxic reaction), asthma, rhinitis and sinusitis, conjunctivitis, or other systemic illnesses.

Irritation of the mucous membranes (eyes, upper airways) and skin after prolonged exposure to moisture-induced microbial growth, especially fungi, is typical. Allergic reactions may include rhinitis, sinusitis, conjunctivitis, asthma, or dermatologic reactions. Toxic health reactions typically are more severe and present with multiorgan abnormalities, including skin reactions; upper and lower airway abnormalities; immunologic dysfunctions (T-lymphocyte or immunoglobulin enumeration or functional abnormalities) resulting in infections and decreased resistance to other pathogens (e.g., pulmonary macrophage dysfunction); and central nervous system abnormalities (headaches, dizziness, mood changes, concentration problems, extreme fatigue). Such complex health disorders may be best described clinically as a **fungal syndrome**.

8. What about microbial contamination of buildings?

Growing epidemiologic and clinical evidence indicates a link between various health problems and exposure to fungi and bacteria in indoor air. In many cases, the exact cause of building-related illnesses cannot be firmly established because of a lack of valid or sensitive scientific methods or appropriate exposure information. Buildings and ventilation systems with water damage, leaks, and condensation problems pose a new challenge to occupational health care because of the great number of involved buildings and the complexity of clinical-epidemiologic investigations, which often require multidisciplinary cooperation. Increasing evidence links allergic, toxic, or inflammatory reactions to indoor exposure to microbial substances such as fungal allergens, endotoxins, mycotoxins, (1-3) β-D-glucan, MVOCs, and other particulates. Associated diseases fall into the category of infection (legionnaires' disease), irritative symptoms (endotoxins, some mycotoxins), allergic disease (fungi), alveolitis (hypersensitivity pneumonitis) or toxic pneumonitis (fungi, actinomyces, endotoxins, (1-3) β-D-glucan), and organic dust toxic syndrome (ODTS). ODTS is closely related to exposure to high amounts of fungal aerosol mixtures, typically in agricultural settings.

Although water-damaged buildings with indoor environmental quality problems may result in exposure to a mixture of microbial agents, some substances and species seem to be more potent and should alert the examining physician. The indoor presence of such fungi as *Aspergillus fumigatus, Aspergillus versicolor, Paecilomyces variotii, Stachybotrys chartarum (atra), Penicillium* spp., and *Fusarium* spp. has been associated with serious toxic or allergic reactions.

9. How is sick building syndrome defined?

Sick building syndrome (SBS) refers to poorly defined physical conditions or nonspecific symptoms (primarily sensory complaints) that are related to a problem building. No definite or specific cause (exposure) can be identified by industrial hygiene evaluation of the work area. Although some clinicians try to avoid the diagnosis because they believe that it can mean many things to many people, it has found widespread use in clinical practice and medical literature. Exposure sources and circumstances may vary considerably from building to building and case to case. SBS is typically a multifactorial problem involving chemical, microbial, physical, and psychosocial factors:
- Building factors (age, defects, and moisture problems)
- Type of ventilation system
- Ventilation rates (i.e., below 10 L/sec per person)
- Volatile organic compounds
- Carpets
- Work organization, job stress and dissatisfaction
- Overcrowded work areas
- Use of video display terminals
- Individual constitutional factors (e.g., preexisting atopy, allergy, or asthma)

Physiologic effects of indoor exposure or conditions and work-related psychological stress factors may interact or be superimposed on each other. Common complaints and symptoms may vary in clinical presentation and prevalence with the time of the building investigation. Typically SBS presents primarily with sensory complaints, mucous membrane irritation, neurotoxic effects, respiratory symptoms, and skin abnormalities.

10. What are building-related illnesses?

Building-related disease or illness refers to a category of clinical diagnoses that are related to an identifiable, known hazardous building exposure. Such illnesses have defined clinical findings and objective laboratory or functional test abnormalities. The pathogenesis of specific building-related illnesses has been related principally to infectious, immunologic, or toxic sources or exposures. In clinical practice, complex historical and physical findings may make it difficult to specify the diagnosis and disease mechanism. Some cases may be a combination of allergic and toxic reactions, particularly reactions related to microbials (i.e., fungi and their metabolites). However, individual susceptibility and exposure circumstances need to be examined carefully because of the great variations from case to case.

Important Building-related Illnesses and Exposure Sources

DIAGNOSTIC CATEGORY	EXPOSURE
Infectious disease	
Legionnaires' disease/Pontiac fever	*Legionella pneumophila*
Viral syndrome/upper respiratory infection	Respiratory viruses, influenza
Tuberculosis	*Mycobacterium tuberculosis*
Allergy/immunologic reaction	
Dermatitis, urticaria	Dust mite, microbial (fungi), carbonless copy
Rhinitis, sinusitis	paper (alkyl phenol novolac resin)
Asthma	Animal antigens, epoxy resins, latex
Extrinsic allergic alveolitis (hypersensitivity pneumonitis)	Microbial (fungi, bacteria, endotoxins, β-glucan, *Actinomyces* spp.)
Humidifier fever	
Organic dust toxic syndrome	Mixed organic dust (bacteria and fungi)
Toxic reaction	
Central nervous system dysfunction	Pesticides, heavy metal (lead, mercury), volatile
Headaches, dizziness, cognitive abnormalities	organic compounds (formaldehyde)
Chronic fatigue syndrome (CFIDS)	
Irritant syndrome	
Eye irritation/conjunctivitis	Glass fibers (man-made mineral fibers), combus-
Mucous membrane irritation (nose/throat)	tion products (CO, NO_2), low humidity (< 25–
Epistaxis	30%)

Sources: Environmental Protection Agency: Indoor Air Pollution. An Introduction for Health Professionals. Washington, DC, Environmental Protection Agency, 1994 (Publication No. 523-217/81322); Hodgson MJ: The medical evaluation. Occup Med State Art Rev 10:177–194, 1995; and Menzies D, Bourbeau J: Building related illnesses. N Engl J Med 337:1524–1531, 1997.

11. Describe the diagnosis of SBS or building-related illnesses.

The clinician can make a correct diagnosis and establish a causal relationship only if suffi-cient and accurate exposure information has been gathered and the patient has objective evidence of disease. In most cases the physician depends on the patient's exposure history and data pro-vided by other health care providers, industrial hygienists, or microbiologists to establish a diag-nosis and treatment plan. Sampling and identification methods of important exposure sources are available, but sampling strategies depend on the goal (medical, legal, or research) and should be conducted by experienced and trained professionals, such as industrial hygienists. Clinicians may contact the American Industrial Hygiene Association (www.aiha.org) or the American Conference of Governmental Industrial Hygienists (www.acgih.org). The medical exam of patients with po-tential occupational or environmental health problems should follow general professional practice guidelines and current medical science. Often the symptoms and signs are nonspecific and multi-ple. No specific tests are "routine" or "necessary"; frequently tests are chosen on a case-by-case basis according to experience and training. Consider what tests are available and required for what purpose (medical diagnostic work-up, legal documentation, or research). Several government agencies and professional organizations provide helpful information for further research and databanks (www.cdc.gov; www.cdc.gov/niosh; www.acoem.org; www.osha.gov; www.ccohs.ca; http://occ-env-med.mc.duke.edu/oem;www-iea.me.tut.fi/cgi-bin/oshweb.pl).

12. Why the big fuss about *Stachybotrys chartarum (atra)*?

The toxigenic fungus *Stachybotrys chartarum (atra)* has been associated with several cases of severe illnesses after intense or prolonged exposure in humans (inhalation) and animals (in-gestion). Widespread contamination has been found after flooding or chronic water leaks in resi-dential homes, farms, offices, hospitals, court houses, and schools. Recent research has applied modern epidemiologic and laboratory tools to address important medical and public health policy issues. One study reported that after ongoing severe fungal exposure, primarily to *S. chartarum*, office workers complained of multiple symptoms that suggested toxic effects on lungs, eyes, skin, mucous membranes, central nervous system, or cardiovascular system. Significant abnormalities affected the humoral and cellular immune system compared with nonexposed controls. A more recent case-control study by the Centers for Disease Control and Prevention and the National Institute for Occupational Safety and Health reported an increased incidence of hemosiderosis/hemorrhagic lung diseases among infants living in an area of Cleveland with massive moisture and flooding problems before the cluster occurrence. Respiratory disorders (including hypersensitivity pneumonitis) were reported in a group of courthouse workers with intense exposure over several months primarily to *S. chartarum* and *Aspergillus versicolor*. *S. chartarum* produces potent trichothecenes (i.e., satratoxin) and spirolactones, which interfere with protein synthesis, DNA, and the immune system. The production of mycotoxins depends on certain environmental and substrate conditions, such as high water and cellulose content. Conventional field sampling and identification relying mainly on cultures appear insufficient to assess toxic exposure relationships. The exact exposure dose and duration required to develop adverse health effects is unknown. Therefore, a zero-level indoor tolerance has been generally accepted by experts. Infants and children may be at an increased health risk (potentially fatal lung disease) with intense exposure to toxic mold.

13. What is a fungal allergy?

An estimated 25–30 million people in the U.S. currently have a diagnosis of allergic rhinitis, and about 10 million have asthma. Allergic rhinitis is a significant factor in asthma, chronic sinusitis, and otitis media. About 13 million workers (approximately 10% of male and 12% of female workers) have allergic rhinitis resulting in about 3.4 million sick days and medical costs of around $10 billion. Allergens involved in the development of occupational or environmental allergies are either low-molecular-weight chemicals (metabolites) or high-molecular-weight plant or animal proteins. Atopy is an important risk factor for asthma and rhinitis caused by fungal allergens. People with elevated IgE-levels (total IgE >100 IU/l) are considered atopic. Mold allergen exposure may be seasonally related (outdoor exposure) or insidious (indoor exposure due to building defects and moisture problems). Allergens may stem from protein materials of the fungal spores or hyphae (fungal structures or mycelial fragments). These antigenic particles are inhaled and deposited, depending on size (2–200 μm). in the upper (>10 μm) or lower (< 10 μm) airways and may result in hypersensitivity reactions. Hypersensitivity is defined as an exaggerated or inappropriate immune response to allergen exposure. A hypersensitivity reaction requires prior contact with an allergen and involves subsequent sensitization. Hypersensitivity has been grouped into four general categories, according to the Gells and Coombs system, that may overlap clinically:

Hypersensitivity type	Manifested disease	Agent
I (immediate type)	Asthma, allergy	IgE antibodies
II (cytotoxic hypersensitivity)	Not important in this context	
III (immune complex-mediated)	Extrinsic allergic alveolitis (hypersensitivity pneumonitis)	Antigen-antibody complex
IV (delayed type)	Contact dermatitis	T-lymphocytes

The term **allergy** is now used primarily for type I hypersensitivity reactions, which are triggered by various substances found in buildings, including dust, animals/anthropoids (cats, mites, cockroaches), and plant or fungal antigens. People with hypersensitivity may react at low levels of exposure. In such situations the workplace exposure limits, often referred to as threshold limit values (TLVs) or permissible exposure limits (PELs), are not applicable. Diesel exhaust particulates (from air intake problems) may act as a powerful adjuvant for IgE production. Extrinsic allergic alveolitis (hypersensitivity pneumonitis) is an immunologic lung disorder representing a mixture of types III and IV reactions; it may result in chronic respiratory problems with peripheral destruction of alveoli and fibrotic lung changes. Hypersensitivity pneumonitis also may be seen in nonatopic people. The clinician should attempt to identify possible allergens based on the history, timing, and environmental conditions. During allergen exposure physical signs may be present.

14. What are the important fungal allergens?

More than 80 genera of fungi have been associated with respiratory tract allergy, including the following:

Alternaria spp. (many important allergenic fractions have been identified; the most important is Alt a1)

Cladosporium spp. (of more than 60 antigens identified, two are major allergens)

Aspergillus spp. *(A. fumigatus, A. versicolor, A. nidulans, A. glaucus)*

Basidiomycetes spp.

Candida albicans (two major allergens have been identified)

Penicillium spp. (i.e., *P. notatum* with 11 IgE-binding proteins)

Fusarium spp.

Helminthosporium spp.

Drechslera spp.

Curvularia spp.

Botrytis cinerea

Epicoccum nigrum

Trichophyton spp.

At present relatively few fungal allergens have been well defined and characterized at the molecular level. In clinical settings great difficulties with fungal allergen extracts and laboratory tests are often encountered. Cross-reactivity of fungal allergens; low-sensitivity, false-negative allergy testing; and variations in laboratory quality are common problems. Diagnosis of fungal allergy is based on clinical signs and symptoms, verifiable exposure to fungi, results of skin testing, radioallergosorbent testing (RAST), or, if necessary, provocation challenge testing. RAST testing is generally considered less sensitive than skin testing. The primary management of allergic conditions is allergen avoidance and symptomatic pharmacologic treatment (antihistamines, antiinflammatory medication, and beta-mimetics [asthma]).

15. What is allergic bronchopulmonary aspergillosis (ABPA)?

ABPA is a complex immunologic reaction to exposure to *Aspergillus fumigatus.* In nonatopic patients, *Aspergillus* hyphae may grow in the lungs and cause the production of an aspergilloma ("fungal balls"). A combination of toxic effect on lung epithelia and an allergic response may be responsible for the clinical and pathologic findings. The most important diagnostic criteria are asthma, central bronchiectasis, total IgE > 500 IU/ml, immediate cutaneous reactivity to *Aspergillus*, and elevated IgE or IgG antibodies to *A. fumigatus*. Other important findings include eosinophilia, x-ray infiltrates, and bronchiectasis. ABPA should be suspected in all patients with asthma who have immediate cutaneous reaction to *A. fumigatus.* Standard chest radiographs may not be sensitive enough, or changes may be transient; other false-negative test findings are also possible. High-resolution CT is optimal to detect bronchiectasis. Physical examination may be normal or reveal crackles and wheezing. Acute flare-ups may present with fever, malaise, sputum production, and wheezing. Irreversible pulmonary fibrosis may develop if the condition is not identified in time and exposure cessation is not instituted. Treatment includes exposure elimination and primarily steroid medication; antifungal antibiotics may be beneficial in some cases. Prevention depends on exposure control and avoidance and adequate building maintenance.

16. What are mycotoxins?

Mycotoxins are metabolites produced by fungi under various environmental conditions; they have toxic effects on both animals and humans. More than 250 different mycotoxins are known to be produced by various fungi, the most important of which are *Stachybotrys, Aspergillus, Penicillium, Fusarium, Claviceps, Alternaria, Myrothecium, Phoma,* and *Trichoderma* species. Some fungi produce well-known antibiotics that are used in medical practice (penicillin, griseofulvin). Not all fungi necessarily produce high amounts of toxin materials when growing on foodstuff or in indoor environments. Production appears to depend on available nutrients, moisture content, and whether competitive organisms are present. Mycotoxins vary widely in toxicity and target organs (gastrointestinal tract, liver, kidney, cardiovascular system, immune system, central nervous system). Aflatoxin produced mainly by *Aspergillus flavus* and *A. parasiticus* is the most potent known carcinogen causing liver cancer. Ochratoxin produced by *Penicillium verrucosum* and *A. ochraceus* is nephrotoxic and has been associated with Balkan nephropathy. *Stachybotrys chartarum* produces trichothecenes, a group of potent protein synthesis inhibitors, as well as other poorly characterized chemicals, that are responsible for cases of mycotoxicosis (stachybotrystoxicosis). Mycotoxins important to food safety and human health include aflatoxin, sterigmatocystins, ochratoxins, citrinin, trichothecenes (macrocyclic and T2-toxin, vomitoxin), patulin, zearalenone, rubratoxins, tremorgens, and ergotoxins.

Clinically Important Fungi and Mycotoxins and Principal Target Organs in Humans and Animals

FUNGI	MYCOTOXIN	TARGET ORGAN
Penicillium (> 150 species)	Patulin	Lung, brain
	Citrinin	Kidney, lung
	Ochratoxin A	Kidney (Balkan nephropathy)
	Citroviridin	Liver
	Gliotoxin	Nervous system
	Verruculogen	Lung disease, AIDS
	Secalonic acid D	Neurotoxic, lung/teratogenic in rodents
Aspergillus spp. (fungal spore size: 2–3.5 μm)		
A. flavus	Aflatoxin (β_1)	Liver cancer, respiratory tract cancer
A. versicolor	Sterigmatocystin	Carcinogen
A. ochraceus	Ochratoxin A	Kidney, liver
A. parasiticus	Patulin	Lung, brain

Stachybotrys chartarum (atra) (fungal spore size: 1–6 μm) (also some *Fusarium* spp.)	Trichothecenes (> 49 known chemical derivatives): T2; nivalenol; deoxynivalenol; diacetoxyscirpenol; satratoxin H, G; other macrocytic trichothecenes	Immune system
		 Upper and lower airways
		 Skin and mucous membranes
		 Cardiovascular system
		 Eyes (irritation)
		 Central nervous system
		 Cytotoxic
		 High dose: acute, lethal (human case reports)
		 Low dose: chronic exposure
		 Opportunistic infections
		 Teratogenic, abortogenic (in animals)
		 Reported special conditions:
		     Alimentary toxic aleukia (ATA)
		     Staggering wheat disease
		     Red mold disease

17. What diagnostic tests are available?

Several laboratory tests are available to support the history and findings in the environmental clinical assessment: complete red and white cell count, erythrocyte sedimentation rate (ESR), chemistry with liver function tests, and urinalysis. Total IgE helps to determine atopic status; specific IgE-allergen tests (RAST) assess various environmental allergens and fungi (based on environmental sampling data); and IgG-antibodies to specific fungal and bacterial agents (*Actinomyces* spp.) may be used as exposure markers. Note that asymptomatic people may exhibit elevated antibody levels; levels do not necessarily correlate with disease severity and status. Acute high-toxicity effects may suppress IgG-antibody development).

No readily available methods reliably detect mycotoxins in humans. Toxic effects need to be assessed based on clinical information, indirect measures of adverse health effects on body organs, and tissue and immunologic markers. If severe allergic or toxic immune system abnormalities are suspected, special studies may be necessary. Clinically useful information can be obtained by studying lymphocyte enumeration (CD 3, CD 19, CD 4 and CD8, NK), lymphocyte function (mitogen transformation test), and immunoglobulins A, M, G, and IgG subgroups. Primarily T-lymphocyte abnormalities have been found in people with significant exposures and illnesses.

Other tests also may be indicated based on clinical findings and special exposure monitoring needs. Examples include pulmonary function tests, bronchoprovocation test (methacholine challenge that causes a drop > 20% in FEV_1 is considered positive), RAST in vitro testing, and allergy skin testing. Skin tests and in vitro testing may have problems with reproducibility and validity; they may produce false-negative results, or cross-reactivity of antigen substances may limit proper identification of offending agents. Allergy skin testing should be performed only by properly trained personnel and experienced clinicians.

18. How do I sample for bioaerosols, including fungi?

Sampling may be necessary to verify microbial exposure, to assess occupational or environmental health risks, or to confirm a clinical diagnosis. Various methods and tools are available to characterize (identification) and quantify (dose) biologic exposures in clinical practice. Preferably they should be done by qualified and experienced technicians and personnel, because collection and analysis procedures are not widely standardized and require knowledge of the appropriate sampling strategy and instruments. Bioaerosols in the work environment are generally complex mixtures of microbial, animal, and plant particles.

Guidelines for proper collection and transportation and laboratory requirements have been proposed by the AIHA, ACGIH, and other professional organizations. A visual inspection of the building is necessary to determine the extent of moisture problems and evidence of microbial growth. Sampling strategies and methods depend on the purpose (medical, legal, public health, research) of the field investigation. Some methods are available only for special research applications, such as ergosterol, beta-glucans, and mycotoxins. New methods and instruments are constantly being developed to improve practicality and to gather more detailed information about the exposure.

The most commonly used detection methods are measurements of viable (identification by culture) and nonviable (microscopic identification) fungi, bacteria, endotoxins, and, more recently, MVOCs. Impactors with various nutrient agar plates (such as the Anderson, RCS, or SAS) are used to collect air samples to identify and measure airborne viable fungi. Fungal or bacterial identification using culture methods tends to be more reliable than microscopic visual inspection of slide deposits, which does not allow subspeciation. Nonviable fungi and particles are collected and quantified using a sticky-surface sampler such as the Burkhard spore trap or Allergenco and Air-O-Cell air sampler methods. Nonviable particles are of great medical importance because they also carry antigens or mycotoxins. Bulk samples are analyzed (by culture and microscopically) by mycologists and useful in identifying sources of fungal air pollution. The results are reported in colony-forming units (air test: CFU/m^3; surface area [bulk]: CFU/m^2) with fractionation of the dominant fungal species.

In indoor-air quality assessments the numbers and species identified are compared with "normal" outside reference samples. In a healthy indoor environment the CFU numbers are usually lower than in the outside environment, and the fungal species are similar. Some fungi are considered by most experts to be unacceptable for indoor environments and require risk management and intervention, especially *Stachybotrys chartarum* and *Aspergillus versicolor*. There are no CFU levels, PELs, TLVs, or other government standards for fungi and bacteria. "The lower the better" is the generally accepted guideline. It is difficult to determine acceptable TLVs because of methodologic sampling limitations, environmental variability, and various health effects and differences in susceptibility. Young and old patients, patients with cancer or organ transplantation, and patients with severe liver or kidney diseases may be more susceptible to adverse health effects of fungi and bacteria. Keep in mind, however, that biologic contaminants are a ubiquitous part of normal daily life and do not necessarily pose a health threat.

19. What are key questions for the treating clinician?

The astute physician asks patients about their occupation, work environment, and indoor environmental conditions. Signs and symptoms related in time and place to certain activities (e.g., farming, composting, wood-working) or problem buildings, such as offices with water damage, flooding, and visible microbial growth (stained walls and ceilings, mildew odor, material degradation), are clues to recognition of environmental diseases. The following questions should be asked:

1. Do you have visible mold or noticeable mildew odor in your home, office, school, or other indoor environment?

2. Do you know of any water or roof leaks, flooding, or ventilation system defects that resulted in wetness of paper or office materials, walls, and ceilings?

3. Do the health problems go away when you discontinue the activity or leave the house or office?

4. What aggravates or improves the health problems (e.g., changes in exposure duration or intensity, personal protective equipment [respirator])?

5. Are other people also affected by the environmental conditions?

6. Are certain people more affected and sicker than others (e.g., children, immunocompromised people)?

20. What about treatment of fungal syndromes?

The primary treatment is exposure control and avoidance. Supportive care and symptomatic medications may be indicated if specific complications are present (e.g., use of bronchodilators, antiallergy medication, or antibiotics). In special cases (including asthma and various constitutional disorders) use of an antifungal medication, such as itraconazole, may be beneficial if possible adverse drug reactions are monitored and avoided and other treatment has not been successful. The primary goals should be correction of building defects and, optimally, total removal of any microbial (fungal) sources that may contribute to indoor air pollution.

21. What are the special prevention and clean-up considerations for toxic fungi?

Clean-up measures depend on the size of the problem. Refer to guidelines established by expert panels, such as the New York City Department of Health (www.bioaerosols.com) and the Canada Mortgage and Housing Corporation.

- In case of floods wait until flood waters have receded below basement level before pumping out the basement area. Floors, walls, and other surfaces contacted by flood waters should be properly disinfected for at least 15 minutes with a chlorine solution of 1 cup of laundry bleach per gallon of water. Caution should be taken not to mix other cleaning agents with the chlorine solution. Proper personal protection (e.g., rubber gloves, goggles, proper ventilation) is mandatory. It is also important to refer to the material safety data sheet (MSDS) for more detail about personal protection.

- Eliminate or correct water problems or leaks associated with any existing source of water damage. Carpets, rugs, furniture, and other items with absorbent material must be removed and discarded if not thoroughly dried within 24 hours.

- Stained ceiling tiles or wall board should be replaced. All accumulated residues should be removed from the area, including corners, edges of floors, and under and around fixtures. Use high-efficiency particulate air (HEPA) vacuum devices.

- Caution should be taken around electrical equipment and fixtures. During clean-up activities, only people doing the clean-up should be in the home. During all clean-up activities a tight-fitting HEPA dust mask and goggles should be worn. Rubber or vinyl gloves and waterproof boots also should be worn during all phases of the clean-up. Open all windows for drying and ventilation.

BIBLIOGRAPHY

1. American Conference of Governmental Industrial Hygienists: Guidelines for the Assessment of Bioaerosols in the Indoor Environment. Cincinnati, OH, American Conference of Governmental Industrial Hygienists, 1989.

2. American Thoracic Society: Achieving healthy indoor air. Report of the ATS Workshop: Santa Fe, NM, Nov. 16–19, 1995. Am J Resp Crit Care Med 156:S33–S64, 1997.
3. Auger PL, Gourdeau P, Miller JD: Clinical experience with patients suffering from a chronic fatigue-like syndrome and repeated upper respiratory infections in relation to airborne molds. Am J Indust Med 25:41–42, 1994.
4. Bernstein DI: Allergic reactions to workplace allergens. JAMA 278:1907–1913, 1997.
5. Bettina V: Mycotoxins. Chemical, Biological and Environmental Aspects, vol. 9. Amsterdam, Elsevier, 1989.
6. Canada Mortgage and Housing Corporation: Toxic mold clean-up procedures (draft). Ottawa, Canada Mortgage and Housing Corporation, 1998 (www.cmhc-schl.gc.ca).
7. Committee on Environmental Health, American Academy of Pediatrics: Toxic Effects of Indoor Molds. J Pediatr, pp 712–714, 1998.
8. Corrier DE: Mycotoxicosis: Mechanism of immunosuppression. Vet Immunopathol 30:73–87, 1991.
9. Dillon HK, Heinsohn PA, Miller JD: Field guide for the determination of biological contaminants in environmental samples. Fairfax, VA, AIHA Biosafety Committee, American Industrial Hygiene Association, 1996.
10. Environmental Protection Agency: Indoor Air Pollution. An Introduction for Health Professionals. Washington, DC, Environmental Protection Agency, 1994 (Publication No. 523-217/81322).
11. Etzel RA, Montaña E, Sorenson WG, et al: Acute pulmonary hemorrhage in infants associated with exposure to *Stachybotrys atra* and other fungi. Arch Pediatr Adolesc Med 152:757–762, 1998.
12. Fink JN: Hypersensitivity pneumonitis. In Patterson R, Grammar LC, Greenberger PA (eds): Allergic Diseases. Diagnosis and Management. Philadelphia, Lippincott-Raven, 1997.
13. Graveson S, Frisvad JC, Samson RA: Microfungi. Munksgaard, Denmark, 1994.
14. Greenberger PA: Allergic bronchopulmonary aspergillosis. In Patterson R, Grammar LC, Greenberger PA (eds): Allergic Diseases. Diagnosis and Management. Philadelphia, Lippincott-Raven, 1997.
15. Hendry KM, Cole EC: A review of mycotoxins in indoor air. J Toxicol Environ Health 38:183–198, 1993.
16. Hodgson MJ: The medical evaluation. Occup Med State Art Rev 10:177–194, 1995.
17. Hodgson MJ, Morey P, Leung WY, et al: Building-associated pulmonary disease from exposure to *Stachybotrys chartarum* and *Aspergillus versicolor*. J Occup Environ Med 40:241–249, 1998.
18. Horner WE, Helbling A, Salvaggio JE, Lehrer SB: Fungal allergens. Clin Microbiol Rev 8:161–179, 1995.
19. Horwitz RJ, Bush RK: Allergens and other factors important in atopic disease. In Patterson R, Grammar LC, Greenberger PA (eds): Allergic Diseases. Diagnosis and Management. Philadelphia, Lippincott-Raven, 1997.
20. Husman T: Health effects of indoor-air microorganism. Scand J Work Environ Health 22:5–13, 1996.
21. International Association for Research on Cancer: IARC Monographs on the Evaluation of Carcinogenic Risks to Humans. Vol 56: Some Naturally Occurring Substances: Food Items and Constituents, Heterocyclic Aromatic Amines and Mycotoxins. Lyon, France, International Agency for the Research on Cancer, World Health Organization, 1993.
22. Jarvis B: Mycotoxins in the air: Keep the building dry or the bogeyman will get you. In Johanning E, Yang CS (eds): Fungi and Bacteria in Indoor Environments—Health Effects, Detection and Remediation. Albany, NY, Eastern New York Occupational Health Program, 1995.
23. Johanning E, Yang CS (eds): Fungi and Bacteria in Indoor Environments—Health Effects, Detection and Remediation. Proceedings of the International Conference, Saratoga Springs, 1994. Albany, NY, Eastern New York Occupational Health Program, 1995.
24. Johanning E, Biagini R, Hull D, et al: Health and immunology study following exposure to toxigenic fungi (*Stachybotrys atra*) in a water-damaged office environment. Int Arch Occup Environ Health 68;4:207–218, 1996.
25. Johanning E, Auger P, Reijula K: Building-related illnesses associated with moisture and fungal contamination—Current Concepts. N Engl J Med 338:1070–1071, 1998.
26. Johanning E: *Stachybotrys* Revisited. Clin Toxicol 36:629–631, 1998.
27. Kaplan AP (ed): Allergy. Philadelphia, W.B. Saunders, 1997.
28. Kreiss K: The epidemiology of building related complaints and illness. Occup Med State Art Rev 4:575–592, 1989.
29. Kwon-Chung KJ, Bennett JE: Medical Mycology. Philadelphia, Lea & Farber, 1992.
30. Lacey J, Crook B, Bai AJ: The detection of airborne allergens implicated in occupational asthma. In Muilenberg M, Burge H (eds): Aerobiology. Boca Raton, FL, Lewis Publisher, 1996.
31. Macher J (ed): Bioaerosols: Assessment and Control. Cincinnati, OH, American Conference of Governmental Industrial Hygienists, 1998.
32. Male DK: Immunology. An Illustrated Outline. St. Louis, Mosby, 1986.
33. Male DK, Champion B, Cooke A, Owen M: Advanced Immunology. New York, Gower Medical, 1987.

34. Menzies D, Bourbeau J: Building related illnesses. N Engl J Med 337:1524–1531, 1997.
35. Montaña E, Etzel RA, Allan T, et al: Environmental risk factors associated with pediatric idiopathic pulmonary hemorrhage and hemosiderosis in a Cleveland community. Pediatrics 99:1–8, 1997.
36. Muilenberg M, Burge H (eds): Aerobiology. Boca Raton, FL, Lewis Publisher, 1996.
37. Patterson R, Grammar LC, Greenberger PA: Allergic Diseases. Diagnosis and Management. Philadelphia, Lippincott-Raven, 1997.
38. Pope AM, Patterson R, Burge HA (eds): Indoor Allergens. Assessing and Controlling Adverse Health Effects. Washington, DC, Institute of Medicine, National Academy Press, 1993.
39. Reijula K: Building with moisture problems—A new challenge to occupational health care. Scand J Work Environ Health 22:1–3, 1996.
40. Rosenwasser LJ, Borish L, Gelfand E, et al: Yearbook of Allergy, Asthma and Clinical Immunology. St. Louis, Mosby, 1997.
41. Rylander R, Jacobs RR (eds): Organic Dusts—Exposure, Effects and Prevention. Boca Raton, FL, Lewis Publisher, 1994.
42. Rylander R: Evaluation of the risks of endotoxin exposure. Int J Occup Environ Health 3(Suppl): S32–S36, 1997.
43. Sharma RP, Salunkhe DK: Mycotoxins and Phytoalexins. Boca Raton, FL, CRC Press, 1991.
44. Skov P, Valbjörn O, et al: The "sick" building syndrome in the office environment: The Danish town hall study. Environ Int 13:339–349, 1987.
45. Skov P, Valbjörn O, Pedersen BV: Influence of indoor climate on the sick building syndrome in an office environment. Scand J Work Environ Health 16:369–371, 1990.
46. Sorenson WG, Lewis DM: Organic dust toxic syndrome. In Howard/Miller (ed): The Mycotica VI. Human and Animal Relationship. Berlin, Springer Verlag, 1996.
47. Sorenson B, Kullman G, Hintz P: NIOSH Health Hazard Evaluation Report. HETA 95-0160-2571. Morgantown, WV, Centers for Disease Control and Prevention, National Center for Environmental Health, U.S. Department of Health and Human Services, 1996.
48. World Health Organization: Indoor Air Pollutants: Exposure and Health Effects. Copenhagen, WHO Regional Office for Europe (Euro Reports and Studies No.78), 1983.
49. Yang CS, Johanning E: Airborne fungi and mycotoxins. In Hurst CJ, Knudsen GR, McInerney MJ, et al (eds): Manual of Environmental Microbiology. Washington, DC, ASM Press, 1997, pp 651–660.

23. BIOLOGIC AND CHEMICAL TERRORISM

David R. Franz, D.V.M., Ph.D.

1. What is biologic terrorism?

Biologic warfare may be defined as the intentional use of microorganisms or toxins to produce death or disease in humans, animals, or plants. Biologic terrorism is distinguished from biologic warfare by the scope of the attack and the number of agents available to the terrorist. Because it is not necessary to kill thousands to achieve the desired impact, the terrorist has a much larger number of agents and targets from which to pick. We have fewer tools and less information to protect citizens from terrorism than to protect a defined military force from classic biologic warfare attacks. Therefore, preexposure prophylaxis of the civilian population from most agents would not be cost-effective. Biologic terrorism can occur almost anywhere at any time and may appear epidemiologically much like an emerging disease outbreak.

2. What is chemical terrorism? How may it differ from a biologic attack?

Much of what is stated above about biologic terrorism applies to chemical terrorism. In most societies, humans are more comfortable with chemicals than with biologic agents; the terrorist, therefore, may be more likely to choose a chemical than a biologic agent. Like the biologic terrorist, the chemical terrorist has a large number of agents from which to select, including commercially available products. However, because of the nature of its effects, a chemical attack would manifest itself much differently from a biologic attack. The latent period from exposure to onset of clinical signs is much shorter for chemicals (minutes) than for biologic agents (hours or days). This fact changes the training, preparation, and response necessary to deal with a chemical attack and shifts the burden from physicians—in the case of a biologic attack—to first responders.

3. What kinds of biologic agents may be used in terrorism?

The biologic terrorist may use one of the 15–20 classical "battlefield" agents (e.g., anthrax, plague, smallpox, or viral encephalitides) or any of hundreds of less effective agents that are found naturally in the environment. To produce a true mass-casualty attack, the terrorist probably will need help. The technical requirements to grow, purify, and dry the agent to a talcum-like consistency that can be easily dispersed as a true respirable (1–10-μ particle) aerosol are not trivial and make state sponsorship almost mandatory, except for highly contagious pathogens. Many other common bacteria or toxins—and possibly viruses—are readily available in the environment and may be dispersed over a small area by a simple device or sprayed on a food bar in a restaurant or supermarket, potentially causing illness in dozens or hundreds of people. Even a hoax such as labeling a harmless package as containing a popular pathogen may serve the terrorists' purposes.

4. What are the symptoms of a biologic warfare-related disease? How may a physician recognize them?

The classic biologic warfare-related diseases present almost universally with flulike symptoms. Fever, myalgia, headache, and respiratory effects are often the first signs in patients exposed to a bacterial or viral aerosol cloud. Following inhalation of toxins, respiratory distress and fever may be most common. Ingestion of enteric pathogens may result in the classic signs of food poisoning and enteritis. More important than the signs and symptoms in individual patients is the pattern of disease in a population. As with emerging disease, the epidemiology of the outbreak probably will be the key to diagnosis.

5. What treatments are available?

Early diagnosis and treatment are critical for the classic lethal agents such as anthrax and pneumonic plague; physicians may have only 24–36 hours after inhalation exposure before treatment becomes much less effective. Commonly available antibiotics (doxycycline, ciprofloxacin, and gentamicin) are indicated for many of these agents. Supportive therapy, analgesics and, in the case of some viral hemorrhagic fevers, the antiviral drug ribavirin may be used. Decontamination of patients or the environment is believed to be much less important for biologic agents than for some of the chemical agents.

6. What are the major potential chemical agents and their actions?

Like biologic agents, chemical agents need not be lethal to serve a major purpose of terrorists: gaining media attention. However, the classic chemical warfare agents (organophosphate nerve agents, cyanide, phosgene, and vesicants such as mustard) are probably the most feared. Many act on the respiratory and/or nervous systems. Most can be lethal, and all are at least incapacitating. Generally, chemical intoxications cause illness almost immediately and require rapid response. The mustards have rapid effects at the molecular level but may not cause clinical disease—manifest as blisters on the skin and pulmonary lesions—for hours. Readily available industrial chemicals are also potential weapons. Compounds such as chlorine, phosgene, cyanide, and other potent industrial chemicals are available commercially and may be used as weapons.

7. What treatments are available?

Preparing medically to respond to a chemical attack is in some ways easier than preparing for a biologic attack. Specific therapies are similar within classes of chemical agents, and symptomatic therapy is more often feasible. Drugs typically available in hospital pharmacies and common equipment for artificial ventilation have broad application. Decontamination with 0.5% sodium hypochlorite or even flushing with water can stop or greatly reduce continued absorption. Atropine, oximes, and anticonvulsants such as diazepam may be used for nerve agent intoxication. Decontamination must be performed immediately for vesicants, which are absorbed in seconds or minutes. Skin, eye, and pulmonary exposure are treated much like thermal burns; infection control and pain management are central to therapy. Cyanide, in high doses, causes death within minutes. However, before cardiac failure, the classic antidotes, sodium nitrite and sodium thiosulfate, are effective. The elapsed time from exposure to treatment is typically much more important for chemical agents than for biologic agents. Care must be provided within minutes rather than hours or days. Therefore, it is the first responder rather than the physician who may diagnose and provide early treatment to chemical exposure.

8. What can physicians do to prepare for a terrorist attack?

Individual clinicians are better prepared to deal with a terrorist attack than most of us believe. The diseases caused by biologic agents, although not seen every day in hospitals, have pathogenic mechanisms similar to disease-causing agents that physicians know well. The most likely used bacterial agents can be treated with antibiotics. Many of the likely used viral agents are not lethal. The biologic toxins, although some are extremely toxic, are difficult to disseminate effectively, and many of the chemical agents may be treated with readily available drugs and artificial ventilation. Clinical diagnosis may be easier for chemicals than for biologic agents. Physicians must familiarize themselves with physical and biologic characteristics of broad classes of agents and think in terms of patterns of disease in populations rather than in individual patients.

9. What should physicians do if they suspect that patients have been exposed to chemical or biologic terrorist agents?

Physicians who observe a group of patients with acute-onset respiratory or neuromuscular signs must consider a chemical agent in the differential diagnosis and be aware of the possibility of continued exposure from either the environment or their patients. For personal protection from the volatile chemicals, one must use a mask containing activated charcoal; for biologic agents, a surgical or painter's mask provides some protection. For highly volatile chemical agents, clinical diagnosis may be the only option for agent identification immediately after an attack. The U.S.

military—and first responders in some major cities—have simple assays for identification of chemical warfare agents, but these field assays are not yet widely available. None of the biologic agents has acute onset, and few are highly contagious; therefore, standard isolation precautions are adequate while diagnosis and early treatment are begun. Nasal swab samples may contain bacteria, virus, or toxin for 24–48 hours after an aerosol attack; however, few field diagnostic kits are available for such agents. When clinical signs occur, blood or serum should be collected for culture, viral isolation, or other diagnostic applications. Information provided to victims and the public, even for nonlethal agents and hoaxes, may be as important as medical treatment. Credible authorities must use the media effectively to explain exactly what risk remains, to answer specific questions about water or food treatment or agent persistence, and, in general, to calm the public.

10. To what governmental bodies should physicians report evidence of chemical or biologic attack?

For a suspected chemical attack, local, state, and national law enforcement agencies will become quickly involved. An effective local response is most important after a chemical attack; therefore, physicians should focus first on reducing further exposure and saving lives and inform local law enforcement authorities. The biologic attack may be subtler. Increased numbers of patients that suggest an outbreak should be reported to state public health authorities, who typically inform the Centers for Disease Control and Prevention. For emergency assistance, physicians may call the U.S. Public Health Service, Office of Emergency Preparedness, at 1-800-USA-NDMS, ext. 0.

11. What lies ahead in terms of chemical and biologic terrorism?

The chemical and biologic terrorist threat to cities worldwide is real. State-sponsored bioterrorism is a concern because, with help, an individual or small group could truly produce mass casualties. But even after an effective attack, the established public health infrastructure within local, state, and national governments could make an enormous difference. At the other end of the spectrum, spraying a diarrhea-causing bacterial preparation on a salad bar or adulteration of food products with a toxic chemical is extremely easy and may cause discomfort to a few hundred people. Effective domestic preparedness must involve efforts on many fronts. In addition to public health capabilities, a responsive research infrastructure with which to deal with the unknown, an effective intelligence program to reduce that which is unknown, solid law enforcement, moderation on the part of the media, and especially education of health-care providers and citizens can effectively reduce the impact of chemical or biologic terrorism. Such an integrated approach serves as a deterrent by increasing the risk to the terrorist and reducing the likelihood of a successful attack.

BIBLIOGRAPHY

1. Baskin SI, Brewer TG: Cyanide poisoning. In Zajtchuk R (ed): Medical Aspects of Chemical and Biological Warfare. Washington, DC, Borden Institute, 1997, pp 271–286.
2. Christopher GS, Cieslak TJ, Pavlin JA, et al: Biological warfare: A historical perspective. JAMA 278:412–417, 1997.
3. Franz DR: Defense Against Toxin Weapons, 2nd ed. Ft. Detrick, MD, USAMRIID, 1997.
4. Franz DR: Jahrling BP, Friedlander AM, et al: Clinical recognition and management of patients exposed to biological warfare agents. JAMA 278:399–411, 1997.
5. Holloway HC, Norwood AE, Fullerton CS, et al: The threat of biological weapons: Prophylaxis and mitigation of psychological and social consequences. JAMA 278:425–427, 1997.
6. Kaufmann AF, Meltzer MI, Schmid GP, et al: The economic impact of a bioterrorist attack: Are prevention and postattack intervention programs justifiable? Emerg Inf Dis 3:83–94, 1997.
7. Lederberg J: Infectious disease and biological weapons: Prophylaxis and mitigation. JAMA 257:435–436, 1997.
8. Roberts B (ed): Terrorism with Chemical and Biological Weapons. Alexandria, VA, Chemical and Biological Arms Control Institute, 1997.
9. Takafuji ET, Johnson-Winegar A, Zajtchuk R: Medical challenges in chemical and biological defense for the 21st century. In Zajtchuk R (ed): Medical Aspects of Chemical and Biological Warfare. Washington, DC, Borden Institute, 1997, pp 677–685.

10. Sidell FR: Nerve agents. In Zajtchuk R (ed): Medical Aspects of Chemical and Biological Warfare. Washington, DC, Borden Institute, 1997, pp 129–179.
11. Sidell FR: Triage of chemical casualties. In Zajtchuk R (ed): Medical Aspects of Chemical and Biological Warfare. Washington, DC, Borden Institute, 1997, pp 337–349.
12. Sidell FR, Urbanetti JS, Smith WJ, et al: Vesicants. In Zajtchuk R (ed): Medical Aspects of Chemical and Biological Warfare. Washington, DC, Borden Institute, 1997, pp 197–228.
13. Torok TJ, Tauxe RV, Wise RP: A large community outbreak of salmonellosis caused by intentional contamination of restaurant salad bars. JAMA 278:389–395, 1997.

24. WORK-RELATED MUSCULOSKELETAL DISORDERS: ERGONOMICS AND TREATMENT OPTIONS

Jonathan Dropkin, M.S., P.T., C.I.E., and
Ellen Kolber, M.S., M.A., O.T.R., C.H.T., C.I.E.

1. What are the risk factors for work-related musculoskeletal disorders (WMSD)?
- Repeated exertions
- Awkward and extreme postures
- Static and confined positions
- Excessive force
- Lack of rest/imbalance between rest and activity
- Psychosocial stressors
- Mechanical stresses
- Vibration
- Cold temperatures

2. What is ergonomics and how is it related to biomechanical stress?
Ergonomics is the application of knowledge about human abilities and limitations to the design of tools, machines, systems, tasks, and environments. Ergonomic design helps prevent injuries by reducing biomechanical stress. Biomechanical stress is the interaction between mechanical properties of human tissue and the response of those tissues to mechanical stresses. Ergonomic design ensures safe and productive human functioning through minimization of this biomechanical stress.

3. What is anthropometry and why is it important to the field of ergonomics?
Anthropometry is the study of measurements of the human body in terms of size, mass, shape, joint properties, physical strength, and joint range of motion. The results include the acquisition of statistical data that describe human size, mass, and form. The development of sophisticated methodologic models that analyze human movement and function are additional outcomes of this research. There are a number of important considerations in regard to anthropometry and ergonomics. Because the design of seating, tools, and space layout tends to be targeted toward the middle 90% of the population, the smallest 5% and the largest 5% of the population have a greater risk of injury and are more likely to have problems functioning in the average space. Retrofit solutions may be effective in compensating for some design inadequacies. Adequate adjustability to accommodate all workers who use a worksite helps address the issue of size variation. Matching strength demands of the job with strength capabilities of the workers is also an important consideration.

4. What are the elements of a successful ergonomics program?
A successful program should include the following:
- Surveillance of health and safety records to determine patterns of work-related musculoskeletal illnesses
- Job analysis to determine worker exposures to ergonomic hazards that cause work-related musculoskeletal illnesses
- Job (re)design to reduce or eliminate ergonomic hazards
- Training of employers and employees in the identification and control of ergonomic hazards
- Medical management of injured workers

5. Who should oversee an ergonomics program?
To actively control work-related musculoskeletal illnesses, a job analysis team should be organized to oversee the ergonomics program. Responsibility and participation by management are needed for an effective job analysis team. Management representatives may include plant

manager, plant nurse, heads of production departments, safety manager, engineering manager, purchasing manager, maintenance manager, and frontline supervisors. Management also should perform routine reviews of the ergonomics program to make sure that team goals are met. Because job analysis teams concentrate on improving the interrelationship between workers and their jobs, employee involvement (safety stewards in plants with unions, production employees in plants without unions) is important in assuring the success of an ergonomics program. Other members of the team may include an occupational health professional (physician, physical therapist or occupational therapist), an industrial hygienist, and an ergonomist.

6. What is the role of the primary care physician in performing an ergonomic job analysis?

Although ergonomists are ideally suited to evaluate the workplace and make recommendations regarding proper ergonomic design, most clinicians do not have access to an ergonomist. In the absence of an ergonomist, it is important for the physician to evaluate the patient's workplace exposures to ergonomic hazards. Much of the information gathered about the patient's job, including work operation(s) and work task(s), can be done in the physician's office. Often this can be performed by using exposure questionnaires and by job simulation. Questions focused on exposure to ergonomic risk factors, including repetitive movements, awkward and/or static postures, forceful exertions, and extremes in temperature, can supply much of the qualitative information that may be required for job analysis. Having the worker bring in tools or equipment, using mock-ups located in the physician's office, and job simulation can assist the physician in gathering data and making recommendations that are appropriate for the individual worker.

7. What specific industries or occupations are particularly at risk for ergonomic illnesses?

A number of occupational factors have been identified as probable causes of ergonomic illnesses, including repetition, prolonged trunk or upper limb intensive activities, forceful exertions, awkward and/or static posture, whole body or segmental vibration, temperature extremes, and localized mechanical stress. Ergonomic illnesses related to these factors have become the most common category of work-related illnesses in the United States, affecting workers in a variety of industries and occupations. Such industries and occupations include building trades workers (e.g., construction workers), food preparation workers (e.g., frozen food packers, fruit and vegetable canning workers, poultry workers), clerical workers (e.g., typists), textile workers (e.g., garment workers), manufacturing workers (e.g., plastics manufacturers, bearing manufacturers, tire and rubber workers), health care workers (e.g., convalescent and nursing home workers, dental hygienists), foundry workers (e.g., iron foundry workers, metal casting workers, iron and steel production workers), lumber production workers (e.g., forestry workers), grocery checkers, industrial workers (e.g., aircraft engine workers), and packing house workers (e.g., fish cannery workers).

8. What methods can be used to prevent injuries caused by poor ergonomics in the workplace?

Modification of potential ergonomic exposures is important to prevent musculoskeletal illnesses. Ergonomic exposures associated with poor ergonomics can be reduced ideally with engineering controls (e.g., changes in machines, tools, and workstation layout). While awaiting the implementation of engineering controls, administrative controls may be used. Administrative controls include changes in work practices and policies, reduction of shift length or overtime, work enlargement through addition of work elements not requiring motions similar to the current work cycle, increases in rest breaks, rotation of workers through strenuous jobs, worker training and education in risk reduction techniques, and changes in patterns of work and time of task. Although administrative controls are less expensive, they should not be considered a substitute for the more effective engineering controls.

9. What general advice may be offered to workers concerning methods to reduce the risk of injury?

• Have the worksite arranged in an optimal ergonomic configuration. Encourage workers to ask for assistance from their superiors, human resources person, or union representative if more information or help is needed.

- Improve body awareness and attention to posture of the the trunk and the extremities. Observe levels of fatigue and discomfort.
- Vary and pace overall work activities. A break schedule of very short duration rest breaks taken frequently is more valuable than long breaks concentrated to one or two periods in the work day.
- Create a habit of making subtle adjustments and readjustments at the worksite to address various task performance needs and size.
- Use postures and muscle tone that minimize strain.
- Create a habit of checking your posture and how tense your muscles are. Incorporate tension-reducing activities intermittently throughout the day.

10. What is the proper set-up for a computer worksite?

Use of a footrest when the keyboard cannot adjust low enough is permissible, although its use introduces overall balance and constraint of position. Worksite guidelines are as follows:

Chair should:
- Provide support for the lower and upper back
- Allow feet to fully contact the floor or footrest
- Allow thighs to be parallel to the floor
- Provide support to lower and upper back
- Allow the user to get comfortably close to work surfaces
- Arm rests are optional but should not confine the user or put pressure on the arms

Monitor should:
- Be positioned so that the top of the screen is at or slightly below eye level
- Be placed directly in front of the user
- Have correct lighting or glare filter
- Be at a distance of about 2 ft away from the user, based on user comfort

Copy should be positioned directly adjacent to or below the monitor with the use of document holders.

Keyboard and mouse should:
- Be positioned in front of and close to the user
- Facilitate elbow positioning of 90° or slightly greater, necessitating a keyboard surface that is generally lower than standard desk height
- Promote the use of straight wrists

Wrist rests may be used with the following proviso: some evidence suggests that while typing it is better to use the rests more as a guide to maintain straight wrists than as a perch to rest on.

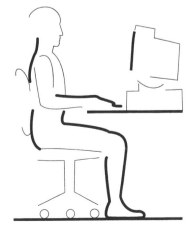

The generally accepted standard for optimal computer worksite configuration.

11. What are some of the common ergonomic problems found in many computer worksites?

Common problems include:

- People incorrectly place their keyboards and mice on their desks, which positions the devices too high for most users. Most people need to have a keyboard and mouse tray or an adjustable table to position these devices at the correct height.
- People often do not account for the placement of the mouse. The keyboard may be positioned correctly, but the mouse is often placed on some distant surface, requiring increased static muscle contraction and frequent long reaches.
- People acquire so-called "ergonomic" keyboards and mice, thinking that they prevent injury. Some of these devices do help limit the effects of assuming certain postures; however, it is more important to address the overall configuration/layout first before dealing with the individual components.
- Even if a perfect ergonomic set-up and computer components are provided, injury will result if the duration of the computer use exceeds the capacity of the tissues.
- People often place the monitor on top of the computer, which tends to position the monitor too high and may lead to neck pain. The computer can be removed and placed elsewhere to allow the monitor to be lowered. Larger monitors make an ideal height more difficult to obtain.

12. Do specific exercises that have been shown to prevent the onset of upper extremity symptoms (e.g., in heavy computer users) exist?

The effective use of exercise as a means of primary prevention is unclear; however, clinical evidence suggests that certain types of exercise enhance soft tissue function. Stretches and light range of motion exercises warm up soft tissue (see figure, top of next page). However, it is highly speculative as to whether strengthening exercise can be effective in fortifying the body to better tolerate ergonomic risk factors. Over-fatiguing muscles may be more risky if zealous efforts of strengthening are combined with a high-risk job.

13. What factors in regard to the use of exercise programs for the treatment of established WMSD cases should be considered?

The performance of exercise should not cause an increase in symptoms. Acute patients should generally be treated with gentle stretches and range of motion exercises of the involved arms or hands. Heavy strengthening exercises of painful upper extremities should be avoided. The strengthening of postural muscles, which include the upper back and stomach muscles, serves to improve posture and metabolic efficiency. Aerobic exercise that can be performed without increasing symptoms may be of benefit as a result of its effect upon microcirculation and healing.

14. What types of treatment modalities do occupational therapists (OTs) and physical therapists (PTs) use with patients who have WMSDs?

General therapy treatment methods include the use of:

- Heat (from hot packs, paraffin, and ultrasound)
- Cold (from ice or cold packs)
- Electrical stimulation (aids in the metabolic activity of muscles)
- Phonophoresis (ultrasound used to introduce a topical antiinflammatory medication such as cortisone)
- Iontophoresis (use of an electrical charge to introduce ions of medication to injured tissue)
- Massage (believed to provide a number of beneficial effects, including increasing circulation to injured tissue and remodeling the collagen [sometimes termed scar tissue] that has been deposited within the injured structure so that it is more like normal noninjured tissue)
- Exercise (see question 13)
- Treatment to improve functional deficits (training in the use of alternate patterns of movement and adaptive equipment to reduce forces to soft tissue)

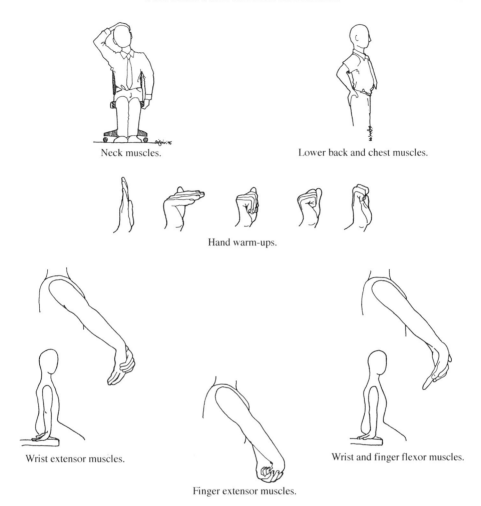

Neck muscles.

Lower back and chest muscles.

Hand warm-ups.

Wrist extensor muscles.

Finger extensor muscles.

Wrist and finger flexor muscles.

Stretches and warm-ups enhance blood flow and the viscoelasticity of muscles and tendons. NOTE: perform carefully and with caution; discontinue exercising if discomfort is felt.

- Provision of orthotics and wearing programs (splints used to rest or position the hand, wrist, and forearm)
- Contrast baths (alternating soaks in warm and cool water, 10–15 minutes each, several times/day, to improve circulation to areas with pain)

15. When should a patient with WMSD be referred to OT and when should the patient be referred to PT?

Deciding which is best may be difficult because the two fields overlap considerably, and differences in philosophy and methods used by individual clinicians within their own disciplines exist. Therefore, knowing the individual therapist's approach is important. However, some referral guidelines do apply:

1. OTs are generally better trained in addressing functional status, such as worksite and return-to-work issues, splint fabrication, and treatment of the smaller muscle groups of the hands.

2. PTs are generally better trained in the use of the electrical modalities described in question 14. They address trunk posture and the larger stabilizing muscles of the body.

Both OTs and PTs can be certified hand therapists (CHTs), an orthopedic specialization that may apply to both disciplines. CHTs focus mainly on acute and subacute injuries of the upper extremities.

16. Are splints helpful in treating injuries of the hand, wrist, and forearm? If so, how should they be used?

Splints are used to rest or position injured forearms, wrists, and hands. Total immobilization, which is required after fracture, for example, is not required for the treatment of WMSDs and may, in fact, be counter-productive. Atrophy and soft-tissue shortening are among the problems of excessive immobilization.

Prefabricated splints may be bought. Splints made by a therapist are known as custom-made splints. For either type, several points should be considered:

1. A very good fit is necessary in order to avoid pressure on bony or soft tissue structures, such as the ulna and radial styloids on distal lateral and medial aspects of the wrist. There should not be any pressure from the splint on the body.

2. They should be effective in limiting unwanted motions and allowing noninvolved joints and structures to fully clear the confines of the splint.

3. A typical splint program prescribes the use of splints at night for positioning and during the day for limited rest periods. A light daytime support may be used for performing daily activities.

4. Wrist splints used during active hand use, such as while using the keyboard and mouse, are not generally recommended because of the effect of the splint on distal joints, general patterns of movement, and on local soft tissue structures.

5. The angle of wrist extension of the type of wrist splint used for carpal tunnel syndrome should not be > 10–15°.

BIBLIOGRAPHY

1. Centers for Disease Control: Occupational disease surveillance. MMWR 38:485–489, 1989.
2. Chaffin DB, Andersson GBJ: Occupational Biomechanics. New York, John Wiley & Sons, 1991.
3. Chapanis A: To communicate the human factors message you have to know what the message is and how to communicate it. Keynote address at HFAC/ACE Conference, Edmonton, Alberta, Canada, 1988. Also reprinted in Hum Factors 34(11):1–4, 1991; 35(1):3–6, 1992.
4. Grandjean E: Ergonomics in Computerized Offices. Philadelphia, Taylor & Francis, 1992.
5. Keyserling WM: Occupational ergonomics: Promoting safety and health through work design. In Levy B, Wegman D (eds): Occupational Health: Recognizing and Preventing Work-Related Disease, 3rd ed. New York, Little, Brown, 1995.
6. Kroemer KHE, Grandjean E: Fitting the Task to the Man. Philadelphia, Taylor & Francis, 1997.
7. Nordin M, Frankel VH: Basic Biomechanics of the Musculoskeletal System. Philadelphia, Lea & Febiger, 1989.

25. HEALTH HAZARDS OF VIBRATION

Martin Cherniack, M.D., M.P.H.

1. What is the difference between whole-body vibration and segmental vibration?

Whole-body vibration refers to vibration transmitted to the entire human body, usually through a supportive structure such as an industrial platform or vehicle seat. Key anatomic sites of resonance occur at relatively low frequencies; for example, in the trunk and torso at 5 Hz and in the head and shoulder at 20–30 Hz. Segmental or hand-arm vibration is associated with specific clinical lesions, involving the fingers, hands, and wrists, originates in the upper extremity from direct contact with vibrating tools and instruments, and is generally associated with higher transmitted tool frequencies (200–500 Hz) that are absorbed below the level of the elbow.

2. What are the major health effects of whole-body vibration?

Whole-body vibration acts as a general stressor with short-term detrimental effects on visual and manual tracking. There are associations between low back disease in interstate truckers and exposure to road vibration. Frequencies below 1 Hz have been associated with motion sickness. Because potential exposures occur over a mixed frequency range and because associated chronic conditions, such as hypertension, have multiple etiologies, a distinct exposure-disease profile is lacking. Although the predominance of biomedical writing and the best-recognized clinic syndromes involve segmental vibration, the largest population of vibration-exposed workers are commercial vehicle drivers, whose exposure is to whole-body vibration.

3. What are the major health effects of segmental or hand-arm vibration?

Well-characterized neurologic and vascular signs and syndromes have been associated with the regular use of hand-held vibrating tools. Examples include damage to unmyelinated nociceptors in the fingertips and to myelinated larger nerve fibers in the fingers, hands, and wrists; cold-induced vasospasm (Raynaud's phenomenon) affecting the fingers; and soft tissue pain, usually affecting the forearms. Hand pain and paresthesias, decreased tactile perception, and symptoms consistent with focal nerve compression are among the most common clinical neurologic signs. A complex pattern of loss of forearm and hand strength also has been noted; its etiology is less clearly defined, but it is a major source of functional incapacity.

4. How does hand-arm vibration syndrome differ from vibration white fingers?

Beginning with the earliest clinical descriptions more than 80 years ago, the most striking clinical feature caused by exposure to hand-arm vibration has been cold-induced finger blanching or Raynaud's phenomenon. Hence, the historical descriptive term **vibration white fingers (VWF)**. By the 1980s it was clear that the neurologic deficits and symptoms produced by hand-arm vibration were objectively quantifiable and could occur independently of vascular symptoms. Accordingly a new clinical rating scheme—the Stockholm Scale—was introduced in 1987 to establish separate grading criteria for vascular and neurologic signs and symptoms. The term **hand-arm vibration syndrome (HAVS)** has been recommended as inclusive of multiple tissue pathologies. In referring only to vasospastic disease, VWF is fully acceptable.

5. What is the distinction between acceleration and frequency—the units used to represent vibration exposures?

Vibration, whether segmental or whole-body, is a mechanical oscillation, the energy content of which is most often expressed in terms of units of **acceleration**. The time component of tool acceleration is referred to as the root mean square (rms) and may be expressed as m/sec^2, g (1 g = 9.8 m/sec^2), or decibels relative to 10^{-6} m/sec^2.

The number of oscillations per second is called the **frequency** and is expressed in Hertz (hz). In almost all occupational settings, several different frequencies occur either simultaneously or sequentially from the same tool, and frequency characterization, as well as translation into units of acceleration, requires an analytic transformation. This transformation is usually done with constant relative band widths, in the form of one-third octave band widths, such as 6.3 Hz, 8.0, and 12.5 Hz. Accelerations at each of these one-third octave bands are then added together to determine the sum of energy from a particular tool over its observed range of oscillations (frequency spectrum). A major controversy involves whether each of the one-third octave band-specific acceleration measurements should be graded equally or whether certain frequencies, considered less injurious, should be discounted (weighting).

6. What occupations are most associated with the development of HAVS? How frequently does it occur?

Workers who use vibratory tools that are either air-powered, such as grinders and impact wrenches, or reciprocating, such as chainsaws, commonly experience upper extremity symptoms. Other hand-held tools producing vibration and implicated in the presentation of HAVS include rock drills, rivet guns, chipping or pneumatic hammers, jackhammers and pavement breakers, brush saws, burring machines, and cutting wheels.

A more subtle finding has been neurologic deficits and occasionally vasospastic disease in users of dental tools, surgical saws and drills, and ultrasound devices. The latter syndromes are intriguing but also problematic because the principal frequencies of biomedical instruments are several thousands Hz above presumed biologic effect.

7. What are the best tests for diagnosing the vascular and neurologic components of HAVS?

The best quantitative test for evaluating the vascular component of HAVS is cold-challenge plethysmography, a highly specialized procedure that uses strain gauges and temperature-regulated occlusion cuffs to detect cold-induced arterial spasm. A traditional visual test involving upper extremity immersion in ice water and observation for Raynaud's attacks is no longer widely used because of cumbersomeness and patient discomfort. Some investigators have recorded finger temperature recovery after water immersion as an index of Raynaud's phenomenon. This test has not been recommended by consensus bodies; therefore, interpretation must rely on local experience and validation.

More testing devices and approaches are applicable to neurologic assessment. Nerve conduction studies remain the best method for evaluating injury to myelinated fiber. Because injuries may occur in the finger and palms as well as at the site of familiar entrapment syndromes (carpal tunnel, canal of Guyon), conventional distal segment sensory measurements are often insufficiently discriminatory. Fractionating or "inching" techniques along the median nerve are more subtle and accurate.

Sensory testing includes new automated and quantitative modalities as well as traditional clinical tests (e.g., pain, light touch, 2-point discrimination, gap detection). The Stockholm Workshop, a regularly convening nongovernmental body that advises on HAVS, recommends vibrotactile testing at single or multiple frequencies as the preferred test. An extensive medical literature focuses on finger receptor deficits in patients exposed to segmental vibration, which are recognized by vibrotactile testing. Other potentially useful but less validated quantitative tests include temperature perception thresholds and current perception thresholds.

8. Does hand-arm vibration cause carpal tunnel syndrome? Is carpal tunnel release surgery helpful?

In many studies of occupationally associated or acquired carpal tunnel syndrome, exposure to vibratory hand tools has been identified as an important risk factor. In addition, patients with documented carpal tunnel syndrome who are also exposed to vibration have a less successful response to surgery and poorer long-term functional outcomes. Two different, although not exclusive, explanations have been proposed for these observations. One explanation stresses biomechanical factors, tightened grip, and awkward tool-handling postures that produce either tension in the flexor tendon digitorum or flexor tendon synovitis and raised intracarpal pressures. In this conventional biomechanical explanation, vibration does not injure the median nerve directly but contributes to a work-practice problem. An alternate view emphasizes direct nerve injury due to leakage and effusion from small blood vessels, edema, and fibrosis—a process more similar to generally distributed neuropathies. In support of this direct neuropathic view are the patterns of digital nerve fibrosis observed in vibratory tool users and direct vibration-induced nerve injury in laboratory animals.

Distinguishing between these two patterns may have important clinical implications. A direct neuropathy is less amenable to surgical release, but it also involves the potential for misdiagnosis and ineffective or harmful treatment. Slowed distal nerve conduction in industrial workers in the absence of clinical signs or symptoms has been described in as many as 40% of symptomatic blue collar workers. Digital paresthesias produced by vibratory damage to small nerve fibers may coexist with clinically benign nerve slowing, leading to a presumption of focal nerve entrapment at the wrist. Without good quantitative sensory testing, differentiation is difficult.

9. How should patients with HAVS be clinically staged and treated?

The Stockholm Workshop has developed a staging system for both neurologic and vascular components of HAVS. Vascular stages reflect the number of involved fingers, and the frequency and severity of attacks. The neurologic deficit scale extends progressively from pain and discomfort to impaired perception and functional performance compromise. Although the scale is useful for longitudinal comparison and clarity of staging, it is probably best appreciated for its independent staging of vascular and neurologic components.

Cessation or attenuation of exposure is a necessary part of any treatment plan, because clinical interventions are suboptimal. For vasospastic disease, calcium channel blockers are usually helpful, but side effects may prove unacceptable in a young workforce. A more conservative intervention involves the use of battery-heated gloves and mittens in cold weather.

In patients with apparent median nerve mononeuropathies, carpal tunnel surgery should be a treatment option only in the presence of a well-characterized focal compression and after diffuse injury to small fibers has been ruled out. Dermatomal specificity of symptoms may be helpful in the differentiation. When intrinsic nerve swelling contributes to symptoms, exposure cessation and splinting or compression may produce dramatic improvement over several weeks.

Injury to small nerve fibers is generally not amenable to treatment. Vitamin B_6 has no evident clinical role. Anticonvulsants should be used as in other pain management applications. Long-term deficits from clinically advanced small fiber injuries are likely to persist.

10. What is vibration weighting? Why does the National Institute for Occupational Safety and Health (NIOSH) recommend against weighting, whereas the International Standards Organization (ISO) and the American National Standards Institute (ANSI) support its use?

The one-third octave band, center frequency-weighted acceleration has been the general measure of vibration exposure levels. Most international standards bodies, including the ISO and ANSI, recommend filtering upper frequencies so that frequencies from 6.3–16 Hz are measured at unity and progressive frequencies from 16–1500 Hz are reduced in the summing of accelerations. This model originates from observations (first introduced 30 years ago) that adverse clinical effect is associated with subjective discomfort. Subjective discomfort is more dominant at lower frequencies. The limitations of this model are widespread and generally recognized. For example, VWF, a vascular disorder, has no etiologic association with perceptions of discomfort. Furthermore, growing evidence indicates that the most damaging frequencies for nociceptive and vascular injury occur in the 200–500 Hz range but are not as subjectively unpleasant as the more heavily weighted lower frequencies. Predictive models that discount higher frequencies tend to overpredict disease from lower frequency tools, such as chainsaws, and to underpredict disease from tools, such as small burring devices, that generate higher frequencies.

Recognizing the deficiencies of the rating scheme, NIOSH has recommended against weighting. But this approach is also problematic. Because many tools produce a frequency spectrum that extends to 5000 Hz and above, the sheer bulk of higher-frequency measurements, many of which probably produce little adverse biologic effect, results in an overwhelming additive effect, producing summed accelerations that are too large and dispersed for practical use. It is likely that an eventual consensus will include weighting, but only above frequencies at which biologic effect is significant. For now, however, the issue remains unsettled.

11. Do high-speed tools such as dental drills and orthopedic saws pose any risk to their users?

Issues related to weighting and high-speed tool risks are pertinent to the preceding question. Several mitigating considerations are involved. In dentists, ergonomic factors, including consequences of tight gloving, may be more significant than drill speeds, given evolving drill technology. Hand problems in diagnostic ultrasonographers are almost certainly due to biomechanical factors. However, the lower frequencies involved in therapeutic ultrasound may prove to be a potential hazard, as reported in some medical literature. Abnormalities in bone harvesters seem better established because of the high degree of quantitation. Although further study is appropriate, biologic likelihood places greater emphasis on ergonomic factors than on pure vibratory exposures. However, this area is underresearched, and people in the above occupations with symptoms of early neuropathy should be assessed with the assumption that incumbent nerve damage is involved rather than a more amorphous cumulative trauma disorder.

12. Does the use of antivibration gloves or protective tool wraps prevent exposures that lead to HAVS?

Various synthetic rubber and elastic materials have been developed and marketed for the antivibration properties. Gloves and tool handle wraps are two of the most common protective applications. Two important factors are effectiveness of the material and its practical force reduction properties, given changes in grip or handling.

Antivibration materials appear to be highly effective in filtering out higher frequencies, but the protective effect is more limited in the predominant range of biologic effect. Overall, effective reduction from antivibration wraps and gloves appears to be in 10–30% range. The effect may be somewhat higher with smaller tools that operate at higher frequencies. Simple bulk wrapping may amplify exposure from lower-frequency inertial tools if the consequence is a tighter reactive grip.

Gloves and wraps are an important part of a vibration reduction program. Wraps, in particular, should be applied by professionals familiar with their use. Antivibration conversion kits are an efficient way to wrap and modify tools, but the caveats about bulky application still apply. Generic tool conversion kits also may alter force planes and other characteristics of exposure.

13. Is noise exposure a contributor to HAVS?

Several reports suggest that noise-induced hearing loss is more frequent among vibration-exposed workers. Hearing loss is certainly not a mechanical effect but appears to involve centrally mediated neurologic phenomena. Because hearing loss seems more common in impact types of pneumatic tools, it is also possible that tool-related noise levels have been inadequately measured. In any case, added attention to noise attenuation is clearly advisable.

14. Does smoking cause HAVS?

Smoking does not cause HAVS and has no clear-cut impact on neurologic symptoms. Because nicotine is a vasoconstrictor, smoking aggravates vascular attacks and increases their frequency. For related reasons, beta blockers used as antihypertensives also may aggravate VWF attacks.

BIBLIOGRAPHY

1. Ahlborg G, Voog L: Vibration exposure and distal compression of the median nerve ("carpal tunnel syndrome"). Lakartidningen 79:4905–4908, 1982.

2. American National Standards Institute: Guide for the measurement and evaluation of human exposure to vibration transmitted to the hand. New York, American National Standards Institute [ANSI S3.34], 1986.

3. Brammer A, Taylor W, Piercy J: Assessing the severity of the neurologic component of the hand-arm vibration syndrome. Scand J Work Environ Health 12:428–431, 1986.

4. Brammer A, Taylor W, Lundborg G: Sensorineural stages of the hand-arm vibration syndrome. Scand J Work Environ Health 13:279–283, 1987.

5. Cherniack M, Mohr S: Raynaud's phenomenon associated with the use of pneumatically powered surgical instruments. J Hand Surg 19A:1008–1015, 1994.

6. Dandanell R, Engstrom K: Vibration from riveting tools in the frequency range 6 Hz to 10 MHz and Raynaud's phenomenon. Scand J Work Environ Health 12:38–42, 1986.

7. Ekenvall L, Gemne G, Tegner R: Correspondence between neurologic symptoms and outcome of quantitative sensory testing in the hand-arm vibration syndrome. Br J Indust Med 46:570–574, 1989.

8. Farkkila M, Pyykko I, Korhonen O, Starck J: Vibration-induced decrease in the muscle force in lumber jacks. Eur J Appl Physiol 43:1–9, 1980.

9. Gemne G, Pyykko I, Taylor W, Pelmear PL: The Stockholm Workshop scale for the classification of cold-induced Raynaud's phenomenon in the hand-arm vibration syndrome. Scand J Work Environ Health 13:275–278, 1987.

10. Gruber G: Relationship between whole-body vibration and morbidity patterns among interstate truck drivers. Washington, DC, DHEW Publication No. (NIOSH) 77-167, 1976.

11. Hagberg M, Nystrom A, Zetterlund B: Recovery from symptoms after carpal tunnel syndrome surgery in males in relation to vibration exposure. J Hand Surg 16A:66–71, 1991.

12. Hjortsberg U, Rosen I, Orbaek P, et al: Finger receptor dysfunction in dental technicians exposed to high-frequency vibration. Scand J Work Environ Health 15:339–344, 1989.

13. Iki M, Jurumatani N, Hirata K, Moriyama: An association between Raynaud's phenomenon and hearing loss in forestry workers. Am Indust Hyg Assoc J 46:509–513, 1985.

14. International Standards Organization: Guide for the Measurement and Evaluation of Human Exposure to Whole-body Vibration (ISO2631). Geneva, International Standards Organization, 1974.

15. International Standards Organization: Mechanical Vibration—Guidelines for the Measurement and the Assessment of Human Exposure to Hand-transmitted Vibration. Geneva, International Organization for Standardization, Ref. No. ISO 5349-1986, 1986.

16. Juntunen J, Matikainen E, Seppalainen A, Laine A: Peripheral neuropathy and vibration syndrome. Int Arch Environ Health 52:17–24, 1983.

17. Juul E, Nielsen SL: Locally induced digital vasospasm detected by delayed rewarming in Raynaud's phenomenon of occupational origin. Br J Indust Med 38:87–90, 1981.

18. Koskimies K, Farkkila M, Pyykko I, et al: Carpal tunnel syndrome in vibration disease. Br J Indust Med 47:411–416, 1990.

19. Lundstrom R, Lindmark A: Effects of local vibration on tactile perception in the hands of dentists. J Low Freq Noise Vib 1:1–11, 1982.

20. Lundstrom R: Effects of local vibration transmitted from ultrasonic devices on vibrotactile perception on the hands of therapists. Ergonomics 28:793–803, 1985.

21. Matoba T, Mizobuchi H, Ito T, et al: Further observations of the digital plethysmography in response to auditory stimuli and its clinical applications. Angiology 32:62–72, 1981.

22. Miwa T: Evaluation methods for vibration effects. Part 6: Measurements of unpleasant and tolerance limit levels for sinusoidal vibrations. Ind Health 6:18–27, 1968.

23. Miwa T: Evaluation methods for vibration effects. Part 4: Measurements of vibration greatness for whole body and hand in vertical and horizontal vibrations. Ind Health 6:1–10, 1986.

24. National Institute of Occupational Safety and Health: Criteria for a Recommended Standard. Occupational Exposure to Hand-Arm Vibration. Washington, DC, DHHS #89-106, 1989.

25. Olsen N: Quantitative diagnostic tests in VWF. In Hand Arm Vibration Syndrome: Diagnostics and Quantitative Relationships to Exposure. Stockholm Workshop, Arbets Milio Institute, 1994.

26. Pelmear PL, Leong D, Taylor W, et al: Measurement of vibration of hand-held tools: Weighted or unweighted? J Occup Med 31:902–908, 1989.

27. Pyykko I: The prevalence and symptoms of traumatic vasospastic disease among lumberjacks in Finland: A field study. Work Environ Health 11:118–131, 1974.

28. Rawlinson R: Are we assessing hand-arm vibration correctly? J Low Freq Noise Vib 14:53–60, 1991.

29. Riddle H, Taylor W: Vibration-induced white finger among chain sawyers nine years after the introduction of anti-vibration measures. In Taylor W, Pelmear PL (eds): Vibration White Finger in Industry. New York, John Wiley & Sons, 1982, pp 169–172.

30. Rosen I, Stromberg T, Lundborg G: Neurophysiological investigation of hands damaged by vibration: A comparison with idiopathic carpal tunnel syndrome. Scand J Plast Reconstr Hand Surg 27:209–216, 1993.

31. Rothstein T: Report of the physical findings in eight stonecutters from the limestone region of Indiana. Washington, DC, Government Printing Office, 1918.
32. Sakakibara H, Hirata M, Haxhiguchi T, et al: Measurement of digital nerve conduction velocity for detecting peripheral neuropathy in vibration syndrome. In Hand Arm Vibration Syndrome: Diagnostics and Quantitative Relationships to Exposure. Stockholm Workshop, Arbets Milio Institute, 1994.
33. Taylor W: Hand-arm vibration syndrome: A new clinical classification and updated British standard guide for hand-transmitted vibration. Br J Indust Med 45:281–282, 1988.

26. NOISE AND HEARING CONSERVATION

Robert D. Madory, M.A.

1. How many workers in the United States are exposed to potentially hazardous levels of noise?

More than 25 million workers in the U.S. are exposed to potentially hazardous levels of noise at their workplace. Because noise is the most frequently occurring noxious agent in the industrial setting, this number should come as no surprise. The above estimate comes from combining the numbers of workers in the construction, manufacturing, military, mining, and transportation industries. No figures have been published for workers exposed to noise in the farming and entertainment industries or in occupations concomitantly exposed to noise and environmental factors with synergistic or additive effects, such as ototoxic chemicals and vibration. Therefore, 25 million people must be viewed as a conservative estimate.

2. What units are used to measure noise?

The loudness of a sound correlates with the amplitude or intensity and is measured in decibels (dB). Pitch correlates with the frequency or cycles per second and is measured in Hertz (Hz).

3. Why does one plus one not equal two in adding decibels?

The decibel is the logarithm of a ratio of two sound powers or pressures. The range of intensities that the human ear is capable of perceiving is enormous. If sound pressure for this range were viewed in terms of an absolute ratio, it would vary from 1 (auditory threshold) to 1,000,000 (threshold of discomfort). Because measurements and calculations with such large numbers would be cumbersome, a nonlinear scale such as the decibel is beneficial. Because of this nonlinearity, one plus one does not equal two. For example, if a worker is in a room with a machine producing 90 db(A) of noise and management decides to add another identical machine with an output of 90 db(A), the total noise in the room will not be raised to 180 dB(A) but rather to 93 dB(A). The reason for the 3 dB-increase becomes evident when the decibel formula for power is considered:

$$dB = 10 \log_{10}(P_1/P_2)$$

where P_1 is the power experienced and P_2 is the reference power level. In the above example of adding two identical sound sources, the output is doubled. By plugging in 2/1 in the power section, the formula becomes:

$$dB = 10 \log_{10}(2)$$
$$\text{Log of } 2 = 0.3$$
$$dB = 10(0.3) = 3 \text{ dB}$$

4. Is it necessary to have a scientific calculator or log tables to add decibels?

Fortunately it is not. If one memorizes a few mathematical relationships, it is possible to make reasonable estimates in adding decibels for outputs in industrial settings.

Frequently Used Multipliers for Adding Decibels

MULTIPLIER	POWER
2	3 dB
3	5 dB
10	10 dB

Continuing with the example from the previous question, if a worker is in a room with three machines with 90-dB(A) outputs, the total level in the room is 95 dB(A). Ten of the same machines in the workspace would increase the output to 100 dB(A).

5. How is a dB(A) different from a dB(B), dB(C), or dB(D)?

The A, B, C, or D frequently seen after the dB notation refers to the weighting scale used in the measurement of the reported noise. These scales represent modifications of the frequency response of the measurement equipment intended to replicate human perception at various loudness levels. The human ear is less sensitive to lower-frequency sounds, and this pattern changes with the input level. The dB(A) scale has been spectrally shaped to respond like the ear at an input of 40 dB, and the B scale was devised for inputs in the range of 70 dB. The C scale is essentially linear across the entire frequency region, and the D scale is similar to B except for a "bump" in the area of 2000 Hz that reflects the relatively greater human sensitivity in this region.

6. If dB(A) is intended for measuring lower-level inputs, why is the A scale almost universally applied to measures in workplace environments that are much louder?

It is unknown to this author why the A scale is so commonly used. The dB(D) is the best scale for measuring the louder levels of noise typically seen in occupational noise settings. However, many years of accumulating noise measures with the A scale have made it the industry standard, and it will continue to be widely used except for a few specific applications.

7. What is a time-weighted average (TWA)?

The TWA is a single number descriptor of a daily noise dose. The Occupational Safety and Health Administration (OSHA) stipulates that if a worker is exposed to an average of 90 dB(A) for 8 hours, his or her dose is 100%. A noise dose of 100% is defined by OSHA as the **permissible exposure level** (PEL). A dose of 50% corresponds to a TWA of 85 dB(A) and is designated as the **action level**. Workers who are exposed at the action level or above in their work day must be enrolled in a hearing conservation program. If the exposure level is at the PEL or above, workers also must be provided with a variety of appropriate hearing protectors. The following table depicts the OSHA guidelines for maximal allowable length of exposure at various exposure levels.

Permissible Lengths of Exposure for Various Sound Levels

SOUND LEVEL [dB(A)]	PERMISSIBLE TIME (HR)
80	32
85	16
90	8 (PEL)
100	4
105	2
110	0.5
115*	0.25
120	0.125
125	0.063
130	0.031

* Exposures in excess of 115 dB(A) are not allowable in the workplace regardless of duration.

8. The above table provides limits for steady-state noise. Do the same rules apply to impulsive or impact types of noise?

No. OSHA presents different guidelines for impact noise. Noise dosimeters do not accurately measure impulse noise, and the repetitions should be measured separately using a sound level meter.

Impulse Noise Peaks and Allowable Repetitions

IMPULSE PEAKS (DB-SPL)	ALLOWABLE REPETITIONS/DAY
> 140	0
140	100
130–139	1000
120–129	10,000
110–119	100,000
100–109	1,000,000

9. How is a TWA obtained?

The TWA or average noise exposure during a workshift for an employee can be estimated with an area survey technique using a sound level meter. This approach can be reasonably accurate if the noise level is predictable or constant. However, the preferred method for obtaining a TWA is a noise dosimeter worn by the worker. As stated above, if impulse noises are present, a combination of dosimetry and sound level meter survey is recommended.

10. Can a patient who is not knowledgeable about such factors as TWA or dB give information that may be useful in determining the level of noise in his or her workplace?

A valuable rule of thumb helps to determine whether a workplace has potentially hazardous noise levels. If one needs to shout to be heard by a person 3 feet away or less, the level of the noise in the environment is probably 85 dB(A) or greater.

11. What are the best hearing protection devices?

The best hearing protection devices are the ones worn consistently. It has been determined that 90% of the industrial noise-exposed population in the U.S. needs only 10 dB of protection.

12. If only 10 dB of protection is necessary, why not use cotton balls, cigarette butts, or silly putty?

Some homemade protectors may work, but clearly the manufactured plugs and muffs provide more consistent protection along with superior comfort and hygiene.

13. How is the best protector prescribed for a worker?

Rarely is only one device appropriate. It is important to provide an employee with a number of suitable alternatives so that he or she can select a system. It is also essential that the employee is personally instructed in the use of the selected system. The following factors should be considered in recommending hearing protectors:

1. Comfort (the device will not be worn if it is not comfortable)
2. Compatibility with other safety equipment
3. Compatibility with the shape of the worker's ear canal and head size
4. Medical status of ear canal, eardrum, and middle ear (if the patient is prone to otitis externa or has a perforated tympanic membrane with discharge, earplugs should not be used)
5. Employee's ability to manipulate and insert the device properly
6. Appropriateness for the climate (e.g., earmuffs will not be worn in hot humid climates)
7. Compatibility with type of work (e.g., if the work is completed in a confined area, earmuffs may get in the way)
8. Employee's understanding of care, maintenance, and replacement intervals
9. Hearing ability (a plug that is too efficient may dangerously reduce the communication abilities of a person with hearing loss)
10. Attenuation characteristics of the protector or noise reduction rating

14. How can a physician find out about the attenuation characteristics of a hearing protection device?

The Environmental Protection Agency (EPA) has mandated that all hearing protection devices must be labeled with a noise reduction rating (NRR). The NRR allows comparison of the attenuation characteristics of hearing protectors, but it is not effective at predicting real word attenuation values for an individual worker. In comparing NRRs, differences of 3 dB or less are not significant.

15. How is a real-world estimate of a hearing protector's effectiveness obtained?

The following formula is frequently used for estimating the amount of exposure while wearing hearing protection:

$$\text{Estimated exposure [dB(A)]} = \text{TWA [dB(A)]} - (\text{NRR-7})$$

For example, if a worker with a TWA of 95 dB(A) uses earplugs with an NRR of 27, the estimated exposure is $95 - (27 - 7) = 75$ dB(A). The calculation for NRR is currently under revision and will represent real-world attenuation values more closely in the future.

16. Are earmuffs better than earplugs?

If one looks only at the NRRs, earplugs have better attenuation values. However, studies comparing the two systems in the workplace indicate that real-world attenuation values are generally higher for earmuffs than for earplugs. Earmuffs provide an average of 10–12 dB of protection, whereas foam earplugs provide 10 dB of attenuation. Nonfoam plugs provide even less protection.

17. Does hearing protection have a positive effect on areas other than hearing?

Yes. Although studies in these areas are less conclusive than studies of hearing-related issues, the following nonauditory benefits of hearing protection are reported in the literature:

1. Fewer on-the-job injuries
2. Reduction of peripheral circulation problems
3. Reduction of cardiac problems
4. Better concentration for tasks requiring accuracy
5. Improved performance on job tasks requiring attention to multiple signal sources
6. Less absenteeism
7. Reduction of adverse psychological effects and overall stress levels

18. What is the greatest misconception among workers about hearing protectors?

Employees often believe that they will not be able to hear fellow workers, alarms, machines, and signals when using hearing protection. Such is not the case. A worker's ability to hear speech actually improves in high-noise environments when ear protection is used. An exception to this rule is workers with hearing loss, who may be penalized with ear protection in a low-noise environment.

19. How does one motivate a patient to use hearing protectors consistently?

It is difficult for patients to change a behavior. Motivating employees to wear hearing protectors consistently certainly falls in this category. Selling the long-term benefits of no hearing loss later in life often does not work. It is frequently more effective to emphasize more immediate factors:

1. Reduction in overall stress level
2. Less fatigue at the end of the day
3. No feeling of aural numbness after workshift
4. No tinnitus

20. If a worker's exposure level is measured and hearing protectors are recommended, how can the effectiveness of the program be monitored?

One of the most powerful ways to monitor a hearing conservation program is annual audiometric monitoring. The first or baseline audiogram must be completed within the first 6 months of work in an environment with exposure levels at or above 85 dB(A). Monitoring must be supervised by an audiologist, otolaryngologist, or physician. Testing does not need to be completed by an audiologist. If an audiometric technician is used, he or she must be certified by the Council for Accreditation of Occupational Hearing Conservation. Testing must be done in a sound-proof room, and the worker should have no noise exposure over the previous 16 hours. Use of hearing protectors before testing may substitute for this requirement.

21. How much of a change in hearing from year to year should be considered significant?
OSHA guidelines state that a standard threshold shift (STS) is defined as an average shift in excess of 10 dB for 2000, 3000, and 4000 Hz in either ear relative to the baseline audiogram. The Hearing Conservation Amendment allows age corrections by use of a standardized table.

22. If an STS is noted with an employee, what actions should be taken?
Once an STS is observed, the employee should be notified within 20 days. The STS must be recorded in the employee's file. The records of all employees demonstrating such shifts should be evaluated by an audiologist or physician. In appropriate cases medical and audiologic referrals should be made.

23. What are the criteria for medical referral?
The American Academy of Otolaryngology (AAO) has suggested the following criteria for outside referral in hearing conservation programs:
Audiologic criteria
1. Baseline audiogram
   - Average loss > 25 dB hearing threshold level (HTL) for 0.5, 1, 2, and 3 kHz in either ear
   - Average difference between ears > 15 dB HTL for 0.5, 1, and 2 kHz and/or > 30 dB HTL for 3, 4, and 6 kHz
2. Annual audiogram
   - Change from baseline in either ear > 15 dB HTL for 0.5, 1, and 2 kHz and/or > 20 dB HTL for 3, 4, and 6 kHz
Medical criteria: history of any of the following symptoms
1. Ear pain
2. Discharge in external ear
3. Severe or persistent tinnitus
4. Sudden, fluctuating, or rapidly progressive hearing loss
5. Fullness or discomfort in ears
6. Cerumen impaction or foreign body visible in ear canal

24. Does a patient with an STS have a compensable hearing loss?
STS and compensable hearing loss are distinctly different issues. Compensable hearing loss is defined by each state's workers' compensation formula. The following formula is used in many states:
1. Calculate average hearing loss for 500, 1000, 2000, and 3000 Hz in each ear.
2. Subtract 25 from the average in each ear.
3. Convert the average from each ear to a percentage by multiplying by 1.5%.
4. Calculate binaural impairment percentage by multiplying the better monaural percentage by 5 and adding the poorer monaural percentage to the total; then divide by 6.
5. Round to the closest whole number at each step.

Example

FREQUENCY (Hz)	500	1000	2000	3000	4000	6000	8000
Right ear (dB HTL)	10	25	40	55	65	55	45
Left ear (dB HTL)	10	25	45	50	70	50	40

Right ear $(10 + 25 + 40 + 55)/4 = 32$ $\qquad$ Left ear $(10 + 25 \neq 45 + 40)/4 = 30$
Monaural percentage: right ear $= (32 - 25)1.5\% = 10\%$; left ear $= (30 - 25)1.5\% = 7$
Binaural percentage: $5(7\%) = 35\% + 10\% - 45\%/6 = 7\%$

25. What is the typical configuration for industrial noise-induced sensorineural hearing loss?

The typical noise-induced hearing loss is bilateral and symmetric; it predominantly affects the higher frequencies (3, 4, and 6 kHz). The configuration in the example used for compensable hearing loss is typical of noise-induced hearing loss.

26. Why does a broad-spectrum noise predominantly affect only the higher frequencies on an audiogram?

Because of the resonance characteristics of the outer and middle ear and the anatomy of the cochlea and basilar membrane, broad-spectrum noise is physiologically filtered in such a way that it predominantly affects the basal or high-frequency sensitive region of the inner ear.

27. Where is the lesion due to noise exposure located in the inner ear?

The outer hair cells in the basal region of the cochlea are the first to be damaged in the presence of noise. With more chronic exposure, the lesion spreads to the apical or lower-frequency regions of the cochlea and eventually damages the inner hair cells.

28. Are all shifts of hearing permanent?

No. Exposure to a loud sound can temporarily numb the ear so that the person experiences a hearing loss that improves after several hours. This phenomenon is known as temporary threshold shift (TTS). Chronic exposure to noise that causes TTS portends eventual permanent threshold shift (PTS). Therefore, temporary hearing loss after exposure to noise is a good sign that hearing protection should have been worn; it also explains why OSHA stipulates that the worker should not be exposed to noise for 16 hours before audiometric testing.

29. Does simultaneous exposure to noise and chemicals or drugs that damage the cochlea pose a greater risk to hearing?

Certain drugs, such as aminoglycoside antibiotics, loop diuretics, salicylates, and chemotherapy agents, are ototoxic. More recently it has been suggested that exposure to industrial chemicals also may be ototoxic. The damaging effects of noise may be exacerbated by concomitant exposure to certain industrial chemicals and nonchemical environmental factors such as vibration or heat. The following factors may enhance the deleterious effects of noise:

Chemical agents with known additive or synergistic interactions with noise

1. Toluene
2. Carbon disulfide
3. Trichloroethylene
4. Trialkyltins (methyl)
5. Carbon monoxide
6. Cigarette smoke

Ototoxic agents either not influenced by noise exposure or interactions not yet known

1. Butyl nitrite
2. Cyanide
3. Hexane
4. Styrene
5. Xylene
6. Butanol
7. Lead
8. Mercury
9. Trialkyltins
10. Trialkyltins (ethyl)

Environmental factors with known interactions with noise

1. Hand-arm vibration (e.g., chainsaw)
2. Whole-body vibration (e.g., tractor)
3. Elevated ambient temperature
4. Elevated body temperature
5. Physical activity that may result in movement of hearing protectors and thus alters attenuation

30. Many solvents and heavy metals listed above affect the central nervous system. Can it be assumed that retrocochlear pathways are at risk?

As stated above, the site of lesions for noise-induced hearing loss is the cochlea. However, many solvents and heavy metals act on the central aspects of the auditory nervous system.

Because a pure-tone audiogram essentially reflects cochlear function, it is important to use other audiologic measures more sensitive to retrocochlear pathologies in evaluating workers exposed to neurotoxic agents.

31. What audiologic tests are used to evaluate retrocochlear function?

Auditory brainstem response (ABR) measures and, to a lesser extent, acoustic reflex assessment with thresholds and decay are currently considered the best audiologic measures of cranial nerve VIII and lower brainstem pathologies. Pathologies at the upper brainstem and cortical levels are evaluated by more elaborate tests using modified speech stimuli and late auditory-evoked potential measures. Such testing is clearly not practical for screening, but for patients in whom retrocochlear damage is possible they certainly must be considered.

32. What areas of current research are most promising?

A new audiologic testing technique called **otoacoustic emission measures** (OAEs) is based on a recent observation that the ear produces sound in response to acoustic stimulation. This emission is not a passive echo but rather a sound generated by an active process at the level of the outer hair cells. The otoacoustic emission is measured with equipment that presents an acoustic stimulus and records the ear's response with a special ear probe connected to a signal-averaging computer. The measures usually take only a few minutes per ear. In essence, OAE testing directly measures outer hair cell function. Because the outer hair cells are the locus of damage during the incipient stages of noise-induced hearing loss, OAE measures may be able to detect subtle cochlear damage that does not register with traditional audiometry, as some initial studies indicate. More research is under way on this topic and other issues, such as predicting individual susceptibility to noise-induced hearing loss. Because of their high correlation with outer hair cell function, speed, and reliability, OAE measures will soon take their place in hearing conservation testing protocols.

33. What are the new and exciting technologic advances in hearing protectors?

1. The materials and design of passive protectors have been improved to provide more attenuation and to allow easier insertion.

2. Systems have used hearing aid circuit designs that monitor input level and allow lower levels of sound to pass unattenuated while louder sounds are electrically compressed.

3. Active noise reduction systems electronically attenuate incoming sounds by using wave cancellation techniques. This technology has been used in the design of sound systems in cars and airplanes and also in over-the-ear types of protectors. At this point active noise cancellation systems work only for lower-frequency sounds (below 500 Hz). However, in the near future the speed of processors will allow active attenuation in higher-frequency regions.

4. FM stereo radios built into earmuffs attenuate outside noise and ensure that the radio will not exceed 85 dB(A).

5. Wireless communication attenuators with microphones located under the earmuff allow the speaker's voice to be picked up at a sufficient level without the interference of outside noise that is typical of an external microphone.

The electronic systems discussed above may cost anywhere from $500–1,000.

34. Lastly, if the TWA exceeds the PEL, will OAEs assist in determining the best NRR to prevent TTS, PTS, and STS?

If you understand this question, congratulations. If you do not, either read this section again or buy a few vowels from Vanna on *Wheel of Fortune.*

BIBLIOGRAPHY

1. American Academy of Otolaryngology–Head and Neck Surgery: Otologic Referral Criteria for Occupational Hearing Conservation Programs. Washington, DC, American Academy of Otolaryngology–Head and Neck Surgery, 1983.
2. Attias J, Furst M, Furman V, et al: Noise-induced otoacoustic emission loss with or without hearing loss. Ear Hearing 16:612–618, 1995.

3. Berger E: Extra-Auditory Benefits of a Hearing Conservation Program. Earlog 6. Indianapolis, Cabot Corporation, 1982.
4. Berger E: The Effects of Hearing Protectors on Auditory Communications. Earlog 3. Indianapolis, Cabot Corporation, 1984.
5. Boettcher F, Gralton M, Bancroft B, Spong V: Interaction of noise and other agents: Recent advances. In Dancer A, Henderson D, Salvi RJ, Hamernick RP (eds): Noise-Induced Hearing Loss. St. Louis, Mosby, 1992, pp 175–187.
6. Fechter L: Potentiation of noise-induced hearing loss by chemical contaminants in the workplace and environment. Pre-clinical studies. In Proceedings from the Hearing Conservation Conference III/XX. Des Moines, National Hearing Conservation Association, 1995, pp 129–136.
7. Franks J, Sizemore C: Cutting-edge developments in hearing protection and communication devices. In Proceedings from the Twenty-first Hearing Conservation Conference. Des Moines, National Hearing Conservation Association, 1996.
8. Kemp D, Ryan S, Bray P: A guide to the effective use of otoacoustic emissions. Ear Hearing 11:93–105, 1990.
9. Lipscomb D: Hearing Conservation in Industry, Schools and the Military. Boston, College-Hill, 1988.
10. Morata T, Dunn D, Kretschmer L, et al: Effects of occupational exposure to organic solvents and noise on hearing. Scand J Workers Environ Health 19:245–254, 1993.
11. Occupational Safety and Health Administration: Occupational noise exposure: Hearing conservation amendment. Final rule. Fed Reg 46:9738–9785, 1983.
12. Pekkarinen J: Noise, vibration, heat and cold: Do they interact? In Proceedings from the Hearing Conservation Conference III/XX. Des Moines, National Hearing Conservation Association, 1995, pp 137–144.
13. Rink T: Hearing protection and speech discrimination in hearing-impaired persons. Sound Vibration 13:22–25, 1979.
14. Rink T: Audiometric testing: A five-year review. In Proceedings from the Twenty-first Hearing Conservation Conference. Des Moines, National Hearing Conservation Association, 1996.
15. Royster L: Report of the NHCH Task Force on Hearing Protector Effectiveness. Rockville, MD, American Hearing and Speech Association, 1996.

III. Special Groups at Risk

27. OCCUPATIONAL HEALTH AND SAFETY FOR CHILD CARE WORKERS

Rene Gratz, Ph.D., Judith A. Calder, M.S., R.N., and Miriam Shipp, M.D., M.P.H.

1. How many workers are employed in the child care industry? What types of settings do they work in?

According to the 1994 fact sheet published by the Center for the Child Care Workforce (CCCW), an estimated 3 million child care teachers, assistants, and family child care providers in the United States care for 10 million children each day. Of the 3 million, 97% are female, 33% of all teaching staff are women of color, and most are in their childbearing years.

Among the 40 million Americans who have no health insurance, child care providers as a group bear a significant burden. A study by CCCW revealed that only 18% of child care centers offered health coverage to teaching staff. When child care providers become ill or injured as a result of worksite exposure, they often do not seek costly medical care because of the out-of-pocket expense; as a result, they may become a source of contagious illness to other children, staff, and families in the child care setting, in addition to compromising their own health.

Child care providers work in a variety of settings, such as larger centers that are generally multi-classroom (e.g., infant centers, preschools, Head Start, and school-aged programs) or family child care settings that operate out of the child care provider's own home (e.g., small homes of 2–8 children or large group homes with 6–12 children). The regulations for centers and licensed family child care homes vary in each state and address the health and safety needs of the children, but rarely are the needs of child care providers addressed. In general, child care providers work in physically and emotionally demanding settings and receive very low pay and few benefits. Men in child care settings often experience a sense of isolation working in a predominately female profession. Additionally, family child care providers may experience isolation because they are usually the lone adult among children each day.

2. What are the specific health concerns faced by child care workers?

Child care providers are at increased risk for exposure to infectious disease. In addition to common diseases such as upper respiratory infections and viral gastroenteritis, child care providers are exposed to hepatitis, cytomegalovirus (CMV), chickenpox, polio, rubella, parvovirus B19, influenza, tuberculosis, *Shigella*, *Giardia*, meningitis, *Streptococcus*, ringworm, scabies, lice, herpes, *Cryptosporidium*, and rotavirus. Some of these diseases may be serious enough to be considered occupational risks. In addition to infectious disease exposure, other health risks to child care workers include stress, burnout, and environmental exposure to excessive noise and chemicals (e.g., disinfecting solution).

3. What types of injuries are commonly seen in child care workers?

Daily routines of lifting, carrying, bending, and sitting on small furniture and the floor provide many opportunities for muscle pulls, strains, and sprains that research cites as the most common occupational injuries. The very few studies conducted to date demonstrate that most child care-related physical injuries occur to the lower back.

Worksite Analysis of the Child Care Work Environment

PROBLEM	RECOMMENDATIONS
Incorrect lifting of children, toys, supplies, and equipment	1. Education on proper lifting and carrying techniques 2. Promote job rotation where possible 3. Encourage independence in children whenever feasible
Inadequate work heights (e.g., child-size tables and chairs)	1. Create a chair that allows staff to slide their legs under the table 2. Use sit/kneel chairs 3. Educate staff on proper body mechanics 4. Provide the staff with adult-size chairs for occasional use
Difficulty lowering and lifting infants in and out of cribs	1. Modify crib sides to enable them to slide down or modify the legs of the cribs to accommodate the staff 2. Educate staff on the proper use of body mechanics
Frequent sitting on the floor with back unsupported	1. When possible, have staff sit up against a wall or furniture for back support 2. Perform stretching exercises 3. Educate staff on proper body mechanics
Excessive reaching above shoulder height to obtain stored supplies	1. Redesign kitchen area, placing heaviest items at waist height 2. Reorganize snacks and supplies to simplify snack preparation procedures 3. Use step stools when retrieving items that are above cupboard height
Frequent lifting of infants and toddlers on and off diaper changing tables	1. Educate staff on proper body mechanics 2. Have toddlers use steps in order to decrease distance staff are lifting
Forceful motions combined with awkward posture are required to open windows	1. Use step stool to allow for better leverage and reduce awkward posture 2. Have maintenance staff improve quality of window slide
Carrying garbage and diaper bags to dumpster	1. Provide staff with cart to transport garbage 2. Relocate garbage cart closer to work area 3. Reduce size and weight of loads 4. Educate staff on proper body mechanics

From Gratz R, Claffey A: Taking care of yourself: The physical demands and ergonomics of working with young children. Presentation at the Annual Conference of the National Association for the Education of Young Children, Dallas, TX, November, 1996.

4. What measures may a child care center take to reduce injuries to child care workers?

Early childhood professionals have spent much time, effort, and study in designing environments to facilitate optimum child development; the workplace also should be studied and designed with the adult's optimal ergonomic health as a priority.

Child care workers spend much of their workday sitting on the floor with the children; they move heavy equipment and furniture regularly; and when they are not sitting on the floor, they may be sitting on child-size chairs that are too small.

Proper lifting of children and equipment in the child care setting should occur in the following sequence: (1) keep lower back bowed in ("curving back like a cat") while bending over; (2) keep the child or object as close as possible to your body; (3) bow back in and raise up with head first; (4) never twist or jerk; (5) put the child or object down by keeping low back bowed in; (6) squat whenever possible; (7) have a stable base of support; (8) do not twist or rotate trunk—if it is necessary to turn, turn with your feet, not your body; (9) whenever possible, stabilize the body against a stationary object such as a wall or cabinet; (10) if getting up from a squat position is difficult, support self on a stable surface (table, chair) and push up with hands in addition to legs; (11) to lower a child or object to the floor, use the same mechanics in the reverse order—have a firm grasp on the child or object, place feet shoulders' width apart, one foot ahead, and keep your back straight as you bend your legs to lower the child; extend arms straight down and do not rotate trunk.

5. Which infectious diseases are of concern to the child care worker?

Many infectious diseases, such as upper respiratory infections, flu, and diarrhea, affect adult workers as well as children in the child care environment. Other diseases may be more readily transmitted from adults to children, such as tuberculosis, pertussis from unrecognized adult carriers, and more recently, diphtheria. Infections such as hepatitis A and giardiasis may not be apparent in children but are in adults, and are thus more readily transmitted. Other diseases may have severe consequences for pregnant adults or for immunocompromised people, such as CMV, rubella, parvovirus B19, and chickenpox.

Some infectious diseases are more serious when contracted by adults. Chickenpox produces more serious disease in nonimmune infected adults. CMV is of special concern for adults or children with immune deficiencies. Young children with hepatitis A (a virus spread by fecal/oral transmission) show few symptoms, but adults become very ill.

Adults infected with parvovirus B19 are at risk of developing arthritis. Many child care professionals have been immunized against polio during their childhood. Unimmunized child care providers may be at rare risk to develop vaccine-associated poliomyelitis if exposed to the live vaccine virus excreted in the stool of recently immunized children.

Hepatitis B is transmitted through blood, by sexual contact, and (rarely) through saliva. It may be transmitted to child care providers through providing first aid to children and through handling body fluids that contain blood, or (rarely) by being bitten by an infected child. The OSHA Bloodborne Pathogen Standard (issued 1991) for employers requires that they inform new employees of this occupational risk, prevention practices, and recommended hepatitis B vaccinations. Unvaccinated employees who have occupational exposure to blood can receive hepatitis B vaccination within 24 hours of a blood exposure. There is no reason to exclude hepatitis B carriers (see question 10).

6. What measures may a child care center take to reduce the risk of infectious disease for child care workers?

Child care workers must understand that preventive health practices not only protect the children in care from infectious disease, but also protect them as well. Critical practices include handwashing, universal precautions, environmental cleaning and sanitation, health checks, and exclusion guidelines for both workers and children.

Factors that increase the risk of transmitting disease to children in child care settings also affect their caregivers, and some may be serious enough to be considered occupational risks:

1. **Adult immune status or susceptibility to disease:** Anecdotal evidence and some empirical data show that caregivers new to child care work get sick more often than longer-employed workers who have experienced more illness and have thus become more resistant. Caregivers lacking antibody resistance to common childhood illness and those with compromised immunity because of disease, disability, allergy, or medication may be more susceptible. Caregivers who are not fully immunized are at risk for vaccine-preventable disease, such as hepatitis B.

2. **Environmental characteristics** (e.g., large facility size, large group size, group mixing, and age of children in care): Child care workers who provide care for younger, diapered, children with undeveloped hygiene habits have more opportunities for exposure to infectious agents.

3. **Routine habits:** Poor hygiene practices, poor environmental sanitation practices, lack of training on disease transmission and prevention, poor monitoring of health practices, and lack of equipment (e.g., gloves, soap) can increase the risk of disease transmission.

4. **Employment policies and benefits:** Lack of employee health assessments, benefits, good working conditions supportive of health, clear policies related to health and safety, and guidelines for the exclusion of child care staff with illness are detrimental to the health of child care workers.

7. What components of a physical health assessment are relevant to child care workers?

Requiring pre-employment health assessments not only identifies caregivers susceptible to infectious diseases but also to other occupational risks, such as back injuries, allergies, and stress. Ideally, health assessments should be performed after a job offer and before contact with children begins. By the mandate of the Americans with Disabilities Act, an individual physical health assessment can be required only if they are required for all applicants who have been extended offers.

Although state child care regulations regarding pre-employment health assessments vary greatly, staff who will have contact with children are recommended to have a health appraisal (see Child Care Staff Health Assessment form on next page) which includes:

1. A health history
2. A physical examination
3. Vision and hearing screening
4. TB screening by the Mantoux method
5. A review of immunization status and history of childhood infectious diseases including measles, mumps, rubella, diphtheria, tetanus, polio, and chickenpox.
6. Assessment of need for immunization against influenza, pneumococcus, and hepatitis B; if worker is of childbearing age or planning pregnancy, risk of exposure to chickenpox, CMV, and parvovirus B19 need to be assessed.
7. Assessment of orthopedic, psychological, neurologic, sensory limitations, or communicable disease that may impair the staff member's ability to perform the job.
8. A review of occupational health concerns (e.g., pregnancy, difficulty being outdoors, allergy to art materials, skin conditions affected by frequent handwashing)
9. Inquiries regarding the status of household members related to communicable disease (e.g., TB vaccination is recommended, especially for family child care providers)

Child care regulations rarely address the need for ongoing health appraisals. Because recommendations for the health screening, TB testing, and immunization of adults vary over time and geographic location, it is always best to check with the local health department regarding current recommendations. (See figure, next page.)

8. What tests and/or immunizations are currently recommended for a child care worker?

Adult immunizations for child care workers to discuss with their health provider include combined tetanus and diphtheria toxoids (dT, given every 10 years), measles-mumps-rubella (MMR, 1 dose if born after 1956), hepatitis B (3 doses), chickenpox (2 doses if adult has never had disease), hepatitis A (2 doses, especially if adult works with diapered children), polio (IPV [inactivated polio vaccine] if unvaccinated). Immunizations for older adults and for people with chronic illness to consider include influenza (every fall season) and pneumococcal vaccine (at age 65 or with chronic disease). Also consider the following serologic tests: vaccine preventable diseases if immunization history is unknown, varicella and hepatitis if illness history is unknown, and CMV and parvovirus B19 in a woman of childbearing age if illness history is unknown.

9. Are current occupational standards (e.g., NIOSH lifting guidelines) adequate to protect child care workers?

Unfortunately, most occupational health standards are more helpful for other occupational settings than for the child care workplace. The NIOSH lifting guidelines set forth an equation that can be used to determine maximum weight to be lifted depending on a variety of factors such as distance of weight from body, frequency of lifts, duration of lifts, and hand location (NIOSH, 1994). Although the revised 1991 lifting equation is an improvement over the 1981 NIOSH equation, it still is not very useful for lifting in the child care setting. This is due to the fact that lifting activities in child care are unpredictable—the "object"—that is, the child is not only asymmetric, but also is not stable (i.e., moving and squirming), and also may be resistant while being lifted.

Other occupational health regulations may be applicable to the child care setting, such as state laws requiring health and safety education in the workplace. However, these regulations are applied

Child Care Staff Health Assessment

****** **Employer should complete this section.** ******

Name of person to be examined: _____

Employer for whom examination is being done: _____

Employer's Location: _____ Phone number: _____

Purpose of examination: ☐ pre-employment (after offer of employment) ☐ annual re-examination

Type of activity on the job (check all that apply):

    ☐ lifting, carrying children   ☐ close contact with children   ☐ food preparation
    ☐ desk work   ☐ driver of vehicles   ☐ facility maintenance   ☐ other

****** **Part I and Part II below must be completed and signed by a licensed physician, nurse practitioner, or physician's assistant.** ******

Based on a review of the medical record, health history, and examination, does this person have any of the following conditions or problems that might affect job performance and require accommodation by employer?

Date of exam: _____

Part I: Health Problems   *(circle)*

visual acuity less than 20/40 (combined, obtained with lenses if needed)? .... yes no
decreased hearing (tested at 20 db for 500, 1000, 2000, 4000 Hz)? .... yes no
respiratory problems (asthma, emphysema, airway allergies, current smoker, other)? .... yes no
heart, blood pressure, or other cardiovascular problems? .... yes no
gastrointestinal problems (ulcer, colitis, special dietary requirements, obesity, other)? .... yes no
endocrine problems (diabetes, thyroid, other)? .... yes no
emotional disorders (depression, drug or alcohol dependency, other)? .... yes no
neurologic problems (epilepsy, Parkinsonism, other)? .... yes no
musculoskeletal problems (low back pain, neck problems, arthritis, limitations on activity)? .... yes no
skin problems (eczema, rashes, conditions incompatible with frequent handwashing, other)? ... yes no
immune system problems (from medication, illness, allergies, and sensitivities to materials)?.... yes no
other special medical problem or chronic disease that requires work restrictions
    or accommodation? .... yes no

Part II: Infectious Disease Status

Consider immunization for:

    dT (every ten years) .... yes no
    MMR (two doses for persons not immune to measles by history or serology) .... yes no
    Hepatitis B (three dose series) .... yes no
    Influenza .... yes no
    Pneumococcus (for those over 65 or with chronic medical conditions) .... yes no
    Hepatitis A (two doses) .... yes no
    Chickenpox (2 doses for adults) .... yes no
    Polio (OPV in childhood or IPV series for adults never previously vaccinated) .... yes no
Female of childbearing age susceptible to CMV, parvovirus, toxoplasmosis or herpes? .... yes no
Evaluation of tuberculosis status shows a risk for communicable TB? .... yes no
    Tuberculosis status must be determined by performing the Mantoux test for persons not
    previously tested positive for tuberculosis infection. Positive Mantoux tests should be
    followed by x-ray evaluation.

Please attach additional sheets to explain all "yes" answers above. Include the plan for follow-up or suggestions for accommodation.

_____   _____   _____
Date   Patient's Signature   Printed last name and title

Phone number: _____

I have read and understand the above information.

_____   _____
Date   Patient's Signature

Child care staff health assessment. Adapted from Aronson S, Smith H, Martin J: Model Child Care Health Policies. Project ECELS, Pennsylvania Chapter American Academy of Pediatrics, 1993.

inconsistently and not sufficiently monitored in most workplaces. They are especially difficult to use in the child care field, because it is principally composed of small and unregulated workplaces. Despite this, clinicians in the child care health field can use NIOSH and other guidelines to help formulate specifications for child care. In order to do this, they must look closely at the tasks required in child care and the training/monitoring possibilities in the child care workplace in order to create sound policies.

10. What aspects of the OSHA Bloodborne Pathogen Standard apply to child care settings?
The OSHA Bloodborne Pathogen Standard requires that every employer develop and implement a plan for the following: universal precautions, blood exposure plan, hepatitis B vaccine, and training on the Bloodborne Pathogen Standard. Child care centers and family child care providers who employ aides, substitutes, or use volunteers must comply with OSHA regulations regarding infection control according to these guidelines: (1) handwashing at appropriate times using appropriate techniques; (2) latex gloves worn by all child care providers when they come in contact with blood or body fluids containing blood; (3) cleaning with disinfectant on a daily basis on all surfaces used by children and on an "as needed" basis on any surface(s) in contact with blood; (4) proper disposal of infectious materials; (5) blood exposure notification within 24 hours to determine infection risk and recommend hepatitis B vaccine if needed and not previously provided; and (6) infection control training held (at least) annually as part of job orientation.

11. What precautions should be taken by a pregnant woman working in a child care setting?
Pregnancy is a common occurrence in a workforce composed primarily of women of childbearing age. As a job that demands close personal contact with infants and young children, child care work poses special considerations. The incidence and severity of the listed effects may vary widely and depend on many factors, most importantly the stage of gestation when the infection is acquired. Common problems for pregnant child care workers include fatigue, exposure to infectious diseases, back problems, frequent urination, swollen feet, and varicose veins. Pregnant child care professionals should consult their own health care provider with any questions and concerns.

Possible Effects, Risk, and Prevention of Illness and Stress in Pregnancy

ILLNESS AND RISK	EFFECT	PREVENTION
Rubella (German measles) (10–20% of young adults lack immunity)	Depends on gestational age at time of exposure; deafness, microcephaly, central nervous system (CNS) disease, heart defects, cataracts	Blood test if immunity uncertain; avoid contact if not immune; vaccinate if not pregnant
Hepatitis B (rarely transmitted in day care setting)	Prematurity, psychomotor retardation, newborn disease	Avoid contact with blood products; vaccinate if not pregnant; pre-employment vaccination or 24 hours after blood exposure
Cytomegalovirus (CMV) (annual rate of infection of day care providers is 8–20%)	Risk for severe disability is small if infected 1st trimester: visual-hearing impairments, cognitive and motor deficits, CNS disease, microcephaly, mental retardation, jaundice, retinitis, stillbirth	Blood test for immunity; handwashing, gloving when handling urine and saliva; if pregnant and not immune, avoid contact with children < 2 years old during first 24 weeks of pregnancy
Varicella zoster (chickenpox) (8% of adults lack immunity)	1st trimester: miscarriage, muscle atrophy, clubbed feet, CNS disease, cataracts Perinatal period: neonatal death	Blood test if immunity uncertain; avoid contact if not immune; vaccinate if not pregnant

Table continued on following page.

Possible Effects, Risk, and Prevention of Illness and Stress in Pregnancy (Continued)

ILLNESS AND RISK	EFFECT	PREVENTION
Fifth disease (parvovirus B19) (approx. 50% of adults lack immunity)	If infected first half of pregnancy, rarely: stillbirths; miscarriage; fetal hydrops; anemia jaundice; enlarged liver	Blood test for immunity; handwashing; avoid shared utensils; consult health care provider if not immune and exposed
Toxoplasmosis (66% of adult women lack immunity)	Infection depends upon stage stage of pregnancy; spectrum of abnormalities similar to CMV	Thorough handwashing after handling raw meat and vegetables, after cleaning a cat litter box or outdoor sandbox, and after gardening
HIV/AIDS (no reports of day care transmission)	Fetal infection	Appropriate precautions handling blood and body fluids
Herpes simplex 2 (different from herpes simplex 1 virus transmitted through oral secretions)	Spontaneous abortions, prematurity, microcephaly, fetal infection	Usually sexually transmitted; handwashing, gloving
Stress	Miscarriage, prematurity, toxemia, preeclampsia, nausea, prolonged labor	Decrease sources of stress; relaxation techniques; good diet and exercise

Adapted from Gratz R, Boulton P: Health considerations for pregnant child care staff. J Pediatr Health Care 8:18–26, 1994. Reprinted with permission.

Common Problems and Recommendations for Pregnant Child Care Staff

PROBLEM	RECOMMENDATION
Fatigue	Always take scheduled breaks Rest on left side during breaks and lunch, or with feet elevated Keep each workday to no more than 8 hours Rest when fatigued
Exposure to infectious diseases	Use frequent and proper handwashing techniques Use of gloves and universal precautions, where appropriate Establish informational network for parents and staff Alert health care provider of child care work and potential for exposure
Back problems	Use proper lifting and carrying techniques Avoid heavy lifting Maintain good standing and seated posture Use adult-size furniture; bring an adult-size, easily movable, comfortable chair from home, if necessary Avoid floor-sitting To avoid constant bending, have children climb up to teacher, if developmentally appropriate Trade strenuous chores of lifting/moving heavy objects with other staff
Frequent urination	Have other staff available to cover room assignment to maintain staff-child ratios
Swollen feet, varicose veins	Wear support hose Exercise Change position frequently Rest with feet elevated

From Gratz R, Boulton P: Health considerations for pregnant child care staff. J Pediatr Health Care 8:18–26, 1994, reprinted with permission.

12. What advances or new developments have occurred recently regarding improving child care work environments?

Over the last 15 years, collaborative work between child care and health professionals has filled the gap in knowledge and practice related to health promotion in child care settings. However, only recently have child care providers themselves benefited from that collaboration. Perhaps the most important development has been the publication of the National Health and Safety Performance Standards "Caring For Our Children" through the joint efforts of the American Public Health Association and the American Academy of Pediatrics (1992). These recommendations, guidelines, and standards represent a consensus among experts in all disciplines that relate to child care as to what constitutes the best health and safety practices for child care programs.

National standards may be used as a reference by caregivers and health professionals, for licensing and regulatory improvements, and by consumers of child care in selecting and improving quality child care. Because the standards are meant to improve the overall health of the child care environment, they also have a positive health impact on the providers themselves.

13. What health and safety training is required for child care workers?

Health and safety training requirements for child care workers vary among states and jurisdictions. For example, child care regulations in one state may encompass and enforce occupational health and safety, whereas child care regulations in other states assume that the regional OSHA is responsible for enforcement. Some states have OSHA requirements that exceed federal standards mandating worker training. For example, California requires all employers, including those in child care, to perform routine hazard identification and correction to inform workers of problem areas and to provide orientation and quarterly staff training to reduce the hazards.

Among the training topics child care programs identify are: proper lifting, carrying, and moving techniques; hazard identification and correction; emergency management; child behavior management; infection control; design and use of physical space; child care curriculum and program planning; first aid; and conflict resolution. All states require employers to provide training on the federal OSHA Bloodborne Pathogen Standard, and most states require training in first aid and CPR and on reducing the spread of disease by use of good personal hygiene, environmental sanitation, and the management of illness. All states also require that policies for the management of emergencies and for safety practices that impact the children are in place.

CONTROVERSY

14. Has the increased use of child care had significant impact on the epidemiology of infectious diseases in the U.S.? What is the cost of the impact on society?

Several studies have shown that children in child care have a higher incidence of infectious disease than those cared for at home. Increased antibiotic use also is prevalent in child care: although antibiotic use increased in general in the U.S. between 1980 and 1992, several studies have indicated that antibiotics are used more frequently in children in child care and for longer durations than in children cared for at home. Thus, increased antibiotic use may contribute to antibiotic resistance: studies demonstrate that the recent increased use of antibiotics is one of the most consistently identified risk factors for developing resistant strains.

The data seem to suggest that there is always an increased incidence of infectious disease and antibiotic among children in child care. Indeed, it has been shown that the increase in infectious disease leads to a larger cost to society in health care costs and days of work lost for parents caring for ill children. However, some evidence suggests that children experience an increase in infectious diseases whenever they enter group care (e.g., at school entrance), and that the incidence of infections decreases after the third year of group care. Therefore, entering child care may simply change the timing of when children acquire infectious diseases. In addition, the practice of some organizations providing care for mildly ill children under strict protocols is on the rise, a factor that also may contribute to a decrease in parent days of work lost. Several such organizations are workplaces that are interested in increased productivity for their employees who are parents.

Vaccine use may reduce some infectious diseases in child care. In most states childhood vaccination coverage is monitored in pre–school-aged children when such children first enter school; thus, it is likely that young children in child care have increased vaccination rates. This is especially likely for vaccines against milder diseases such as varicella.

It is important to acknowledge that infectious disease and antibiotic resistance for children and adults in child care can be reduced by a cooperative effort of child care providers, health care providers, and parents. Child care providers can reduce infection by following the national recommendations mentioned previously, which have been shown to reduce the spread of infectious diseases. Health care providers can learn more about the child care environment in order to reinforce these guidelines and educate families about infectious disease in child care, and to help prevent increased antibiotic resistance by avoiding prescribing antibiotics unless absolutely necessary. The development of new vaccines for children, such as those against pneumococcus, meningococcus, and influenza, also will help to reduce the incidence and cost of infectious disease in child care.

15. How does the provision of health care and social services affect the child care workforce?
The provision of health and social services affects child care programs in two ways. The first is the increasing demands to care for children for which providers believe they are not qualified to provide care, which is the result of two major policy developments: (1) the change in the welfare system that is placing more mothers with young children into the workforce and more children in poverty into child care programs, and (2) the enactment of the Americans with Disabilities Act, which ensures that children with disabilities have access to child care services when reasonable accommodation can be made. Health systems and services must extend services to children on-site at the child care program to meet such demands and reduce worker stress.

Secondly, as mentioned above, child care providers are over-represented in the nation's uninsured. Despite their high exposure to illness and injury, employers provide child care workers with little or no health insurance and even fewer offer pension plans. Parents' tuition payments alone cannot cover the costs for quality child care and adequate teacher benefits. The dilemma is: who pays for improved child care worker benefits and improved working conditions?

RESOURCES FOR CHILD CARE WORKERS AND CLINICIANS

Caring for Our Children (available as a manual or video)
American Public Health Association and the American Academy of Pediatrics, American Academy of Pediatrics, 141 Northwest Point Blvd., PO Box 927, Elk Grove Village, IL 60009-0927, 1-800-433-9016.

National Resource Center for Health and Safety in Child Care
University of Colorado, School of Nursing, C-287, 4200 E. 9th Avenue, Denver, CO 80262, 1-800-598-KIDS. The center acts as a clearinghouse for child care health and safety information with extensive on-line services.

Healthy Child Care America
Child Care Bureau, Administration on Children, Youth and Families, (202) 690-5641, and the Child Care Bureau, Health Resources and Services Administration, (301) 443-6600. This campaign outlines ten steps communities can take to improve health and safety in child care and provides resources to states for implementation.

Center for the Child Care Workforce
733 15th Street, NW, Suite 1037, Washington, DC 20005-2112, (202) 737-7700. Types of information/services provided include surveys of salaries and working conditions, research on child care staffing issues, technical assistance on staff training and leadership development, grassroots organizing, and mentoring programs.

National Association for the Education of Young Children (NAEYC)
1509 16th St. NW, Washington DC, 20036-1426, 1-800-424-2460. This early childhood professional association encompasses all aspects of child care and early childhood education.

BIBLIOGRAPHY

1. Applications Manual for the Revised NIOSH Lifting Equation (DHHS (NIOSH) Pub. No. 94–110), 1994.
2. Aronson S: Health concerns of caregivers—Infectious diseases and job stresses. Child Care Exchange 54:33–37,1987.
3. Brown MZ, Gerberich SG: Disabling injuries to childcare workers in Minnesota, 1985 to 1990. An analysis of potential risk factors. J Occup Med 35:1236–1243,1993.
4. Calder J: Occupational health and safety issues for child-care providers. Pediatrics 94:1072–1074, 1994.
5. Caring for Our children. National Health and Safety Performance Standards: Guidelines for Out-of-Home Child Care Programs. Washington, D.C., American Public Health Association and American Academy of Pediatrics, 1992.
6. Fleming DW, Cochi SL, Hightower AW, et al: Childhood upper respiratory tract infections: To what degree is incidence affected by daycare attendance? Pediatrics 79:55–60, 1987.
7. Gratz R: Wisconsin Early Childhood Professionals Occupational Health Survey: Preliminary Report and Recommendations from the Pilot Study. Department of Health Sciences, University of Wisconsin-Milwaukee, 1994.
8. Gratz R, Boulton P: Health considerations for pregnant child care staff. J Pediatr Health Care 8:18–26, 1994.
9. Gratz R, Claffey A: Adult health in child care: Health status, behaviors, and concerns of teachers, directors, and family child care providers. Early Childhood Research Quarterly 11:243–267, 1996.
10. Gratz R, Claffey A: Taking care of yourself: The physical demands and ergonomics of working with young children. Presentation at the Annual Conference of the National Association for the Education of Young Children, Dallas, TX, November, 1996.
11. Holmes SJ, Morrow AL, Pickering LK: Child-care practices: Effects of social change on the epidemiology of infectious diseases and antibiotic resistance. Epidemiol Rev 18(1):10–28, 1996.
12. Hurwitz ES, Gunn WJ, Pinsky PF, et al: Risk of respiratory illness associated with day-care attendance: A nationwide study. Pediatrics 87:62–69, 1991.
13. King P, Gratz R, Scheuer G, Claffey A: The ergonomics of child care: Conducting worksite analyses. WORK: A Journal of Prevention, Assessment & Rehabilitation 6:25–32, 1996.
14. Markon P, LeBeau D: Health and safety at work for day-care educators. Université du Quebec, Chicoutimi, Quebec, Canada, 1994.
15. Pennsylvania Chapter of the American Academy of Pediatrics: Model Child Care Health Policies. Bryn Mawr, PA, Project ECELS, 1993.
16. Reves RR, Jones JA: Antibiotic use and resistance patterns in day care centers. Semin Pediatr Infect Dis 1:212–221, 1990.
17. Reves RR & Pickering LK: Infections in day care centers as they relate to internal medicine. Annu Rev Med 41:383–391, 1990.
18. The Americans with Disabilities Act: Employing People with Disabilities in Child Care. San Francisco, Child Care Law Center, 1996.
19. Wald ER, Guerra N, Byers C: Frequency and severity of infections in day care: Three-year follow-up. J Pediatr 118:509–514, 1991.

28. WOMEN WORKERS

Jeanne Mager Stellman, Ph.D.

1. What are the major occupations held by women workers?

Although the past several decades have seen enormous growth in the numbers of women who are gainfully employed outside their homes, most women continue to be employed in the same traditional occupations. Men hold a much wider variety of occupational titles. The 20 following occupations were most frequently held by women in the 1990s:

1. Secretaries, stenographers, and typists
2. Teachers
3. Bookkeepers and accountant clerks
4. Salesworkers
5. Cashiers
6. Registered nurses
7. Nursing aides and attendants
8. Receptionists
9. Sales supervisors
10. Waitresses
11. Sewers and stitchers
12. Sales representatives, especially real estate
13. Cooks
14. Hairdressers and cosmetologists
15. Janitors and cleaners
16. Assemblers and manufacturing hand workers
17. General office clerical workers
18. Mail and message distributors, especially postal workers
19. Social, recreation, and religious workers, especially social workers
20. Maids

2. Do women workers differ from men workers from an occupational health perspective?

Virtually no hazards are known to affect only women workers, with the possible exception of agents that can cross the placental barrier or be sequestered in breast milk. But even most of these agents exhibit some toxicity in men as well. The major gender-based differences relevant to occupational health are attributable to the different jobs and tasks of men and women, even within the same workplace and job title. As a result, they usually have different exposures. Women tend to be overrepresented in jobs that are repetitive and routine. A well-defined occupational health program seeks to discover and to address these differences. Many of the tools and equipment that women use at work may be designed to accommodate the average man and thus may be difficult for women to use. For example, hand tools may be too large, and work station tables may be too high. Application of basic ergonomic principles to workstations and tools avoids problems for both sexes.

3. Do women workers exhibit special traits or characteristics that make them more suitable for particular kinds of work?

For many years "experts" in job design and occupational health maintained that women were better suited to jobs requiring fine finger agility and that they had more patience for routine, repetitive work. No biologic evidence supports these assertions.

4. What jobs predominantly held by women are associated with occupational dermatoses?

Skin diseases are the most widely recognized occupational illnesses. Conditions associated with occupational dermatoses include exposure to irritants and sensitizers and cold and/or wet conditions. Occupations in which irritants, sensitizers, and cold or wet are combined are associated with higher risk of dermatoses. Many of the jobs that women hold involve exposures to these risk factors. Examples include cooks (sensitizers in foodstuffs and wet conditions, cuts and injuries); janitors and cleaners (cleaning agents and wet conditions); nurses and nurses' aides (frequent handwashing and sensitizers such as disinfecting agents and drugs); sewers and stitchers (formaldehyde in permanent press, dyes and flame retardants); jobs involving paper handling, particularly carbonless copy paper; and hairdressers and cosmetologists (wet conditions and assorted cosmetic chemicals).

5. Do women workers have particular cancer risks?

There are no known gender-based differences in risk for occupational disease—merely differences in occupational exposures that may increase the risk for cancer. Dry cleaning industries and laundries (chlorinated hydrocarbons), electronics industries (exotic chemicals, chlorinated hydrocarbons), health care work (sterilants, some drugs, x-rays), agriculture (pesticides), textile work (formaldehyde and some dyes), and arts and crafts (metals, solvents) are examples of occupations with potential risks.

6. Are women workers more likely to sustain repetitive strain injuries than men?

Carpal tunnel syndrome has reached epidemic proportions among women in some occupations. Meat and poultry workers and women who assemble small machines are at particular risk. High rates of repetitive strain injuries (RSIs) have been found in data entry clerks and workers who use video display terminals (VDTs) for long periods. Repetitive strain injuries in women are the fastest growing occupational injury reported in workers' compensation data. Women are more likely to sustain carpal tunnel syndrome, whereas men suffer from other types of RSIs.

7. What infectious agents are particularly relevant to women workers?

Women work in a variety of industries where infection hazards are present. In health care industries, for example, women are about 80% of the workforce. Blood-borne diseases are a common risk, particularly various forms of hepatitis. HIV infection also may occur, but the rates of transmission are considerably lower than for hepatitis. Tuberculosis, particularly resistant strains, also poses a risk. Women in contact with children, particularly in lower school grades and child-care work, are at risk for respiratory and diarrheal infections. Meat and poultry workers are at risk for infections and warts. Data about other likely infections, such as salmonellosis, are inadequate. Jobs involving contact with the public involve a risk for airborne transmission of contagious disease.

8. Are lifting and carrying occupational health risks for significant numbers of women workers?

Back injuries are the major occupational injury in health care industries, which are dominated by women workers and a leading cause of disability for both sexes. Patient handling is the main cause of injury in health care. Waitresses, janitors, and cleaners also may be routinely required to carry heavy loads, often with improper training and inadequate equipment. Child-care workers may have to carry small, but comparatively heavy children. On average, women have smaller frames than men. Untrained women, on average, cannot lift as much weight as the average male worker. With appropriate training, the lifting and carrying ability of women can be greatly enhanced. Inadequate data are available for assessing the gender-based limits of weightlifting. In general, automated and/or assisted methods for lifting and carrying are preferable for both sexes.

9. Is sedentary office work associated with occupational health risk factors?

Excessive sitting, particularly in a poorly designed, ill-fitting chair, may lead to lower back pain. Sedentary work, if not compensated by exercise regimens, can lead to overweight. Blood circulation in the lower body may impaired by excessive sitting.

10. What hazards for women are associated with VDT usage?

Eyestrain may result from excessive VDT use, particularly if corrective lenses are not adjusted for VDT viewing distance. Bifocals may cause neck strain by inappropriate tilting of the head to view the screen. Poor lighting design may lead to glare and eyestrain. Excessive sitting and repetitive strain from data entry are discussed elsewhere in this chapter. Little evidence suggests that radiation or reproductive health risks exist.

11. Do the multiple off-the-job roles of most women workers affect their health? What remedies are available?

Women continue to have the major responsibility for housework and child care, even as their gainful employment outside the home increases. In 1997 nearly 70% of women with children under the age of 6 years were employed outside the home. Younger women with multiple responsibilities are often found to be the most "stressed" in research studies. Long-term health effects are not known. Remedies include improved opportunities for child care (both well- and sick-child care) and elder care. Nutritious, affordable prepared foods also may help.

12. Can sexual harassment affect a woman's health?

Many experts consider sexual harassment to be capable of inducing stress-related health effects, but no definitive studies have been done. Data show that harassment is widespread, but its long-term effects are not well studied.

13. What is mass psychogenic illness? Are women more likely to be involved in episodes than men?

Mass psychogenic illness (mass hysteria) refers to the widespread occurrence of symptoms in a workplace that cannot be related to specific, measurable causes. Indoor air pollution is commonly associated with mass psychogenic illness; not surprisingly, it has been found to occur more frequently among women, who are the majority of indoor office workers. Instances have occurred in schools, where the demographics are similar. Some experts believe that such episodes are purely psychological, whereas others believe that industrial hygiene techniques and exposure standards are inappropriate or inadequate for assessing white-collar environments such as schools and offices.

14. Can the menstrual cycle be affected by working conditions?

Research on menstruation is insufficient in general and with respect to occupational hazards in particular. Various studies establish that the menstrual cycle can be affected, but few agents have been identified. Some solvents, such as carbon disulfide, xylene, and toluene, have been associated with disruption of the menstrual cycle. Jobs that involve interference with the normal circadian cycle, such as shiftwork, also may affect normal cycling. Workers in the explosives/munitions industries have experienced menstrual dysfunction, and affects have been reported with some phosphate fertilizers.

15. Do differences in male/female physiology influence the effects of exposure to toxic substances?

Because women have a higher percentage of fat as total body weight than men, some experts believe that the toxicity of lipophilic solvents is greater for women. Only anecdotal data are available, and no controlled studies of the range of fat composition by gender of typical workforces, which would include obese men and women with low-fat bodies, have been done to determine the practical meaning of the gender-based difference in body fat for occupational health practitioners.

16. Which traditional women's jobs involve long periods of standing? Can standing affect health?

Many women must stand for long periods at work. Sales workers, cashiers, nurses, and nurses' aides stand for much of the work period. Excessive standing has been associated with an increased risk for varicose veins. More research is needed, along with job redesign to allow periods of sitting during the work day.

17. Is the quality of indoor air an occupational health hazard for women?

Indoor air-quality complaints were the single largest category of complaints received by the National Institute for Occupational Safety and Health (NIOSH). The long-range health effects of poor indoor air quality are not well understood. Women workers represent the majority of indoor office workers.

18. Are employers permitted to exclude women workers from jobs that they believe are too hazardous?

No. The only way in which an employer can legally exclude women is to demonstrate that no men are at risk from the same hazards. To date no such gender-specific hazards are known. The Supreme Court has ruled that this principle also holds for reproductive hazards (*UAW v. Johnson Controls*).

19. Are women as likely to enjoy the same level of fringe benefits as men (e.g., health insurance and employer-paid pension)?

No. On average women still earn 59–70% of the wages that men earn in the same professions. On average they also have less insurance coverage and lower pensions.

CONTROVERSY

20. Are women more likely to have medical complaints, seek medical attention, and be absent from the job? Are women more sickly than men? Are they less effective employees for this reason?

Women have higher rates of absenteeism and seek medical care more frequently than men. Many experts attribute the attendance differences to family-related causes (e.g., women take time from work to care for sick children and relatives and to meet other family obligations). Studies that controlled for child care-related absence have found no differences in male/female attendance. Many experts also believe that women are more health-conscious and respond to symptoms at an earlier stage than men, thus accounting for the difference in utilization rates. When men seek health care, they are generally sicker than women and require more extensive medical treatment. No evidence indicates that women are less effective employees than men.

BIBLIOGRAPHY

1. Collins BS, Hollander RB, Koffman DM, et al: Women, work and health: Implications for worksite health promotion. Women Health 25:3–38, 1997.
2. Headapohl DM (ed): Women Workers. Occup Med State Art Rev 8(4), 1993.
3. Messing K: One-Eyed Science: Occupational Health and Women Workers. Philadelphia, Temple University Press, 1998.
4. Messing K: Women's occupational health: A critical review and discussion of current issues. Women Health 25:39–68, 1997.
5. Paul M (ed): Occupational and Environmental Reproductive Hazards. Baltimore, Williams & Wilkins, 1993.
6. Pottern L, Zahm S, Sieber S, et al: Occupational cancer among women: A conference overview. J Occup Med 36:809–813, 1994.
7. Stellman JM, Warshaw LJ: Work and workers. In Stellman JM (ed): Encyclopedia of Occupational Health and Safety, 4th ed. Geneva, ILO, pp 24.1–24.17, 1998.

IV. Diseases

29. CARDIAC TOXICOLOGY

Neal L. Benowitz, M.D.

1. Atherosclerosis is the most common type of cardiovascular disease in the general population. It also may present as a manifestation of chemical toxicity from what agents?

Carbon disulfide, arsenic, and combustion products, including environmental tobacco smoke, appear to accelerate atherosclerosis. Chronic lead exposure also may accelerate atherosclerosis by elevating blood pressure.

2. What are the usual industrial sources of carbon disulfide exposure?

Carbon disulfide is used in the manufacturing of viscose rayon and various chemicals. It also is used as a solvent for rubbers, fats, oils, and resins. Inhalation is the major route of exposure, but carbon disulfide also may be absorbed through the skin.

3. What clinical features suggest carbon disulfide-induced atherosclerotic vascular disease?

Acute intoxication, evidenced by episodes of dizziness and headaches, or chronic intoxication, which may include encephalopathy, polyneuropathy, paresthesias, and/or psychosis, is suggestive, but neither is necessary for the development of cardiovascular disease. Clinical features of carbon disulfide-induced cardiovascular disease are generally nonspecific, including hypertension, hypercholesterolemia, and hypothyroidism. Fundoscopic examination may reveal microaneurysms and hemorrhages, resembling diabetic retinopathy but in a nondiabetic patient. Many of the cardiovascular abnormalities are reversible once exposure to carbon disulfide is ended. Carbon disulfide also may produce cerebral, renal, and peripheral vascular disease.

4. What are the key elements for a diagnosis of carbon disulfide-induced cardiovascular disease?

Carbon disulfide-induced cardiovascular disease is suggested in a worker who has been exposed to carbon disulfide for 5 or more years and presents with atherosclerotic vascular disease, particularly in association with abnormal retinal microcirculation in the absence of diabetes.

5. What are the cardiovascular manifestations of chronic arsenic exposure?

Several case-control studies suggest a 2–3-fold increase in mortality from ischemic heart disease in workers exposed to arsenic, including copper smelters and vintners working with arsenic-containing insecticides. Chronic exposure to arsenic in drinking water produces peripheral vascular disease, which may present as dry gangrene and autoamputation of the lower extremities. Gangrene due to chronic arsenic exposure, called "blackfoot disease," has been endemic in some areas of Taiwan, Chile, and Mexico, where arsenic levels in drinking water are high. The pathology of blackfoot disease involves thickening and fibrinoid necrosis of arterioles. Acute arsenic poisoning also has been associated with cardiac arrhythmias, including polymorphous ventricular tachycardia with Q-T interval prolongation (torsade de pointes).

6. What noncardiovascular clinical features suggest chronic arsenic poisoning?

Signs and symptoms of chronic arsenic poisoning including gastrointestinal disturbances; dermatitis, often with hyperpigmentation; and peripheral neuropathy (mixed sensory and motor).

Such signs and symptoms help to make the diagnosis but usually are not present in people with arsenic-induced cardiovascular disease.

7. What chemical causes are suggested by the development of ischemic heart disease in the absence of atherosclerosis?

Nonatheromatous coronary heart disease (angina pectoris, acute myocardial infarction, or sudden death due to coronary spasm) may be seen after withdrawal from chronic exposure to organic nitrates. Exposure in the workplace usually involves nitroglycerin or ethylene glycol dinitrate, which are used in construction (blasting) and munitions manufacturing.

8. What is "Monday morning angina"? Why does it occur?

Monday morning angina implies the development of chest pain 1–3 days after the last exposure to organic nitrates. In people who work Monday through Friday, it often occurs on Sunday or Monday and is relieved by return to nitrate exposure at work. Some workers have learned to relieve symptoms by wearing bandannas or hats that they wore during work. Relief of symptoms results from continued absorption of nitrate that previously impregnated headgear worn in the workplace. Monday morning angina is thought to be a rebound effect after prolonged exposure to nitrates. Nitrate exposure induces vasodilation, which is then opposed homeostatically by sympathetic neural and angiotensin-mediated vasoconstriction. When nitrate exposure is withdrawn, unopposed vasoconstriction results in coronary spasm.

9. The most ubiquitous industrial and environmental chemical toxin is carbon monoxide, which is produced by combustion. What are the major cardiovascular consequences of excessive carbon monoxide exposure?

Carbon monoxide exposure may occur in any workplace that uses equipment powered by combustion engines, such as forklifts; foundry workers, fire fighters, and workers in automobile garages, among others, are also at risk. Low-level exposure (carboxyhemoglobin concentrations of 5% or lower) may reduce maximal exercise capacity in healthy people as well as patients with chronic angina pectoris, chronic obstructive lung disease, or peripheral vascular disease with claudication. Severe carbon monoxide poisoning may present with acute myocardial infarction or sudden death. Acute carbon monoxide poisoning sufficient to cause myocardial infarction is usually associated with a depressed level of consciousness, including coma. However, in some people, particularly workers with underlying coronary heart disease who are exercising, exposure to lower levels of carbon monoxide has produced myocardial infarction without depression of consciousness.

10. What clinical features suggest carbon monoxide intoxication?

At low levels of exposure (up to 20–30% carboxyhemoglobin), people experience headache, nausea, dizziness, fatigue, and dimmed vision. Hypertension and hyperventilation are also common. At higher concentrations one sees depression of consciousness and coma. Laboratory findings include elevated carboxyhemoglobin levels (usually levels > 30–50% are required before severe symptoms develop), respiratory alkalosis, and/or respiratory acidosis. Arterial blood gases generally reveal a normal oxygen tension, but the oxygen content of the blood is reduced.

11. What chemical exposures should be considered in patients who present with cardiomyopathy and cardiac failure?

Chemicals of concern include cobalt, arsenic, lead, antimony, and organic solvents.

12. What are the clinical features of cobalt cardiomyopathy?

Cobalt cardiomyopathy was seen in epidemic form in Quebecois beer drinkers in the 1960s. Cobalt was added to beer to stabilize the foam. Cobalt cardiomyopathy occasionally has been reported in workers exposed to cobalt-containing dusts, such as may be seen in tungsten carbide workers. The syndrome in Quebecois beer drinkers resembles the syndrome seen in thiamine deficiency (beriberi heart disease). Cobalt poisoning interferes with energy metabolism in a manner biochemically similar to that of thiamine deficiency. Clinical symptoms include congestive cardiomyopathy with low cardiac output, venous congestion, pericardial effusion, and polycythemia. The electrocardiogram typically shows low voltage, ST-segment depression, T-wave inversions, and, in some cases, Q-waves suggestive of myocardial infarction.

13. A worker describes palpitations and episodes of dizziness at work, suggesting cardiac arrhythmias. What industrial chemicals should be considered as potential contributors to cardiac arrhythmias?

Arrhythmias are reported to occur with exposure to halogenated hydrocarbons, organophosphate insecticides, arsenic, and arsine. Carbon monoxide is also potentially arrhythmogenic in people with underlying coronary heart disease because it may aggravate ischemia.

14. How do halogenated hydrocarbons produce cardiac arrhythmias? What are the implications of the pathogenetic mechanisms for treatment?

Halogenated hydrocarbons include many solvents used in dry cleaning, degreasing parts, and painting and chemical manufacturing, as well as fluorocarbons used as refrigerants and propellants in various products. Hydrocarbons sensitize the heart to the effects of catecholamines. Experimental studies show that the dose of epinephrine required to produce ventricular tachycardia or fibrillation is reduced after solvents are inhaled. The combination of asphyxia and hypoxia produced by high levels of solvents, along with sensitization of the myocardium to the effects of catecholamines, are believed to underlie the development of ventricular arrhythmias, including ventricular fibrillation and sudden death. At high doses, solvents also may produce sinus bradycardia, cardiac arrest, or atrioventricular block, which may predispose to escape ventricular rhythms.

The major implication for treatment is that behavioral agitation or activity of the exposed person should be minimized to reduce catecholamine release. Medical treatment obviously should avoid the use of catecholamines; when tolerated, beta blockers are appropriate.

15. Organophosphate insecticides are commonly used in agriculture. What cardiovascular disturbances are most commonly seen with organophosphate intoxication?

Acute intoxication with organophosphates and carbamate insecticides produces diverse cardiovascular disturbances, including hypotension, sinus tachycardia, sinus bradycardia, varying degrees of heart block, prolonged Q-T interval, ventricular premature beats, and ventricular tachycardia, often of the torsade de pointes type. In one published series, 40% of patients with severe organophosphate poisoning had one or more cardiac arrhythmias.

16. What are the noncardiac clinical features of organophosphate poisoning? What is the most life-threatening feature of organophosphate poisoning?

The signs of organophosphate poisoning result from cholinergic stimulation and include small pupils, diaphoresis, salivation, lacrimation, increased bronchial secretions, and muscle fasciculations. Symptoms may include weakness, headache, sweating, nausea, vomiting, abdominal cramps, and diarrhea with mild poisoning and chest discomfort, dyspnea, inability to walk, and blurred vision with severe poisoning. The most severe cases may be associated with severe muscular weakness, paralysis, convulsions, or coma. Chest radiograph may show apparent pulmonary edema, which actually represents markedly enhanced pulmonary secretions. Electrocardiography may show Q-T interval prolongation and nonspecific ST- and T-wave changes.

The most life-threatening manifestations of organophosphate poisoning are respiratory failure or fatal cardiac arrhythmias. Intensive cardiac and respiratory monitoring is recommended for several days after moderate-to-severe intoxications. The development of hypoventilation is a warning of impending respiratory failure, which may require assisted ventilation.

17. Ventricular tachycardia of the torsade de pointes type has been reported after exposure to organophosphates as well as arsenic and various medications. How should torsade de pointes due to chemical exposure be treated?

Ventricular tachycardia of the torsade de pointes type is typically recurrent and self-limited but may degenerate to ventricular fibrillation and cause death. Emergent treatment includes intravenous magnesium and, if the patient is hypokalemic, potassium. Another treatment option is intravenous isoproterenol, which may suppress recurrent ventricular tachycardia by increasing heart rate. When the duration of recurrent ventricular tachycardia is likely to be long, such as after organophosphate or arsenic poisoning, definitive treatment is transvenous cardiac pacing. A temporary pacemaker should be placed with use of overdrive pacing at a rate adequate to suppress recurrent ventricular tachycardia.

18. What cardiovascular and other toxicity may be seen in workers with excessive lead exposure?

Occupational exposure to lead-containing dust and fumes occurs in lead smelters, foundries, and in industries such as battery manufacturing, construction work, demolition, and vehicle radiator repair, in which lead compounds are used. The most common cardiovascular manifestation is elevation of blood pressure, which occurs in proportion to blood lead concentrations, even without overt lead toxicity. Hypertension increases the risk of coronary heart disease and stroke. Excessive lead exposure has been associated with accelerated peripheral vascular disease as well as renal insufficiency, anemia, and peripheral neuropathy. Excessive exposure to lead is confirmed by finding elevated blood lead levels, usually greater than 35 μg/L.

BIBLIOGRAPHY

1. Allred EN, Bleecker ER, Chaitman BR, et al: Short-term effects of carbon monoxide exposure on the exercise performance of subjects with coronary artery disease. N Engl J Med 321:1426–1432, 1989.
2. Ben-David A: Cardiac arrest in an explosives factory worker due to withdrawal from nitroglycerin exposure. Am J Ind Med 15:719–722, 1989.
3. Benowitz NL: Cardiotoxicity in the workplace. Occup Med State Art Rev 7:465–478, 1992.
4. Jarvis JQ, Hammond E, Meir R, Robinson C: Cobalt cardiomyopathy. J Occup Med 34:620–636, 1992.
5. Sweetnam PM, Taylor SWC, Elwood PC: Exposure to carbon disulphide and ischaemic heart disease in a viscose rayon factory. Br J Ind Med 44:220–227, 1987.
6. Tseng CH, Chong CdK, Chen CJ, Tai TY: Dose-response relationship between peripheral vascular disease and ingested inorganic arsenic among residents in blackfoot disease endemic villages in Taiwan. Atherosclerosis 120:125–133, 1996.
7. Wilcosky TC, Simonson NR: Solvent exposure and cardiovascular disease. Am J Ind Med 19:569–586, 1991.

30. OCCUPATIONAL ASTHMA

William S. Beckett, M.D., M.P.H.

1. How is occupational asthma different from preexisting asthma?

Other than the fact that something in the workplace either worsens preexisting asthma or actually causes it de novo, occupational asthma looks, acts, and is treated medically the same as other forms of asthma. Just as in cases of asthma caused or exacerbated by home allergens or irritants, the first principle of treatment is to interrupt the inflammatory process by reducing exposure to the offending substance. No reliable population-based prevalence estimates of occupational asthma are available. Experienced observers have estimated that 5% or more of all cases of adult-onset asthma may be occupational in origin.

2. What features in an asthmatic's history suggest occupational asthma?

New-onset asthma in a working adult or worsening of asthma with a new job or workplace exposures should prompt questions about occupational causes. Perhaps the most useful question is, "Does your asthma get better on weekends, vacations, or other times when you are away from work?" A "yes" answer is highly suggestive of an occupational component. On the other hand, a "no" answer does not rule out occupational asthma, because in some cases, well-established disease does not improve until a period away from exposure has elapsed. Asthma that improves during a prolonged period away from work and promptly gets worse on return to work strongly suggests an occupational source.

Usually an airborne substance—most often a dust—is found in the workplace air of people with occupational asthma, although careful questioning may be required to identify it. The duration from onset of exposure (i.e., new job, or new materials in the air) may vary strikingly from as little as a few weeks to as much as several years.

3. What occupational exposures cause asthma?

Over 200 different substances have been demonstrated to cause occupational asthma. Workplace inhalation of substances in the following categories frequently causes asthma:

- Isocyanate chemicals (used in polyurethane paints and foams)
- Acid anhydrides (used in epoxy resins)
- Formaldehyde, glutaraldehyde
- Amines, aliphatic and heterocyclic
- Metal dusts
- Animal proteins (e.g., guinea pig, cat, cow, chicken)
- Insects
- Flours
- Wood dusts or barks
- Enzymes
- Pharmaceuticals

4. How should a case of suspected occupational asthma be approached?

The approach to the patient with suspected occupational asthma may be divided into three phases:

1. **Is it asthma?** Asthma is an episodic, remitting illness characterized by the symptoms of wheezing, chest tightness, cough, and dyspnea; reversible airflow obstruction (as evidenced by wheezing on physical examination and reduction in FEV_1/FVC ratio on spirometry), and airway hyperresponsiveness to nonimmunologic stimuli, such as cold air, exercise, or methacholine challenge.

2. **Is it occupational asthma?** A functional definition of occupational asthma is that it is worsened by one or more factors at work that are not active in the patient's home environment. This can be demonstrated clinically by physical deterioration at work or after a workday and stabilization of asthma while away from work, and also may be characterized by worsening symp-

toms, physical findings, expiratory airflow, or increased airway reactivity temporally related to work exposures. In many cases, the diagnosis will be abundantly clear from the patient's history in relation to workplace exposures to a known asthma-inducing substance (for a comprehensive listing of substances known to cause occupational asthma, see reference 4).

When further information is needed, a **stop/resume work test** (2 weeks off of work followed by a return to work with multiple self-administered peak-flow measurements or spirometry) can confirm or refute the clinical suspicion.

Intradermal allergy skin prick tests for immediate wheal-and- flare testing (available in allergists' offices) or blood RAST (radioallergosorbent test, available from commercial laboratories) are of similar sensitivity in demonstrating the presence of specific IgE to a suspected workplace sensitizing agent, but are available for only selected causes of occupational asthma.

Methacholine challenge test in the pulmonary function laboratory can demonstrate the degree of current airway reactivity if the diagnosis of asthma is uncertain. Methacholine challenge test is positive in the majority of patients with active asthma, whether occupational or nonoccupational.

3. **What specific agent is causing the occupational asthma?** Specific inhalational challenge (quantitative inhalation of low concentration of the allergen followed by serial spirometry to detect an asthmatic response in the sensitized individual) is considered the gold standard for diagnosis of occupational asthma. Unfortunately, specific inhalational challenge is currently available as a clinical test in only a handful of centers in North America. Assignment of a specific causative agent thus relies on identifying a workplace exposure known to cause occupational asthma or—when available—the demonstration of specific IgE to high–molecular-weight agents by intradermal skin test or RAST. In most cases, a thorough review of the asthmatic patient's exposures by comparing Material Safety Data Sheets with a comprehensive listing of known causes or an industrial hygiene walk-through of the workplace will identify one or more likely causative agents.

5. What is the difference between high–molecular-weight and low–molecular-weight occupational asthma?

Most cases of occupational asthma are caused by large biologic molecules such as those that cause house dust mite, cat, or pollen allergy. The mechanism of high–molecular-weight asthma, which produces antigen-specific IgE and subsequently releases inflammatory mediators, is better understood. Wheal-and-flare skin tests or RAST for specific IgE may be helpful in diagnosis; associated allergic phenomena (particularly allergic rhinitis) frequently occur, and patients with a previous allergic disposition are at higher risk than nonatopic individuals for developing occupational asthma to such substances.

Low–molecular-weight asthma is caused by smaller molecules; usually there is no specific IgE and thus no skin test or RAST to aid diagnosis. The mechanisms for most of these forms of asthma remain uncertain, and atopic and nonatopic people appear to be at equal risk for becoming sensitized. Intradermal skin testing and RAST is available for the following partial list of high–molecular-weight substances that are known to cause occupational asthma:

Animal substances	Food substances
Horse, cow, dog, and cat dander;	Egg white, wheat, oat, soybean,
Goose and chicken feathers	rye, barley, rice, buckwheat

6. What is methacholine challenge testing, and what is its role in the work-up of occupational asthma?

Methacholine is a pharmacologic cholinergic agonist and functions as a bronchoconstricting agent. Asthmatics have airway hyperresponsiveness and usually bronchoconstrict to lower inhaled concentrations of methacholine than nonasthmatics (dose-response curve shifted to the left). By constructing a person's dose-response curve to progressively increasing inhaled concentrations of methacholine, airway reactivity can be measured. It is important to realize that airway responsiveness is a dynamic physiologic attribute; in a normal person it is often temporarily increased by a recent viral bronchitis, and when an asthmatic resolves clinically due to reduction in exposure, airway reactivity may improve into the normal range. Serial methacholine challenge testing can sometimes be useful in documenting changes in airway reactivity, although there can be marked variability over time in normal, nonasthmatic subjects.

7. After occupational asthma is diagnosed, how is it treated?

Although avoidance of the offending substance is the mainstay of treatment, many occupational asthmatics will need temporary or long-term pharmacotherapy. The principles of treatment are the same: inhaled corticosteroids for maintenance antiinflammatory activity; inhaled beta-agonists as needed for occasional symptoms or rescue therapy during an acute exacerbation; additional drugs as needed for control; and short courses of oral corticosteroids to manage severe exacerbations.

8. Does immununologic hyposensitization therapy have any role in occupational asthma?

Although it is useful in selected cases of allergic asthma (e.g., selected cases of cat allergy), immunotherapy has not been demonstrated to have a significant role in the management and treatment of occupational asthma. Because the offending allergen can be avoided through job modification, avoidance is key.

9. How long does it take for a patient to get better? What is the prognosis?

Most patients experience some improvement within weeks to months of stopping exposure. Some will have a complete remission of their disease and become free of symptoms and the need for medications. However, long-term follow-up studies have shown that a significant proportion—in some series the majority—will continue to have some asthma impairment or disability, requiring medication and medical follow-up for years after diagnosis.

10. Is reactive airways dysfunction syndrome (RADS) a form of occupational asthma?

Yes. RADS is defined as an asthma-like condition of symptoms and airway hyperreactivity that lasts at least 1 year after a single, acute inhalation exposure to a potent lung irritant. Most cases occur after an exposure to severe smoke inhalation, a spill, explosion, or accident (e.g., involving a strong acid or base). The single episode causes chronic airway injury, inflammation, and hyperreactivity, which may necessitate chronic or intermittent asthma medications. Occupational asthma may be categorized as asthma with latency (implying recurrent exposure to a sensitizing agent before asthma occurs) or without latency (indicating a single causative exposure, as in RADS).

11. What should be considered in the differential diagnosis of occupational asthma?

1. Nonoccupational asthma
2. Airway symptoms due to inhaled irritants without airway hyperreactivity or airflow obstruction
3. Industrial bronchitis: cough with mucus production caused by inhaled occupational substances (pathophysiologically identical to the chronic bronchitis of cigarette smokers)
4. Hypersensitivity pneumonitis: an allergic interstitial occupational lung disease that may have an airway component (cough, chest tightness, wheeze, and airflow obstruction), but also has lung parenchymal involvement and is usually associated with fever, crackles on chest examination, peripheral blood leukocytosis, and fleeting pulmonary infiltrates on chest x-ray.

12. What workplace interventions are effective in workers with occupational asthma?

Because fatal status asthmaticus has occurred in patients with occupational asthma who were not removed from exposure, a strong rationale prevails for assisting the patient with complete removal from exposure to the sensitizing agent. This approach has been validated in many cases by the recurrence and progression of asthma in individuals whose exposures were reduced but not eliminated. In some instances, the use of respiratory protective devices (masks or respirators) may be effective in preventing asthma attacks during occasional exposure (e.g., for the laboratory animal handler who must venture occasionally into the animal facility for only a few minutes at a time). Workers' compensation regulations in many states protect the employment of sensitized workers if the employer has suitable work for the individual's skills that is completely away from exposure. When no exposure-free employment is available (e.g., for an isocyanate-exposed spray painter in a small auto-body shop), the occupational asthmatic may be forced to seek work elsewhere. Workers' compensation should pay for lost time and medical bills relating to the occupational asthma. Vocational retraining supported by workers' compensation insurance may be the most realistic alternative for workers whose trade would involve re-exposure to the offending substance in any similar workplace.

13. Is preemployment testing of nonasthmatics useful in preventing occupational asthma?

No. To date it has not been demonstrated to be useful in practice. People with a previous history of allergies or asthma are at higher risk for developing occupational asthma to some (high–molecular-weight) allergens. Tests such as allergy skin or methacholine challenge tests have such a high rate of positivity in the general population that their use would unfairly exclude many individuals from a position that may never result in asthma. Moreover, in many situations such tests may not accurately identify people who will go on to develop asthma. The most reasonable approach at present may be to alert patients with an allergic history to the possibility of further sensitization to high–molecular-weight allergens so that they can be removed from exposure promptly if sensitization occurs.

14. What are the criteria for disability due to asthma for workers' compensation and Social Security?

In general, impairment and disability for occupational asthma are evaluated in the same manner as other forms of asthma. Permanent removal from exposure to an identified cause of asthma is usually considered a specific work restriction rather than a permanent disability. The rating for disability is based on the severity of the continuing asthma **after** removal. In many cases a prolonged period of medical management after removal is needed to determine the degree of maximal improvement. A committee of the American Thoracic Society has published guidelines for evaluation of impairment/disability in asthma with special considerations for workers with occupational asthma (see reference 1).

The *Guides to the Evaluation of Permanent Impairment*, published by the American Medical Association, are the most widely used criteria for workers' compensation in states that do not have their own guidelines, indicates that when pulmonary function tests fall in the severely impaired range on three successive tests separated by at least one week, the patient should qualify for disability in spite of optimal medical therapy. The criteria that the Social Security disability rating use is the occurrence of 6 asthma episodes per year (or one episode every 2 months) that requires intravenous or inhaled medication in the hospital or emergency room, in spite of optimal medical therapy.

BIBLIOGRAPHY

1. American Thoracic Society Ad Hoc Committee on Impairment/Disability Evaluation in Subjects with Asthma: Guidelines for evaluation of impairment/disability in patients with asthma. Am Rev Respir Dis 147:1056–1061, 1993.
2. Chan-Yeung M, Lam S: State of the art: Occupational asthma. Ann Rev Respir Dis 133:686–703, 1986.
3. Chan-Yeung M, Malo J-L: Current concepts: Occupational asthma. N Engl J Med 333:107–112, 1995.
4. Malo J-L, Cartier A: Key references in occupational asthma (Appendix B). In Harber P, Schenker M, Balmes J (eds): Occupational and Environmental Respiratory Disease. Philadelphia, W.B. Saunders, 1996.

31. INTERSTITIAL LUNG DISEASES

Feroza Daroowalla, M.D., M.P.H., and Gregory R. Wagner, M.D.

1. What is interstitial lung disease (ILD)?

Interstitial lung disease encompasses a large group of entities characterized by involvement of the interstitial space of the lung, which is the space in the walls of the alveoli between the basement membrane of the alveolar epithelium and the basement membrane of the capillary endothelium. It contains fibroblasts, macrophages, and collagen and noncollagen proteins. The interstitial space is the gas exchange surface of the lung; in some forms of ILD, alterations in the small airways, alveolar ducts, respiratory bronchioles and terminal bronchioles also may be seen.

2. What is meant by pulmonary fibrosis?

Pulmonary fibrosis is the pathologic end-result of the various chronic disease processes involved in ILD. Fibrosis begins with the development of an initial alveolar injury after inhalation of a gas, fume, or dust. This initial insult is followed by a cascade of protective responses characterized by tissue inflammation. If inflammation becomes chronic or recurrent, proliferation of smooth muscle, fibroblasts, and collagen ensues with accompanying architectural distortion. Fibrosis is a process of progressive scarring with associated distortion.

3. How common is ILD?

Current estimates for the annual incidence of ILD are of 40–80 cases per 100,000 in the general population, Occupational exposures are believed to cause 25–50% of cases (20 cases in 100,000 in males and 0.6 cases in 100,000 in females). However, this percentage may be an underestimate because of difficulties in making a conclusive diagnosis of ILD and in tracing workplace exposures over the entire working life of patients.

4. What are the causes of ILD?

ILD in immunocompetent hosts may be grouped according to cause or syndrome:

Inhalation causes (occupational and environmental): inorganic dusts leading to asbestosis, silicosis; organic dusts or aerosols leading to hypersensitivity pneumonitis, as in machine workers, farmers, pigeon breeders.

Idiopathic disease: sarcoidosis, histiocytosis X, idiopathic pulmonary fibrosis.

Inherited causes: familial idiopathic pulmonary fibrosis, tuberous sclerosis, neurofibromatosis.

Collagen vascular disease/pulmonary renal syndromes: pneumonitis with systemic lupus erythematosus, ILD with rheumatoid arthritis, Wegener's granulomatosis, Goodpasture's syndrome.

Other specific entities: bronchiolitis obliterans, lymphangioleiomyomatosis, eosinophilic pneumonia.

5. What exposures may result in occupational interstitial lung disease (O-ILD)?

Exposures to inorganic dusts in the workplace may result in ILD. Examples are free silica, asbestos, coal, beryllium, and hard metal (tungsten carbide with cobalt). Less common causes include exposures to tin, aluminum, or iron. Exposure to organic dusts or aerosols (thermophilic bacteria, fungi, animal proteins) may result in hypersensitivity pneumonitis. ILD also may result from toxic pneumonitis due to chemical or gas exposure. Industries in which such exposures occur and the disease outcomes are listed in the table below.

Occupational Interstitial Lung Diseases

INDUSTRY	DISEASE	AGENT
Mining	Coal worker's pneumoconiosis, silicosis	Coal dust, silica
Insulating, ship-working, steam-fitting, plumbing	Asbestosis	Asbestos
Airplane, spacecraft manufacture	Chronic beryllium disease	Beryllium particulate
Machine working	Hypersensitivity pneumonitis	Metal-working fluids
Machining, sawing, filing,	Hard metal disease: interstitial pneumo-nitis and hypersensitivity pneumonitis	Cobalt
Farmwork, silo work	Farmer's lung	Bacterial and fungal proteins in moldy hay or grain

6. What are the symptoms of O-ILD?

Most patients with O-ILD report some level of dyspnea, initially with exertion and in later stages with minimal activity. Some patients complain of tiredness or fatigue and inability to accomplish tasks that they previously performed. Initially they may attribute their limitations to normal aging. Cough is a common symptom; usually it is not accompanied by phlegm unless a component of bronchitis is involved. Chest pain may occur in patients with accompanying pleural disease. Although hemoptysis may occur in cases of ILD associated with vasculitis or diffuse alveolar hemorrhage syndrome, it is not a usual feature of uncomplicated O-ILD and should prompt an evaluation for carcinoma, tuberculosis, or other complications.

7. How can patients with O-ILD be identified?

Patients with O-ILD may present with dyspnea and cough. Others may be identified through changes on chest radiograph (see question 11) without symptoms or with impairment that they attribute to aging or other causes. For some patients the first finding may be an abnormality on spirometry, such as a reduction in vital capacity.

8. What are common findings on physical examination of a worker with O-ILD?

Early and even advanced ILD may be unremarkable on physical exam. More commonly, however, physical findings include bibasilar end-inspiratory crackles (Velcro rales) on lung auscultation. In addition, the patient may be tachypneic or tachycardic, at rest or with mild exertion; patients in later stages may show signs of cor pulmonale and pulmonary hypertension. Examination also should be made for findings that accompany nonoccupational ILD, including skin, joint, and ocular findings associated with connective tissue disease, vasculitis, or sarcoidosis. In rare cases of advanced ILD, clubbing of the digits may be seen.

9. What are the usual findings of pulmonary function testing?

Lung volume measurements, such as vital capacity, residual volume, functional residual capacity, and total lung capacity, are reduced in ILD. Air flow rates, such as the ratio of forced expiratory volume in 1 second to forced vital capacity (FEV_1/FVC), are usually normal because the FEV_1 is reduced in proportion to reduction of vital capacity. This pattern, termed restrictive disease, is classic for ILD. A mixed pattern of restriction and obstruction or a pattern primarily of obstruction (FEV^1 and FEV_1/FVC ratio reduced) is frequently seen in workers with ILD as a result of occupational dust exposure or smoking on the airways. Reduction in carbon monoxide diffusion in the lung (DL_{CO}) is common because of loss of gas exchange units and ventilation-perfusion mismatch. However, the level of reduction in DL_{CO} does not match the severity of disease.

10. What are the findings of arterial blood gas (ABG) measurements?

ABG measurements at rest may reveal no abnormalities or hypoxemia (decreased partial oxygen pressure [PO_2]); partial pressure of carbon dioxide (PCO_2) may be normal or decreased. A normal resting PO$_2$ should prompt a check for hypoxemia during exertion or sleep. One of the best ways to follow disease progression in ILD is to assess resting and exercise gas (O$_2$) over time.

11. What are the expected findings of chest radiography?

Up to 20% of patients with asbestosis or coal worker's pneumoconiosis and up to 10% of patients with hypersensitivity pneumonitis may appear to have a normal chest radiograph. Therefore, patients with symptoms or abnormal pulmonary function tests (PFTs) should be evaluated completely despite a normal initial radiograph. In patients with radiographic abnormality a high-quality film reveals common patterns of specific occupational ILDs (see below). A common feature of late-stage disease is honeycombing, which represents fibrous change in the lung parenchyma.

Silicosis: diffuse rounded reticulonodular densities with upper zone predominance; irregular opacities, possibly massive fibrosis with advanced disease; eggshell calcification of hilar nodes unusual.

Coal worker's pneumoconiosis: diffuse reticulonodular densities; large opacities.

Asbestosis: diffuse densities of irregular shape with lower zone predominance; pleural findings may accompany parenchymal asbestosis: pleural plaques, diffuse pleural thickening, pleural effusions.

12. What is the ILO system for classifying chest radiographs in workers with O-ILD?

Chest radiographs in workers with pneumoconiosis (silicosis, coal worker's pneumoconiosis, and asbestosis) are categorized using a standard method devised by the International Labour Organisation (ILO). The system, called the International Classification of Radiographs of Pneumoconioses, consists of 22 standard radiographs that illustrate the parenchymal opacities and pleural changes associated with pneumoconiosis. These radiographs are used to classify the size, shape, profusion (concentration or density), and extent of parenchymal opacities and pleural changes on posteroanterior (PA) radiographs. The classification is not designed to correlate with the pathologic severity of disease. The system, last updated in 1980, is currently undergoing revision; an updated classification scheme should be released in early 1999.

13. What is the utility of computed tomography (CT) in ILD?

Both conventional CT (resolution of 8–10 mm of lung tissue per slice) and high-resolution CT (HRCT, in which the images resolve tissue slices 1–3 mm in thickness) may be used to evaluate the interstitium, pleura, and airways in O-ILD. Conventional CT has been found to be superior to chest radiography for evaluation of pulmonary masses and pleural plaques (due to asbestos exposure). HRCT allows better identification of thickened lobular interfaces, nodular abnormalities, and loss of volume associated with pulmonary fibrosis. In addition, HRCT is useful for selecting the appropriate area for biopsy. However, CT scanning is not necessary for the evaluation of O-ILD in a patient with a history of exposure and consistent chest radiographic findings. Furthermore, there is no widely accepted standardized method for categorization of O-ILD using CT.

14. What blood tests may be helpful in evaluating O-ILD?

Blood tests are usually nonspecific in O-ILD and are best used for excluding nonoccupational causes of ILD, such as a connective tissue disorder. Potentially useful tests for evaluating the presence of nonoccupational causes of ILD include immunoglobulin levels, rheumatoid factor, antinuclear antibodies, and erythrocyte sedimentation rate. An exception to the above generalization is beryllium-related disease, in which a specific peripheral lymphocyte transformation response helps to detect workers who have developed an immune response to beryllium after exposure. Blood tests also may play a role in evaluating hypersensitivity pneumonitis in which the presence of serum precipitins (IgG antibodies) denotes exposure to a specific antigen.

15. How is lung tissue obtained for pathologic examination?

Various microscopic and staining techniques are used to examine lung architecture, cellular components, and foreign inhaled bodies (ferruginous bodies). Bulk analysis, in which the tissue is digested, is used to analyze the mineral and dust content of the tissue. Open lung biopsy, video-assisted thoracoscopic biopsy, and transbronchial biopsy are the three ways to obtain tissue for examination. Open lung biopsy and video-assisted thoracoscopic biopsy require surgery and inpatient stays. Transbronchial biopsy obtains specimens through a bronchoscope and is less invasive but provides a smaller sample that may not reveal tissue architecture, which may be useful for making a specific diagnosis.

Tissue biopsy is not routinely needed for the diagnosis of O-ILD if the clinical and radiologic patterns are consistent with a history of exposure to a known etiologic agent. However, biopsy has a role in excluding neoplastic or infectious processes and allows assessment of disease severity and response to treatment.

16. What histologic patterns are commonly found in O-ILD?

The histologic patterns typically associated with particular exposures are listed below.

Granulomatous lesions: beryllium, organic dusts
Diffuse fibrosis (usually interstitial pneumonitis): asbestos, hard metal
Macules: coal, tin, aluminum
Nodular fibrosis: coal, silica
Bronchiolitis obliterans: fumes and gases

17. What is the role of bronchoscopy in the diagnosis of ILD?

Bronchoscopy is usually an outpatient procedure during which a fiberoptic scope is introduced into the trachea and main airways through the nose or mouth. It is used for visualizing the airways, taking transbronchial biopsies (TBB), and obtaining lavage fluids (washings). Lavage fluid has been used for cellular immunophenotyping to determine the diagnosis, course, and prognosis of disease, but this use remains controversial. The small tissue samples procured through TBB are most helpful in the diagnosis of granulomatous interstitial processes in which abnormal tissue is found in the peribronchiolar region (e.g., sarcoidosis, beryllium disease, hypersensitivity pneumonitis). Many cases of O-ILD can be diagnosed by history, radiograph, and PFT findings; bronchoscopy should be used as needed for clarification or confirmation.

18. What is the recommended diagnostic pathway for ILD?

Although the approach to diagnosis of ILD varies on a case-by-case basis, the path starts with history, physical exam, chest radiograph, and PFTs to establish that ILD is in the differential diagnosis. These evaluations should be followed by an in-depth assessment of environmental or occupational exposures and exclusion of systemic connective tissue disease, pulmonary renal syndromes, and vasculitis. If the diagnosis remains in question, bronchoalveolar lavage and transbronchial biopsy may be helpful. If neither is diagnostic, open biopsy or thoracoscopic biopsy guided by HRCT should follow.

19. What are the complications of ILD?

Many but not all types of ILD are chronic with progressive loss of lung function and disability. Progressive hypoxemia may require chronic oxygen supplementation. ILD (more specifically, fibrosis) has been found to increase the risk for development of lung cancer independently of the risk conferred by exposure to agents such as asbestos or silica.

20. What is the prognosis of ILD?

ILD related to asbestos, coal, or silica exposure is generally slowly progressive and irreversible, eventually leading to disability and sometimes death. Disease often progresses even after cessation of exposure. In some cases the disease is more rapidly progressive (e.g., acute silicosis, which has a fatal course in a short period). Other types of ILD, such as hypersensitivity pneumonitis, may stabilize or improve after removal from exposure to the offending agent.

21. When should a worker be evaluated for ILD?

All workers exposed to agents known to cause an ILD are candidates for evaluation. Exposed workers who are healthy should be enrolled in surveillance programs in which lung function and radiographs are monitored regularly for changes over time. Many ILDs, including asbestosis, silicosis, and coal worker's pneumoconiosis, involve long latency periods between first exposure and appearance of detectable signs of disease. Workers may not show signs of disease until after discontinuation of exposure; therefore, it is important to evaluate workers with a history of exposure. The latency period between exposure and disease (which ranges from months to 20 or more years) makes it necessary to continue to monitor the health of retired workers. In addition, latency is important to keep in mind in evaluating the current health of workers at a particular workplace. Although the current worker group may appear to be free of disease, current exposures may still be hazardous, causing disease that will not become apparent for years to come. Current healthy workers must be protected from excessive exposure to prevent future disease. Guidelines for determining whether exposures are excessive include the permissible exposure limits (PELs) enforced by the Occupational Safety and Health Administration (OSHA), the recommended exposure limits (RELs) published by National Institute for Occupational Safety and Health (NIOSH,) and the threshold limit values (TLVs) published by the American Conference of Governmental Industrial Hygienists.

22. How is O-ILD managed?

A primary focus of management is removal of the offending exposure in the work or home environment. Treatment of hypoxemia, preventive care with influenza and pneumococcal vaccinations, screening for mycobacterial infection with purified protein derivative (PPD) testing, early treatment of infections, counseling for smoking cessation, and patient and family education about self-care strategies are important components of care for patients with chronic and progressive pulmonary disease such as asbestosis or silicosis. Prevention is critical because the disease is irreversible. In cases of O-ILD with evidence of ongoing inflammation and alveolitis, such as hypersensitivity pneumonitis, a course of corticosteroids and cytotoxic drugs may slow disease progression.

23. How can O-ILD be prevented?

Prevention of ILD in the workplace begins with recognition of the hazardous exposure. **Primary prevention**, which reduces the occurrence of disease, is achieved by eliminating excessive exposure to the hazardous agent. The agent may have to be eliminated entirely and an appropriate replacement found. For example, crystalline quartz (sand) must be eliminated and replaced in abrasive blasting because of the high risk to workers. If an agent cannot be eliminated entirely, exposure in the workplace must be minimized with engineering changes such as ventilation and confinement. To supplement engineering controls and to protect against intermittent high-exposure events, workers may be further protected by educational programs and use of respiratory protective equipment.

Secondary prevention involves methods of early detection and benefits affected workers by reducing the risk of progression. Examples include screening of exposed workers with PFTs or chest radiographs on a regular basis. Screening tests must be accompanied by an ongoing monitoring program to identify workers who exhibit early signs of disease or ill effects due to exposure. Effective interventions must be included.

Physicians evaluating a patient with O-ILD have a role in preventing future cases by reporting the case and ensuring proper workplace evaluation and follow-up. Many state health departments or departments of labor provide this service, as do OSHA and the Mine Safety and Health Administration (MSHA) for workplaces under their jurisdiction. Occupational health professionals or government public health offices are good sources of information for a physician attempting to develop a follow-up plan for a patient with suspected disease and excessive exposure in the workplace.

BIBLIOGRAPHY

1. Coultas DB, Zumwalt RE, Black WC, Sobonya RE: The epidemiology of interstitial lung diseases. Am J Respir Crit Care Med 150:967–972, 1994.
2. Davis GS, Calhoun WJ: Occupational and environmental causes of interstitial lung disease. In Schwarz MI, King TE (eds): Interstitial Lung Disease. St. Louis, Mosby, 1993.

3. International Labour Organisation: Guidelines for the use of ILO international classification of radiographs of pneumoconiosis. Occup Safety Health, Series 22 (rev), 1980.
4. Raghu G: Interstitial lung disease: A diagnostic approach. Are CT scan and lung biopsy indicated in every patient? Am J Respir Crit Care Med 151:909–914, 1995.
5. Raghu G (ed): Interstitial lung diseases: Part I. Semin Respir Med 14:5, 1993.
6. Redlich CA: Pulmonary fibrosis and interstitial lung diseases. In Harber P, Schenker MB, Balmes JR (eds): Occupational and Environmental Respiratory Diseases. St. Louis, Mosby, 1996, pp 216–227.
7. Rose C: Hypersensitivity pneumonitis. In Harber P, Schenker MB, Balmes JR (eds): Occupational and Environmental Respiratory Diseases. St. Louis, Mosby, 1996, pp 201–215.
8. Wagner GR: Screening and Surveillance of Workers Exposed to Mineral Dusts. Geneva, World Health Organization, 1996.
9. Wagner GR, Attfield MD, Parker JE: Chest radiography in dust-exposed miners: Promise and problems, potential and imperfections. Occup Med State Art Rev 8:127–141, 1993.

32. OCCUPATIONAL LUNG CANCER

Robert L. Keith, M.D.

1. What proportion of lung cancer is attributable to occupational exposures?

Occupational exposure is believed to account for 5–27% of all lung cancers, depending on the study, location, and specific industry. Lung cancer is the number-one cause of cancer death in both men and women in the U.S., and in 1998 approximately 170,000 new cases will be diagnosed. As many as 15% of lung cancers are occupationally related (range: 3–17%). Most studies control for smoking and have included predominantly men. As the gender distribution of certain occupations changes, more occupational lung cancer will be observed in women. A recent extensive study from the Netherlands found asbestos exposure to account for 11.6% of lung cancer in men.

2. Name the top three occupational exposures associated with lung cancer.

1. Asbestos
2. Radon
3. Involuntary (passive) smoking

3. What other major occupational exposures are associated with lung cancer?

In evaluating patients for lung cancer, a thorough occupational history is required and should focus on the industries listed in the table below. Exposures may have a long latency period and may include exposures in the home; the occupational history should include all jobs held, areas of the country in which the patient resided, and type of dwelling (i.e., was there a basement?).

Agents Linked to Occupational Lung Cancer

COMPOUND	EVIDENCE	INDUSTRY
Acrylonitrile	Limited	Petrochemical and plastics production
Arsenic	Adequate	Copper smelting, pesticide manufacturing
Asbestos	Convincing	Workers exposed to insulation, brake linings
Beryllium	Limited	Metal processing, ceramics, aerospace equipment
Bis-chloromethyl ether	Adequate	Chemical manufacture
Cadmium	Adequate	Smelting, battery manufacturing
Chloromethyl methyl ether	Adequate	Chemical manufacture of ion-exchange resins
Chromium (hexavalent)	Adequate	Pigment manufacturing, electroplating
Diesel engine exhaust	Limited	Mechanics, drivers, bus garage workers
Fiberglass	Limited	Insulation installation
Mustard gas	Convincing	Weapons manufacture and storage
Nickel	Adequate	Smelting, electrolysis, refining
Passive smoke	Adequate	Home, restaurants
Polyaromatic hydrocarbons	Adequate	Rubber or aluminum production, coke ovens
Radon	Convincing	Mining (especially uranium and hard rock)
Silica	Limited	Mining, masonry, pottery making, sandblasting
Vinyl chloride	Adequate	Production of polyvinyl chloride

Based on Steenland K, Loomis D, Shy C, Simonsen N: Review of occupational lung carcinogens. Am J Indust Med 29:474–490, 1996, and Whitesell PL, Drage CW: Occupational lung cancer. Mayo Clin Proc 68:183–188, 1993.

4. What environmental factors interact with occupational exposure to increase lung cancer risk?

The major confounding factors are cigarette smoking and air pollution (i.e., degree of industrialization). Many early studies did not control for the contribution of concomitant smoking. The effects of smoking may be multiplicative; for example, asbestos-related lung cancer is 8–10 times more prevalent in smokers.

5. What is radon? What is the source of most exposures?

Radioactive radon is an inert gas formed during the decay of uranium (^{238}U) to lead. The carcinogenicity of radon originates from alpha particles emitted during the formation of radon daughters (radioactive decay products). Radon daughters adhere to airborne particles, are inhaled, and damage DNA in bronchial epithelial cells. Radon may migrate from rocks and soil and accumulate in enclosed areas such as underground mines and homes. The average residential radon exposure in U.S. homes ranges from 0.8–1.5 picoCuries (pCi)/L. The Environmental Protection Agency has set a residential radon action level of 4 pCi/L, a level found in 5–10% of U.S. homes. Radon testing kits are commercially available for residential testing. For extensive details about radon, the reader is referred to chapter 14.

6. Has silica exposure been linked to lung cancer?

Numerous epidemiologic studies have been conducted with inconsistent results. Silica exposure is common among miners and highly dependent on the silica content of the ore. High doses of silica are required to cause silicosis (characterized by extensive fibrosis); scarred areas may be a nidus for carcinoma formation.

7. To what substances are welders exposed? Do they increase lung cancer rates?

The welding plume (a mixture of gases, particulates, and fumes) contains cadmium, hexavalent chromium, and nickel. The plume also contains carbon dioxide, nitrogen gases, and ozone. Although male welders as an occupational group have higher rates of cigarette smoking, epidemiologic studies have failed to reveal consistently excessive lung cancer-related mortality.

8. Exposure to environmental tobacco smoke (ETS) in nonsmokers is most often associated with what histologic subtype of lung cancer?

Passive smoking increases the rates of all lung cancer types in nonsmokers, but adenocarcinoma is the most common. It has been estimated that ETS may account for 3,000–4,000 lung cancer deaths annually.

9. Where is malignant mesothelioma located? What are the known causes?

Malignant mesothelioma is a rare tumor originating from mesothelial cells lining the pleural and peritoneal cavities. Malignant mesothelioma is virtually pathognomonic for asbestos exposure and typically is associated with a latency period of 30 years. All types of asbestos fibers, with the exception of anthophyllite, have been implicated. The Cappadocian region of Turkey has an unusually high incidence of mesothelioma (1% of all deaths), which is thought to originate from elevated atmospheric zeolite levels. Zeolite is a hydrated aluminum silicate used to soften "hard" water.

10. Which carcinogens require medical monitoring of exposed workers?

The Occupational Safety and Health Administration requires medical monitoring (history, physical examination, and periodic chest radiograph) for workers exposed to asbestos, arsenic, acrylonitrile, vinyl chloride, bis-chloromethyl ether, cadmium, coke oven emissions, and silica. Sputum cytology is suggested in arsenic and coke oven-emission exposure. Like all patients, potentially exposed workers should be counseled to abstain from smoking.

CONTROVERSIES

11. Can results from radon exposure in miner studies be generalized to residential exposures?

Direct application of the miner-based models suggests that 11–13% of lung cancer deaths among residents of single-family dwellings (10% of all lung cancer cases) may be attributable to radon exposure, but this figure is generally regarded as an overestimate. Problems arise from lack of epidemiologic support in multiple studies due to gross imprecisions in exposure estimates. In fact, miners may have other carcinogenic exposures that potentiate the effect of radon (for example, arsenic, silica, or diesel fumes). More detail is provided in chapter 14.

12. Do electromagnetic fields affect lung cancer rates?

Heavily radar-exposed U.S. naval personnel had a two-fold increase in lung cancer rates in one study (not controlled for smoking). Other studies among military and telecommunication employees have failed to support this finding.

13. Have most occupational lung carcinogens been determined?

No. Only a small minority of compounds in the workplace have been classified as human carcinogens. Many authorities believe that no sensitive or systematic approach has been taken to discover occupational exposures that increase the lifetime cancer risk. Difficulties arise in determining exposures and applying in vitro and animal evidence to humans. Prospective, placebo-controlled, randomized trials of carcinogenicity cannot be performed; therefore, most human studies are epidemiologic.

BIBLIOGRAPHY

1. Doll R: Mortality from lung cancer in asbestos workers. Br J Indust Med 12:81–86,1955.
2. Figueroa WG, Raszowski R, Weiss W: Lung cancer in chloromethyl methyl ether workers. N Engl J Med 288:1096–1097, 1973.
3. Fontham ETH, Correa P, Reynolds P, et al: Environmental tobacco smoke and lung cancer in nonsmoking women: A multicenter study. JAMA 271:1752–1759, 1994.
4. Little JB: What are the risks of low-level exposure to α radiation from radon? PNAS 94:5996–5997, 1997.
5. Lubin JH: Invited commentary: Lung cancer and exposure to residential radon. Am J Epidemiol 140:323–332, 1994.
6. Lubin JH, Boice JD Jr, Edling C, et al: Lung cancer in radon-exposed miners and estimation of risk from indoor exposure. J Natl Cancer Inst 87:817–827, 1995.
7. Robinette CD, Silverman C, Jablon S: Effects upon health of occupational exposure to microwave radiation (radar). Am J Epidemiol 112:39–53, 1980.
8. Rom WN (ed): Environmental and Occupational Medicine, 3rd ed. Philadelphia, Lippincott-Raven, 1998.
9. Sferlazza SJ, Beckett WS: The respiratory health of welders. Am Rev Respir Dis 143:1134–1148, 1991.
10. Steenland K, Loomis D, Shy C, Simonsen N: Review of occupational lung carcinogens. Am J Indust Med 29:474–490, 1996.
11. van Loom AJM, Kant IJ, Swaen GMH, et al: Occupational exposure to carcinogens and risk of lung cancer: Results from the Netherlands Cohort Study. Occup Environ Med 54:817–824, 1997.
12. Wells AJ: Lung cancer from passive smoking at work. Am J Public Health 88:1025–1029, 1998.
13. Whitesell PL, Drage CW: Occupational lung cancer. Mayo Clin Proc 68:183–188, 1993.

33. HYPERSENSITIVITY PNEUMONITIS AND OTHER DISORDERS CAUSED BY ORGANIC AGENTS

Cecile S. Rose, M.D., M.P.H.

1. What is meant by the term *organic agent?*

Substances of animal and vegetable origin are generally referred to as *organic agents.* Airborne organic agents are called *bioaerosols*, which are airborne particles, large molecules, or volatile compounds that are living or were released from a living organism. Sources of common bioaerosol components capable of causing human diseases include bacteria, fungi, protozoa, viruses, algae, green plants, arthropods, and mammals. For example, saliva bioaerosols from cats can cause asthma and rhinitis in cat-sensitive individuals. The necessary conditions and events required to produce aerosolization of an organism or its parts are the presence of a reservoir, amplification (increase the numbers or concentration), and dissemination (aerosolization). Human hosts are reservoirs for some organisms, for example, *Mycobacterium tuberculosis*. Others are found in environmental reservoirs that act as amplifiers or disseminators, such as *Legionella* bioaerosol dissemination from cooling towers.

2. Describe the spectrum of diseases caused by exposure to organic agents.

• Hypersensitivity pneumonitis
• Rhinoconjunctivitis
• Asthma
• Inhalation fevers, such as grain fever, organic dust toxic syndrome (ODTS), and humidifier fever
• Infections, such as legionella pneumonia or unusual infections from outbreaks in laboratory workers
• Chronic airflow limitation and accelerated decline in lung function, such as the decline in FEV_1 often found in workers exposed to cotton dust, grain workers, and animal confinement workers

3. What industries or occupational groups are most likely to be affected by exposure to organic agents?

The most well-recognized occupation associated with exposure to organic agents is the agricultural industry, in which the effects of exposure to grain dusts have been recognized since antiquity. The world produces more than 1.5 billion tons of grain annually, and the United States is a major producer and the greatest exporter of grain in the world.

Farmer's lung disease was the first form of hypersensitivity pneumonitis (HP) described. It is typically associated with inhalation of thermophilic bacteria and fungal contaminants in hay and grain. Mushroom workers, cheese workers, and wood workers are occupational groups in whom hypersensitivity lung diseases, including both HP and asthma, have been described. Proteins capable of causing hypersensitivity pneumonitis are also present in the serum and droppings of birds and can cause "bird breeder's" hypersensitivity pneumonitis.

Health care professionals are at risk of exposure to bioaerosols at work. The risk of occupational infectious illnesses such as tuberculosis has been widely reported, including multidrug-resistant tuberculosis. Laboratory animal workers are at risk for unusual infections such as Q fever (caused by *Coxiella burnetii*) and hypersensitivity lung diseases such as occupational asthma from exposure to aerosolized proteins present in the urine of laboratory animals.

More recently, bioaerosol exposures have been described in a wide variety of environmental settings. For example, organic agents in hot tub mists, contaminated humidifiers in office buildings, and agents associated with decaying wood and damp walls in inner city dwellings have been associated with individual cases and outbreaks of hypersensitivity pneumonitis.

4. What pathophysiologic mechanisms occur in the diseases caused by organic agents?

Organic agents are capable of causing disease by both immune and nonimmune mechanisms. Hypersensitivity pneumonitis results from a cascade of inflammatory and immune mechanisms, the most important of which is a cell-mediated (Type IV) T-lymphocyte activation. Bronchoalveolar lavage typically shows an increase in the total number of white blood cells, with a marked lymphocytosis. Rhinoconjunctivitis and allergic asthma from exposure to organic agents are associated with an IgE-mediated, immediate-type hypersensitivity reaction. The inhalation fevers associated with exposure to organic agents are noninfectious, nonallergic febrile responses to inhalation of high concentrations of grain dusts and some microbial bioaerosols. The chronic airflow limitation and chronic bronchitis associated with organic agents is also probably not an immune-mediated process, but rather a toxic effect from exposure to a variety of organic dust contaminants, probably including endotoxins from the cell walls of gram-negative bacteria.

5. Describe the symptoms and signs of disease caused by exposure to organic agents.

Hypersensitivity pneumonitis (allergic alveolitis) is characterized in its acute form by recurrent pneumonia with fever, chills, cough, chest tightness, shortness of breath, and myalgias. The subacute or chronic forms of HP are manifested by insidious and progressive dyspnea, fatigue, cough, weight loss, and decreased appetite.

Asthma is characterized by symptoms of wheezing, chest tightness, cough, and shortness of breath. Symptoms may occur immediately after exposure or may be delayed 6–12 hours. Diagnosis usually relies on the patient's history, wheezing on examination, or reversible airflow limitation on pulmonary function testing, including methacholine challenge testing.

Allergic rhinitis is diagnosed by history, physical examination, the finding of eosinophils on nasal smear, elevated total or specific IgE antibody levels, and immediate skin prick testing to relevant aeroallergens.

Inhalation fevers are characterized by fevers, chills, malaise, and muscle aches but no prominent pulmonary symptoms or signs. Symptoms usually occur within 48 hours after exposure and subside within 24–48 hours, with no long-term effects.

6. How is the diagnosis of HP established?

Diagnosis is based on a careful clinical and exposure history followed by appropriate diagnosis testing. Results of pulmonary function testing may show restrictive, obstructive, or mixed abnormalities, sometimes with a decreased diffusion capacity for carbon monoxide. Gas exchange abnormalities are often present with exercise. The chest radiograph may be normal in early stages of disease but typically reveals small, discrete, scattered 1–3 mm nodules, often predominantly in the lower lobe. Diffuse, patchy infiltrates or a ground glass appearance may be present. Radiographic abnormalities in acute illness typically regress or resolve over 4–6 weeks if further exposure is avoided. In the subacute or chronic form of HP, linear interstitial markings become more distinct, often associated with progressive loss of lung volume. Although CT scan is more sensitive than chest x-ray, a high resolution CT (HRCT) scan may be normal if disease is diagnosed early. The predominant HRCT pattern is poorly defined centrilobular micronodules, often with ground glass attenuation. These findings probably reflect the histologic findings of cellular bronchiolitis, noncaseating granulomas, and active alveolitis.

7. Are precipitating antibodies useful in the diagnosis of HP?

The finding of specific precipitating antibodies in the serum of a patient with suspected HP indicates exposure sufficient to generate a humoral immunologic response; this may be a helpful diagnostic clue. Precipitins do not appear to have a role in disease pathogenesis but serve as markers of antigen exposure. Precipitins are often found in antigen-exposed individuals without clinically evident disease. Additionally, specific precipitating antibodies are frequently not demonstrable in patients with HP. Results may be negative because of poorly standardized commercial antigens or the wrong choice of antigen.

8. What information should be included in the occupational and environmental histories of patients with suspected exposure to organic agents?

The most important approach to diagnosis of diseases caused by organic agents is a high index of suspicion and careful occupational and environmental history-taking. The occupational history should contain a chronology of current and previous occupations, a description of job processes and specific work practices, and a list of specific exposures. Improvement in symptoms away from work or worsening of symptoms with specific workplace exposures can be a helpful diagnostic clue when present. Additionally, the presence of persistent respiratory or constitutional symptoms, or both, in exposed coworkers can be helpful in identifying exposure-related disease.

The environmental and home history should include:
- A list of pets and other domestic animals
- Hobbies and recreational activities that may involve exposures to organic dusts
- Use of hot tubs, saunas, or indoor swimming pools
- Presence of leaking or flooding in a basement or occupied space
- Presence of humidifiers, dehumidifiers, swamp coolers, or cool mist vaporizers
- Water damage to carpets and furnishings
- Visible mold or mildew contamination in the occupied space
- Use of feathers in pillows, comforters, or clothing

9. Is sick building syndrome (SBS) caused by exposure to organic agents?

No. SBS is not included in the spectrum of diseases caused by exposure to organic agents. SBS is defined as an excess of nonspecific symptoms—including mucous membrane irritation, headache, and fatigue—associated with building occupancy. Specific causes of SBS are unknown and probably vary from building to building. Previous assumptions that SBS results from insufficient outdoor air are not well substantiated by existing epidemiologic studies. The possibility that SBS is associated with indoor exposure to bioaerosols has been raised. European studies suggest that SBS is associated with air conditioning systems with or without humidification. Additionally, occupant activities and furnishing can affect indoor air quality and complaint rates in buildings. Different buildings probably have different sources of poor indoor air quality; thus, SBS probably has several causes.

SBS is included along with building-related illnesses in the broad category of building-associated illnesses. Building-related illnesses (BRI) are distinct clinical entities such as asthma, hypersensitivity pneumonitis, allergic rhinitis, contact urticaria, infections, and toxic syndromes (for example, carbon monoxide poisoning) that result from building exposures. BRIs broadly overlap with the diseases that stem from exposure to organic agents.

10. How many people are affected by diseases resulting from exposure to organic agents?

The number is not known, but probably many more are affected than are clinically recognized. Our understanding of disease incidence and prevalence is hampered by the lack of a national database and reporting system, the nonspecificity of the symptoms associated with exposures to bioaerosols and other organic agents, and the fact that the symptoms mimic many other diseases, such as viral illnesses and chronic bronchitis.

Most of the population-based studies of HP focus on the prevalence of illness among agricultural workers. In Scotland, the prevalence of farmer's lung in three agricultural areas ranged from 2.3–8.6%. A questionnaire survey of western Wyoming dairy and cattle ranchers elicited a history typical of acute farmer's lung disease in 3% of those surveyed. The prevalence of HP among bird hobbyists is estimated to range from 0.5–21%.

11. Describe the treatment options available for diseases caused by exposure to organic agents.

For the hypersensitivity diseases (rhinoconjunctivitis, asthma, and hypersensitivity pneumonitis), early recognition and removal from exposure to the antigen-containing environment is key in disease management. In some cases, removal will result in complete resolution of symptoms and physiologic and radiographic abnormalities. In patients with asthma or hypersensitivity pneumonitis who have severe abnormalities at presentation or persistent symptoms despite removal from exposure, short-term (2–3 months) treatment with oral corticosteroids may be helpful. No treatment for the inhalation fevers has been identified because these disorders are self-limited. Prevention of recurrent episodes is recommended because little information is available on the natural history of recurrent attacks.

12. How is antigen exposure eliminated in disease caused by bioaerosols?

Once a bioaerosol-related disease is diagnosed, eliminating antigen exposure is the most challenging part of the treatment. In some cases, an investigation aimed at assessing the bioaerosol status of the building or home can be undertaken. Although it is often difficult to prove the connection between specific exposures and disease, it may be possible to demonstrate bioaerosol reservoirs, amplifiers, and disseminators during an on-site inspection. The presence of potential bioaerosol sources may be sufficient to permit recommendations for remedial action without further investigation. If additional documentation of exposure is required, quantitative bioaerosol sampling can be considered. The primary objective of air sampling is to identify the source of bioaerosol components so that effective corrective action can be undertaken. Dose-response information is generally not available. Positive results may document the presence of a specific source; however, negative results are usually inconclusive with respect to confirming the presence or absence of sources. An exposure may be considered potentially significant when overall levels of the bioaerosol are at least an order of magnitude higher than those in outdoor air or when the types of bioaerosols differ between the control environment and the complaint environment. The mere presence of an unusual organism or antigen in an environment does not prove a causal relationship between the exposure and the illness.

13. Can diseases caused by organic agents be prevented?

There is little research on the prevention of these diseases. Appropriate design and maintenance of building heating, ventilation, and air conditioning systems is important in limiting microbial amplification and dissemination. Indoor microbial contamination is often related to problems with moisture control. Source control includes preventing leaking and flooding, removing stagnant water sources, eliminating aerosol humidifiers and vaporizers, and maintaining indoor relative humidity below 70%. Contaminants can be diluted by an increase in the amount of outdoor air in a building, and high efficiency filters can be added to the ventilation system to clean recirculated air. Complete elimination of indoor allergens is probably impossible, and it is often necessary to relocate immunologically sensitized individuals once hypersensitivity lung disease has occurred.

The efficacy of various types of respirators in preventing antigen sensitization and disease progression is unknown. Helmet-type powered air purifying respirators have been used to prevent episodic exposure in individuals with previous acute episodes of farmer's lung. Prolonged wearing of respiratory protection is limited by the fact that most respirators are hot and cumbersome; moreover, they may be expensive. Dust respirators offer incomplete protection against organic particulates and are not recommended once sensitization has occurred.

BIBLIOGRAPHY

1. Ando M, Suga M, Nishiura Y, et al: Summer-type hypersensitivity pneumonitis. Intern Med 34:707–712, 1995.
2. Burrel R, Rylander R: A critical review of the role of precipitins in hypersensitivity pneumonitis. Eur J Respir Dis 62:332–343, 1981.

3. Colby TV, Coleman A: Histological differential diagnosis of extrinsic allergic alveolitis. Prog Surg Pathol 10:11–26, 1989.
4. Drent M, Grutters JC, Mulder PG, et al: Is the different T helper cell activity in sarcoidosis and extrinsic allergic alveolitis also reflected by the cellular bronchoalveolar lavage fluid profile? Sarcoidosis Vasc Diffuse Lung Dis 14:31–38, 1997.
5. Embil J, Warren P, Yakrus M, et al: Pulmonary illness associated with exposure to *Mycobacterium avium* complex in hot tub water: Hypersensitivity pneumonitis or infection? Chest 111:813–816, 1997.
6. Hansell DM, Kerr IH: The role of high resolution computed tomography in the diagnosis of interstitial lung disease. Thorax 46:77–84, 1991.
7. Lynch DA, Rose CS, Way D, King TE Jr: Hypersensitivity pneumonitis: Sensitivity of high-resolution CT in a population-based study. Am J Roentgenol 159:469–472, 1992.
8. Niimi H, Kang EY, Swong JS, et al: CT of chronic infiltrative lung disease: Prevalence of mediastinal lymphadenopathy. J Comput Assist Tomogr 20:305–308, 1996.
9. Richerson HB, Bernstein IL, Fink JN, et al: Guidelines for the clinical evaluation of hypersensitivity pneumonitis. J Allergy Clin Immunol 839–844, 1989.
10. Rose C, King TE Jr: Controversies in hypersensitivity pneumonitis [editorial]. Am Rev Respir Dis 145:1–2, 1992.
11. Rose CS, Martyny J, Newman LN, et al: "Lifeguard lung": Endemic granulomatous pneumonitis in an indoor swimming pool. Am J Public Health 88:1795–1800, 1998.
12. Semenzato G, Zambello R, Trentin L, Agostini C: Cellular immunity in sarcoidosis and hypersensitivity pneumonitis. Chest 103:139S–143S, 1993.
13. Vandenplas O, Malo JL, Saetta M, et al: Occupational asthma and extrinsic alveolitis due to isocyanates: Current status and perspectives. Br J Ind Med 50:213–228, 1993.
14. Zacharisen MC, Kadambi AR, Schlueter DP, et al: The spectrum of respiratory disease associated with exposure to metal working fluids. J Occup Environ Med 50:640–647, 1998.

34. WORK-RELATED CARPAL TUNNEL SYNDROME

Robin Herbert, M.D., and Jaime Szeinuk, M.D.

1. What is carpal tunnel syndrome?

Carpal tunnel syndrome (CTS) is a condition in which the median nerve is compressed as it passes though the carpal tunnel in the wrist. The median nerve and nine flexor tendons of the hand pass through the carpal canal, which is bounded by the bony carpus and carpal ligament. Because the tunnel is not distensible, its contents are vulnerable to increases in hydrostatic pressure (e.g., inflammatory conditions of the flexor tendons), which may lead to compression of the median nerve and cause carpal tunnel syndrome.

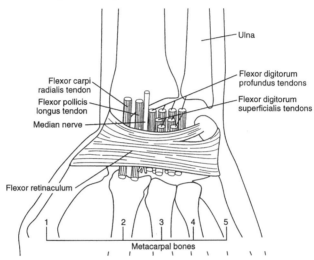

Carpal tunnel syndrome: Carpal tunnel syndrome occurs following compression of the median nerve as it passes through the carpal canal in the wrist. (From Murphy DC: Ergonomics and the Dental Care Worker. American Public Health Association, p 379, 1998, with permission.)

2. What is work-related carpal tunnel syndrome?

Work-related carpal tunnel syndrome (WRCTS) is one of a group of medical conditions known as work-related musculoskeletal disorders (WMSDs), which are sometimes called cumulative trauma disorders or repetitive strain injuries. WRCTS is carpal tunnel syndrome caused by workplace exposures to repetition, force, vibration, or to a combination of expsoure to these factors and/or nonneutral joint posture.

3. How common is WRCTS?

WMSDs have become the most common category of work-related illness in the United States. In 1996, 281,000 disorders due to repeated trauma were reported in U.S. workplaces, representing nearly 64% of all occupational illness cases reported to the U.S. Bureau of Labor Statistics. Of these, CTS has been reported as the most common disabling condition, with almost 30,000 cases requiring days away from work in 1996 alone.

The National Institute for Occupational Safety and Health (NIOSH) estimates that 5–10 workers per 10,000 will miss work each year due to WRCTS, and the estimated prevalence of

CTS in 1988 was 5.3 cases per 1000 current workers. However, the prevalence of WRCTS in high-risk occupations is much higher. High-risk occupations include meat, fish, and poultry processing, sewing machine operation, leather tanning, and both heavy and light manufacturing. The prevalence of WRCTS is these groups may be as high as 15%.

4. How serious is WRCTS?

Although it is not a lethal condition, WRCTS is one of the most disabling and costly of the upper extremity WMSDs. WRCTS is a major cause of lost work days and workers' compensation costs in the United States. In 1995 the median time away from work due to carpal tunnel syndrome was 30 days; 48.5% of all patients with CTS were away from work more than 31 days. Because of the highly disabling nature of WRCTS, medical management should focus on disability prevention, which includes early case identification with prompt medical and/or surgical treatment as well as prompt workplace ergonomic intervention.

5. What are the causes of WRCTS?

In a recent review by NIOSH, which evaluated the relationship between physical workplace factors and CTS, a positive association was found between development of CTS and exposure to highly repetitive work, forceful hand work, or hand/wrist vibration. In addition, NIOSH found strong evidence of a positive association between CTS and exposure to a combination of risk factors (repetition, force, awkward postures, and hand/wrist vibration). Workers found to be at increased risk for developing CTS include garment workers, grocery checkers, food processing workers, forestry workers, manufacturing workers, building trades workers, workers using computer keyboards, dental hygienists, and musicians.

6. What are the nonoccupational causes of CTS?

A number of systemic medical illnesses have been associated with CTS, although the primary literature supporting many of these factors is limited and often contradictory. Among systemic diseases, hypothyroidism, diabetes mellitus, collagen vascular disease (such as rheumatoid arthritis), and uremia are generally considered to be established risk factors for CTS. Pregnancy is another well-established risk factor for CTS. CTS due to pregnancy is a reversible condition, unlike CTS associated with collagen vascular disease and uremia. Other conditions, such as history of oophorectomy and/or estrogen hormone replacement, have been less consistently associated with CTS. Patients with hobbies and sport activities that involve exposure to forcefully repetitive hand activities similar to those experienced in the workplace also may be at risk for CTS.

7. Can CTS be caused by work and medical illness simultaneously?

Few studies have evaluated the possibility of interaction between underlying systemic illness and WRCTS. Nonetheless, workers who have a systemic illness associated with CTS and who are occupationally exposed to ergonomic stresses may be at greater risk of developing WMSDs than coworkers without systemic illnesses. Similarly, it is important to consider the possibility of underlying systemic illness in workers with CTS and inciting ergonomic exposures. An increasing body of evidence suggests that WMSDs, like many other disorders, are multifactorial in origin.

8. How is WRCTS diagnosed?

It is important first to make the diagnosis of carpal tunnel syndrome. Classic symptoms include numbness, tingling, burning, or pain in at least two of digits 1, 2, or 3 with or without pain in the palm. In some cases symptoms may be limited to one of digits 1, 2, or 3. The most accurate way to diagnose CTS is with electrodiagnostic studies in the presence of classic CTS symptoms. Once CTS is diagnosed, work-relatedness is ascertained by a comprehensive occupational history to determine whether the patient's work exposes him or her to any of the biomechanical factors associated with CTS.

9. What other conditions can mimic CTS?
Conditions that may cause symptoms of upper extremity pain similar to those of CTS include cervical radiculopathy, peripheral neuropathy, hand/arm vibration syndrome, and various soft-tissue disorders. Electrodiagnostic testing is necessary to differentiate CTS from other conditions, especially C6–C7 radiculopathy.

10. What activities may exacerbate CTS?
Typically, symptoms are exacerbated by activities that increase postural load on the tendons in the canal. Examples include holding a newspaper, driving a car, or using hand tools such as hammers, screwdrivers, or drills. Frequently patients report nocturnal awakening due to symptoms. Advanced cases may be associated with denervation of abductor pollicis brevis, which abducts the thumb. Such patients typically report difficulty in performing activities that require abduction, such as turning keys, opening jars, and opening door handles.

11. What are the physical examination findings in patients with CTS?
The classically described provocative maneuvers for CTS are Phalen's test, in which paresthesias are reproduced after 1 minute of wrist flexion, and Tinel's sign, in which an electric shocklike feeling occurs in the fingers after tapping the palmar surface of the wrist. However, their specificity for CTS is poor. Most clinicians believe that Phalen's test and Tinel's signs alone are of limited utility in clinical evaluation of CTS; generally, the diagnosis should be based on the presence of the symptoms described in question 8 and electrodiagnostic testing compatible with CTS. In addition, to avoid misdiagnosis, it is critical to conduct a thorough examination of the musculoskeletal system from the neck to the hands and to evaluate the patient for the possibility of other and/or additional musculoskeletal disorders, such as cervical radiculopathy. In addition, it is important to conduct a thorough neurologic evaluation, which should include evaluation of strength, particularly of the abductor pollicis brevis muscle, and assessment of sensation in all digits. It is also important to inspect the hands for evidence of thenar atrophy, which is highly suggestive of advanced or severe CTS.

12. What diagnostic tests should be performed in patients with suspected CTS?
The gold standard diagnostic test is electrodiagnostic studies, including nerve conduction velocities and electromyography. A standard procedure for conducting these studies was published by the American Association of Electrodiagnostic Medicine in 1993. CTS typically is associated with prolongation of the distal motor and/or sensory latencies of the median nerve; slowing of the median sensory and/or motor conduction velocities across the wrist; and/or denervation of the abductor pollicis brevis muscles. Such findings in conjunction with symptoms consistent with CTS are the most valid method of diagnosis. Once CTS has been diagnosed with electrodiagnostic studies and symptoms, it is important to evaluate the patient for possible concomitant systemic medical illnesses that may be associated with CTS. Therefore, all patients should be screened for systemic illness with a complete blood count; blood chemistries, including determination of fasting blood sugar (to rule out diabetes mellitus) and renal function; sedimentation rate (to screen for collagen vascular disease); and levels of thyroid-stimulating hormone (to assess for hypothyroidism). In addition, patients in whom history and physical examination suggest the possibility of rheumatoid arthritis or other collagen vascular disease should be screened with appropriate serologies.

13. What other elements should be included in the history of patients with possible WRCTS?
1. **Personal characteristics**, including age, gender, and dominant hand.
2. **History of the present illness.** A detailed history of symptoms should be obtained to determine the anatomic location of pain and/or neuritic symptoms and to assist in determining whether the condition is due to nerve entrapment, inflammation of tendons and tendon sheaths, or other disorders. The physician should ask about the nature of the symptoms as well as the location, duration, radiation, and exacerbating and alleviating factors. It is important to ask about

prior treatment. The past medical history should focus on information about prior musculoskeletal or neurologic disorders that may be related to the present condition. In addition, the physician should ask about history of trauma or surgery to the upper extremity or neck.

3. **Past medical history.** The history should screen for predisposing conditions, such as diabetes mellitus, collagen vascular disease, hypothyroidism, uremia, malignancy, granulomatous disease (e.g., tuberculosis, sarcoidosis), or infiltrative diseases (e.g., amyloidosis).

4. **Family history.** The presence or absence of neurologic or connective tissue diseases among family members should be investigated.

5. **Social history.** The social history should include a history of smoking and alcohol consumption. It is important to ask about factors in the workplace that may affect elements of treatment, such as emotional stress at work and economic factors that render the patient unable to take time off from work for physical therapy or rest breaks. The physician also should ask about avocational activities with potential exposure to ergonomic hazards. The history should routinely include queries about the home environment, including the amount of housework performed, need to care for young children, hobbies, and recreation.

14. What specific questions should be asked about the patient's workplace in evaluating the possibility of WRCTS?

The occupational history should focus on whether the patient is exposed to repetition (frequent movements of the hands and wrists), forceful exertion involving the hands, awkward wrist posture, vibration, and inadequate rest periods. The physician should ask the patient to describe a typical work day. When possible, a demonstration of all movements performed by the patient in the course of his or her work should be obtained. The rate at which movements are performed should be approximated, and the frequency and duration of rest breaks as well as typical work hours should be noted. In addition, a description of workstations and equipment should be obtained. The patient's posture, including the position of the upper extremities when performing work, should be noted. It is often helpful to have the patient bring in a picture of himself or herself at the workstation to see how well the workstation accommodates the patient or how well tools fit the patient's hand. A description of the work pace also should be obtained. Because treatment of WRCTS often initially requires slowing work pace or initiation of rest breaks, it is important to ask about factors such as piece rate work or productivity requirements that may impair successful treatment plans. The number of years in the current job and previous jobs with similar exposures should be recorded.

15. How is WRCTS treated?

Treatment involves both appropriate medical therapy and modifications in the workstation, work process, and/or work pace to eliminate or decrease exposure to ergonomic stresses. The primary goals of treatment are to prevent disease progression and to allow patients to remain employed or to enable them to return to work as quickly as possible while reducing or eliminating symptoms. In general, cases of mild and moderate carpal tunnel syndrome can be managed nonsurgically, at least initially. Typically nonsurgical management includes use of neutral wrist splints at night; avoidance of inciting occupational and nonoccupational ergonomic exposures; hand therapy (performed by a certified physical therapist or occupational therapist); nonsteroidal antiinflammatory agents; and/or corticosteroid injection into the carpal tunnel. Surgical treatment should be considered in patients who fail to respond to conservative treatment over a 2–6-month period or who have moderately severe to severe carpal tunnel syndrome, as evidenced by clinical or electrodiagnostic evidence of denervation of the abductor pollicis brevis muscle on EMG.

CONTROVERSY

16. Can pre-employment screening for subclinical CTS help to identify high-risk people?

Some employers have begun preemployment "screening" for subclinical CTS to avoid placement of high-risk employees in jobs with exposure to risk factors associated with development of

CTS. This practice is discriminatory and, in fact, has no scientific basis. Preemployment nerve conduction velocities have been shown not to be predictors of subsequent development of WRCTS.

BIBLIOGRAPHY

1. American Association of Electrodiagnostic Medicine: Practice parameters for electrodiagnostic studies in carpal tunnel syndrome. Muscle Nerve 16:1390–1414, 1993.
2. Bureau of Labor Statistics, U.S. Department of Labor, 1998, www.stats.bls.gov.
3. Chammas M, Bousquet P, Renard E, et al: Dupuytren's disease, carpal tunnel syndrome, trigger finger, and diabetes mellitus. J Hand Surg 20A:109–114, 1995.
4. DeKrom MCTFM, Kester ADM, Knipschild PG, Spaans F: Risk factors for carpal tunnel syndrome. Am J Epidemiol 132:1102–1110, 1990.
5. Franzblau A, Werner RA, Johnston E, Torrey S: Evaluation of current pereception threshold testing as a screening procedure for carpal tunnel syndrome among industrial workers. J Occup Med 36:1015–1021, 1994.
6. Heathfield K: Neurological complications of the rheumatic diseases. Rheumatol Rehabil 12:2–21, 1973.
7. National Institute for Occupational Safety and Health, Centers for Disease Control and Prevention: Musculoskeletal Disorders and Workplace Factors: A Critical Review of Epidemiologic Evidence for Work-related Musculoskeletal Disorders of the Neck, Upper Extremity and Low Back. Washington, DC, National Institute of Occupational Safety and Health, 1997.
8. Remple D, Evanoff B, Amadio PC, et al: Consensus criteria for the classification of carpal tunnel syndrome in epidemiologic studies. Am J Public Health 88:1447–1451, 1998.
9. Sivri A, Celiker R, Sungur C, Kutsal YG: Carpal tunnel syndrome: A major complication in hemodialysis patients. Scand J Rheumatol 23:287–290, 1994.
10. Stevens JC, Beard CM, O'Fallon WM, Kurland LT: Conditions associated with carpal tunnel syndrome. Mayo Clin Proc 67:541–548, 1992.
11. Tanaka S, Wild DK, Cameron LL, Freund E: Association of occupational and non-occupational risk factors with the prevalence of self-reported carpal tunnel syndrome in a national survey of the working population. Am J Indust Med 32:550–556, 1997.

35. OCCUPATIONAL AND ENVIRONMENTAL NEUROLOGY

Jonathan S. Rutchik, M.D., M.P.H.

BRAIN CANCER

1. List common characteristics of chemicals associated with brain cancer.

Chemicals that are nonpolar and lipid-soluble readily cross the blood-brain barrier and may be associated with neoplasia specific to the brain. The brain is protected from substances without these properties.

2. What chemicals and industries are associated with brain cancer?

Excessive brain tumor risk has been associated with occupational chemical exposures in many studies involving numerous industries, but specific chemicals are not always implicated. Workers occupationally exposed to synthetic rubber, polyvinyl chloride, crude petroleum, formaldehyde, cutting oils, polycyclic aromatic hydrocarbons, chemical production, agriculture chemicals, and electronics production and maintenance may have an excessive risk of brain cancer. Measures of association vary with the form of the studies, each of which has its own inherent strengths and weaknesses.

- One study reported a fourfold risk of mortality from brain cancer with at least 5 years' employment in the tire assembly department of the rubber industry, where exposures included hexamethylenetetramine, drum resins containing coal tar, and carbon tetrachloride.
- A study of deceased active and retired members of the Oil, Chemical and Atomic Workers International Union in Texas indicated an elevated frequency of deaths (proportionate mortality rate [PMR] = 2.11) from brain tumors among white male hourly employees of three oil refineries in the Texas Gulf coast area.
- Three studies found elevated brain cancer rates associated with employment in chemical plants producing polyvinyl chloride.
- A case-control study conducted in three areas of the U.S. with a heavy concentration of petroleum refineries indicated a slightly increased risk (odds ratio = 1.5) of deaths due to astrocytic brain tumor among men employed in production or maintenance jobs.
- Elevated brain cancer risk was noted among 2307 members of the Royal College of Pathology and among 2317 members of the American Association of Anatomists.

3. Based on animal data, what other chemicals may be associated with brain cancer in humans?

Brain cancer has been experimentally induced in laboratory animals by a number of chemicals. Only bis-chloromethyl ether, vinyl chloride, and acrylonitrile are known industrial agents. In inhalation studies, bis-chloromethyl ether and vinyl chloride have produced neuroblastomas, and acrylonitrile has produced gliomas in rats. Ingestion of acrylonitrile also induced gliomas in rats. Methyl chloroform has been shown to cause nonmalignant astrocytic cell changes in laboratory animals.

4. What difficulties are involved in identifying causation of brain cancer in case clusters?

Human population studies have assessed occupational exposures in many industries and to many agents, but such studies involve many problems. The lack of specificity for disease terminology, definition, and classification leads to inclusion of undefined or improperly defined cases or exclusion of true cases. When "malignant" is not written on death certificate, the "unspecified" classification may be recorded. Although "benign" and "unspecified" classifications are often not considered in epidemiologic cancer studies, many have been found to be primary malignant brain tumors. Furthermore, exposures may vary within study populations. Cohorts may be mixtures of white-collar and blue-collar employees, whose jobs and exposures are very different. Misclassification may underestimate brain tumor risk. In addition, the small number of cases of brain cancer in many studies limits ability to determine relative risk and odds ratios. Lastly, most studies report glial tumors only, such as astrocytoma and glioblastoma, which represent 70% of central nervous system tumors in white men. Together these factors limit the ability of researchers to reach strong conclusions and identify statistically significant associations.

CEREBELLAR SYNDROMES

5. What are the signs of cerebellar syndromes by history and clinical neurologic examination?

Difficulty with walking steadily or a sense of imbalance may be associated with cerebellar syndromes. An assessment of cerebellar function includes the following:
- Observation of gait: base of the gait stance, tendencies to fall, and tandem gait
- Finger-nose-finger and heel-knee-shin maneuvers
- Check response: the ability of a patient to sustain a steady, standing posture when outstretched arms are thrust downward by examiner
- Eye movements
- Other neurologic aspects, such as motor tone and tremulousness

MRI is the imaging study of choice for visualizing the brainstem and cerebellar structures. Brainstem audio-evoked responses evaluate mainly brainstem structures but may be useful when cerebellar symptoms include vertigo, double vision, tinnitus, and hearing abnormalities. The vestibulooculomotor reflex, assessed by an electronystagmograph of eye movements, is useful to measure the effects of the cerebellum on nystagmus and eye movements. Posturography and otoneurologic test batteries also may assess cerebellar influences on balance.

6. What agents have been associated with acute cerebellar syndromes after short-term exposure?

All solvents may cause symptoms of cerebellar dysfunction due to intoxication. Aluminum, bismuth, manganese, thallium, zinc, tin, and lithium, as well as organophosphates, organochlorines, carbon monoxide, and methyl chloride also have been associated with symptoms suggestive of cerebellar dysfunction after acute exposures. Acrylamide acute and subacute exposure has led to intoxication ataxia. Volunteers exposed to styrene for 1 hour were noted to have different saccadic eye movement speeds, suggesting a blocking of cerebellar inhibition of the vestibulooculomotor pathway. Workers exposed to xylene have been tested with posturography, but no consistent results were noted. Concomitant use of alcohol was noted to be an occupational hazard.

7. What agents have been associated with persistent cerebellar syndromes after long-term exposure?

Chronic toluene abuse has led to cerebellar ataxia. Autopsy findings noted cerebellar atrophy in a man with a 12-year history of inhaling paint thinner that contained mixed solvents. Studies of long-term occupational exposure to toluene and other organic solvents have revealed inconsistent results. Chronic methyl mercury exposure has led to lesions in the cerebellum. Posturography was used to assess both children and adults with elevated blood lead levels; more than one study found evidence of effects on vestibular mechanisms. Subclinical changes in vestibulocerebellar functioning were noted in one study at a blood level of 18 μg/100 ml; persistent changes in functioning occurred at mean levels of 47.7 μg/100 ml.

CRANIAL NERVE DISORDERS

8. What aspects of the history and physical examination suggest brainstem or cranial nerve disorders?

Symptoms may pertain to specific cranial nerves (CNs):

- CN I: lack of the ability to smell (anosmia)
- CN II: decreased visual acuity
- CN III: pupillary abnormalities
- CNs IV and VI: double vision
- CNs V and VII: facial pain or numbness
- CN VII: facial weakness or dysarthria (difficulty with speaking)
- CN VIII: difficulty with hearing or imbalance
- CNs VII, IX, X, and XI: difficulty with swallowing or taste (dysgeusia)
- CN XII: difficulty with tongue movements

The light reflex (performed by flashing light into one eye and noting the response of both eyes, then swinging the light into the other eye and noting the same) assesses the arc that includes the afferent fibers in the optic nerve and the efferent fibers from the Edinger-Westphal nucleus (the parasympathetic aspect of CN III). Flashing light into one eye should constrict both eyes equally. The corneal reflex assesses the function of both the afferent CN V and the efferent CN VII of the face. This functional blink reflex test is performed by stroking the cornea with a soft piece of cotton. The cranial nerve examination should assess all of these functions.

9. Which cranial neuropathies have been associated with occupational or environmental exposure?

Symptoms associated with cranial neuropathies are frequently part of the multitude of symptoms experienced by workers with low-level chronic or high-level acute exposures to organic solvents in occupational or environmental settings. Dizziness and blurred vision are common, and occasionally dysarthria is seen. Such symptoms may be nonspecific or associated with brainstem dysfunction. Anosmia is often a complaint of workers chronically exposed to organic solvents, but some workers are not aware of this symptom. Anosmia may make a work environment dangerous because odorants, which are added to chemicals to warn when exposures approach levels associated with ill health effects, may not be noticed. Dysgeusia is reported by workers exposed to high levels of metal fumes, such as zinc oxide, manganese, and other heavy metals. Epidemiologic studies in various populations have used neurophysiologic tests to detect many of these symptoms.

Cranial neuropathies involving the optic, oculomotor, auditory, facial, and vestibular nerves have been noted with chronic exposure to arsenic, along with hypo- and hyperosmias. Acute organophosphate poisoning leads to miosis, lacrimation, and salivation. Cranial nerve palsies, including external ocular, facial, and palatal palsies, have been reported with intermediate syndromes, in which symptoms begin 24–96 hours after exposure.

Trichloroethylene, an organic solvent used in many industries as a degreasing agent, has been associated with trigeminal neuropathy; in the past it was used to treat facial pain or trigeminal neuralgia. It has been associated with low-level chronic occupational and environmental exposures.

Chronic exposure to toluene has been associated with dose-related neurobehavioral abnormalities, including eye movement disorders, anosmia, and hearing changes.

10. Which neurophysiologic tests examine specific aspects of cranial nerve function?

- Chemosensory evoked responses for ability to smell (CN I)
- Pupillometer for CN III
- Electronystagmogram (ENG) for CNs III, IV, VI, and VIII as well as cerebellar function
- Blink testing and facial nerve conduction velocity testing for CNs V and VII
- Audiometry and brainstem-evoked responses for CN VIII and cerebellar and central pathways

11. What is the usefulness of brainstem auditory evoked responses (BAERs)?

Many occupational and environmentally exposed populations have been tested with BAER to assess its complex pathway. Results are often not clearly interpretable. Studies compare populations and controls and report differences in mean latencies. Individual results are mainly normal. Hearing, cochlear nerve function, vestibular-ocular pathways, and other brainstem, cerebellar, and central pathways are evaluated by scoring wave latencies. Workers exposed to aluminum, arsenic, carbon disulfide, lead, perchloroethylene, toluene, xylene, and other agents have been tested with BAER.

12. Describe the anatomy and physiology of taste.

CNs VII, IX, and X are involved with innervating the taste buds of the proximal aspect of the digestive tract. CN VII innervates the anterior two-thirds of the tongue, CN X innervates the posterior one-third of the tongue, and CN IX innervates the soft palate and pharyngeal, laryngeal, and epiglottic areas. Salivary proteins influence the ability to taste; zinc-containing gustins help to determine the capacity to identify ingested flavors. Over 13 chemical taste receptors analyze sweet, sour, bitter, and salty. Simultaneous stimulation of odor and taste receptors leads to the complete perception of taste. Taste impairment is usually due to direct damage to taste buds, inability to regenerate taste buds, interference with direct contact of a substance with taste buds, or impairment of CN VII, IX, or X.

13. What are chemosensory evoked potentials? How have they been used to assess smell and taste?

This test has been used to measure the response to chemical stimulation of the olfactory or trigeminal nerve in workers exposed to volatile organic solvents. An elevated threshold has been noted in workers exposed to xylene, styrene, and a mixture of the two compared with controls. Receptor-specific saturation was hypothesized. Olfactory fatigue or adaptation occurs with repeated exposures and may lead to hypoosmia or anosmia.

14. What is chemical odor intolerance?

Chemical odor intolerance (cacosmia) is defined as a negative hedonic response to and adverse symptoms from low levels of chemicals that are tolerated by most people. Solvents and pesticides have been noted to be initiators, but many chemicals have been found to be eliciting agents (e.g., tobacco smoke, perfumes, cleaning products, automotive exhaust, gasoline, natural gas, new carpets). Patients have been noted to have decreased total sleep and sleep efficiency, impaired reaction times on a divided attention task, and abnormal patterns on continuous visual memory tests. Cacosmia has been hypothesized to be a manifestation of neural sensitization. Affected people have been noted to be sensitizable. Sensitization is the progressive amplification of host responses to an initially novel stimulus by the passage of time between the first and later stimuli.

Kindling is a process in the limbic system by which a repeated intermittent stimulus that is initially incapable of causing a seizure subsequently elicits a full convulsion. Because many substances have been found to elicit electroencephalography findings in chemically intolerant patients, this hypothesis has been considered to be one explanation for multiple chemical sensitivity.

15. How does one approach a patient with suspected neurologic illness due to an occupational or environmental exposure?

- Complete medical, occupational, and environmental history, including past employments and exposures, past residences, natural landmarks near residence, and water sources.
- Complete medical and neurologic examination by thorough practitioner, with observation of skin, gums, and nails.
- Collect exposure data when possible.
- Refer to neurologist for confirmation of any evidence of neurologic dysfunction and secondary neurophysiologic and neuropsychological testing.
- Devise a differential diagnosis.
- Consider the role of specific chemicals in exposure. Review literature, and plan testing to assess possible involved organ system. For example, arrange for color vision testing if color vision is noted to be abnormal in workers exposed to specific chemical.
- Obtain biologic exposure indices from blood or urine.
- Consider removal of patient from exposure source.
- Consider other more common etiologies for diagnoses.

- Repeat neurophysiologic and neuropsychological tests to assess whether improvement is noted after removal from environment.
- Is there significant support in the literature to associate the exposure (at the specific dose level and duration and by the specific method of exposure, such as ingestion, inhalation, or dermatologic absorption) with the neurologic diagnosis?

VISUAL TOXICOLOGY

16. What are the components of the neuroophthalmologic evaluation?

The evaluation includes color vision and visual field testing and assessments of retinal and oculomotor structure and function. It normally complements evaluation of the eye.

17. What neuroophthalmologic tests have been used to evaluate populations exposed to occupational and environmental hazards for subclinical dysfunction?

Many tests have been used for each aspect of the evaluation. Abnormalities in color vision are screened by using testing plates, including Ishihara and relative subjective color saturation testing. However, the Lanthony and Farnsworth-Munsell color vision tests have been used successfully in field studies to screen for subclinical dysfunction. Color fundus photography, direct and indirect ophthalmoscopy, fluorescein angiography, and electroretinography have been used to evaluate the retina. Saccadic eye movement testing, electrooculography, pendicular eye tracking tests (PETT), electronystagmogram (ENG), and brainstem audiometry have been used to screen for oculomotor dysfunction. Direct confrontation and formal visual field assessments as well as visual evoked potentials (VEPs) also have been used on exposed populations. Critical flicker fusion and contrast sensitivity have been used as research tools.

Dyschromatopsia (Color Vision Loss)

18. Which specific industries and agents have been associated with dyschromatopsia?

Population studies have revealed subclinical abnormalities in color vision after exposure to mixed solvent solutions in microelectronics industries, print shops, and paint manufacturing; perchloroethylene in dry cleaning industries; styrene in fiberglass and plastics manufacturing and ship building; carbon disulfide in viscose rayon production; mercury in precision instrument manufacturing; and n-hexane in adhesive bandages production and vegetable oil extraction processing plants.

19. What is Kollner's rule?

Color vision theory is based on the premise of Kollner's rule (1911), which states that blue-yellow color loss localizes dysfunction to the retina, whereas red-green color loss localizes dysfunction to the optic nerve.

20. How is dyschromatopsia differentiated?

Color vision loss is currently divided into three types, based on the character of loss and visual acuity. From Kollner's rule localization can be inferred. Type I (Protan) is associated with only red-green loss and moderate visual acuity loss localizing to proximal optic nerve structures; it is most commonly seen in congenital dyschromatopsia. Type II (Deutan) refers to a mixture of blue-yellow and red-green loss (more severe) with moderate-to-severe loss of visual acuity and is localized to more internal retinal layers. Type III (Tritan) loss refers to blue-yellow loss with normal-to-moderately impaired visual acuity and is localized to the external layers of the retina.

21. Describe the usefulness of the Ishihara, Farnsworth-Munsell, and Lanthony color vision tests.

Ishihara pseudoisochromatic plates test primarily for red-green color loss and are thus useful in assessing for congenital dysfunction. In one study, Ishihara color vision plates testing revealed no significant differences between workers exposed to toluene or tetrachloroethyelene and controls.

The **Farnsworth-Munsell 100 (FM-100) Hue Test** assesses the specific character of acquired color vision loss. It measures the ability to line up 85 colored caps that span a color spectrum in order of color hue. The three types of dyschromatopsia can be ascribed to specific patterns of results.

The **Lanthony D15 (L-D15) desaturation panel** is a simpler and more contemporary method of testing acquired color vision loss and has been used to evaluate most people assessed in industry. Like the Farnsworth D15 (F-D15) panel test, a concise version of the FM-100, the L-D15 test, assesses the ability of a subject to arrange 15 colored caps, but it uses caps with lower saturation.

22. What is the color confusion index?

Results of testing also may be expressed in terms of a color confusion index (CCI), which is the sum of the color differences of adjacent caps divided by the ideal score. A perfect score is one; scores greater than one indicate increasing color vision loss. Because acquired dyschromatopsia may be monocular, testing must be done monocularly. The CCI is the average value for the two eyes.

Retinal Abnormalities

23. Which specific industries and agents have been associated with abnormalities in the structure of the retina?

Workers in the viscose rayon industry, where carbon disulfide exposure is common, have been diagnosed with retinal abnormalities. Abnormalities also have been found in workers in adhesive bandage factories and vegetable oil extraction processing plants using n-hexane.

24. Explain the difference between carbon disulfide (CS_2) retinopathy and diabetic retinopathy.

Fluorescein angiography reveals differences between the two entities. Both involve saccular microaneurysms. In cases of CS_2-induced retinopathy, saccular microaneurysms with diameters of 20–80 μm develop around the posterior pole. In addition, CS_2 retinopathy is characterized by ellipsoid and loop-shape microaneurysms. Flourescein leakage from vessel and prolongation of fluorescein staining along the vessel wall are not observed in CS_2 retinopathy, suggesting that the blood-brain barrier is not disturbed. Atrophic degenerative changes in the pigmentary epithelium are also characteristic of CS_2-induced retinopathy. The avascular areas around microaneurysms and shunt vessel formation are not frequently found in either retinopathy. Unlike diabetic retinopathy, the prognosis for CS_2 retinopathy is good, and proliferative changes, such as preretinal new vessel formation and proliferation fibrous retinitis, do not occur. In addition, there is no laterality in the side of the eye in which microaneurysms first appear.

25. What is the significance of an electroretinogram?

The electroretinogram (ERG) is a useful, noninvasive experimental method to assess the functional integrity of retinal cells. The ERG a wave primarily reflects activity of photoreceptors in the outer (distal) layer of the retina, whereas the b wave reflects the activity of the depolarizing bipolar cells and Müller glial cells of the inner nuclear layer. Flash stimulus may localize damage to the retina because an injured optic nerve does not affect the ERG wave form. ERG has been used mainly in animal studies. Heavy metals selectively affect rods and scotopic vision as opposed to the photopic cone-mediated visual system. A decrement in b wave amplitude was noted in lead factory workers. The authors suggest that this decrement may be an early indicator of lead toxicity in occupationally exposed workers.

Oculomotor Dysfunction

26. What industries and agents have been associated with oculomotor dysfunction?

Battery storage workers exposed to lead, plastic boat manufacturing workers exposed to styrene, torpedo factory workers exposed to 1,2-propylene glycol dinitrate, workers in plants producing inorganic mercury, and environmental exposure to methyl mercury in Japan and Iraq have been associated with oculomotor dysfunction.

27. What types of testing have been used to assess the oculomotor aspect of the visual system?

Extraocular muscle testing may be conducted by assessing the range of motion of each eye. Useful secondary tests include electronystagmography, electrooculography, and evaluation of saccadic eye movement.

28. What volunteer studies have assessed the effects of exposure to chemical agents?

Volunteers were exposed to styrene and trichloroethylene in inhalation chambers in three studies. ENG-recorded eye movements revealed abnormalities suggesting an effect on the vestibuloocular system. In other studies, volunteers exposed to alcohol, marijuana, nitrous oxide, and benzodiazepines were found to have abnormalities in oculomotor function. The effects of alcohol overshadowed those of marijuana.

Visual Field Deficits

29. What types of visual field deficits have been noted in populations exposed to toxic substances?

Central scotoma (absence of vision at the apex of fixation) suggests a lesion to the optic nerve, whereas a retinal lesion is evidenced by an enlarged blind spot. Constriction of a binocular visual field suggests central localization. All three types of abnormalities have been noted in patients and populations exposed to toxic chemicals.

30. What was the significance of the disasters in Minamata Bay and Baghdad?

Major epidemics of organomercury poisoning occurred in Minamata Bay (Nigata), Japan, and Iraq in the 1950s and continued into the 1970s. In Japan the hazard originated when metallic mercury was discharged into the bay as waste sludge. Elemental mercury was converted to methyl mercury by biotransformation. Between 1965 and 1974, 520 patients were identified with evidence of organomercury toxicity. In Iraq, seed farmers using organomecurial fungicides brought about the disaster. More than 6000 people were admitted to hospitals, and 459 died. Sixty percent of 53 patients from Japan and 100% of 2111 Iraqi patients had visual disturbances. Constriction of visual fields was a consistent finding.

31. What agents and industries have been associated with visual field abnormalities?

Lead has been associated with visual field abnormalities in the polyvinyl chloride pipe production industry. Methyl mercury exposure from the environmental disasters in Japan and Iraq led to visual field abnormalities. In addition, visual field abnormalities were found in workers in the viscose rayon industry exposed to CS_2.

Neurophysiologic Testing

32. What is a visual evoked potential (VEP)?

A VEP is a neurophysiologic response to visual stimuli measured by brain electrodes in the occipital cortex. Responses are evoked by flashes, reversing checkerboard pattern, or sine wave gratings. Flash evoked potentials (FEPs) may be used in many different animal species, because keen acuity and precise fixation are not critical. Animals are placed in a small chamber surrounded by mirrors and then stimulated at suprathreshold intensity. Stimulus intensity, pupil diameter, and level of light adaptation may affect the recordings. However, the dilation of pupils and use of supramaximal intensity are easy to control.

The pattern-reversal evoked potentials (PREPs) are more useful clinically than responses from diffuse flashes. FEPs have large inter- and intrasubject variability and are insensitive to functional disorders of the visual system. PREPs reveal primarily foveal or cone activity in humans. Optic nerve damage produces increased P1 latency that is detectable preclinically. Amplitude and latency vary systematically with pattern check size, reversal rate, contrast of dark and light checks, and other stimulus patterns. P1 latency increases and amplitude decreases as the discriminability of the display diminishes. P1 measures vary with subject variables such as pupil diameter, state of light adaptation, and focus on the stimulus display. Without focusing, abnormal amplitude and latency are obtained.

A third type of VEP is sine wave grating (SWEP). Different populations of neurons in the visual system can be selectively stimulated by varying the spatial or temporal frequency, orientation, or contrast of sine wave gratings. The checkerboard patterns used to generate PREPS are complex stimuli that drive heterogeneous neuronal populations. SWEPs offer greater specificity and diagnostic utility than FEPs and PREPs. Individual components of SWEPs for both humans and rats reflect specific functional processes, such as pattern and motion detection. Low spatial frequency gratings primarily stimulate the motion detection processes, whereas high spatial frequency stimulates the pattern recognition processes. When SWEPs are recorded for several spatial frequencies, systematic changes in component amplitudes are observed. Inter- and intra-subject variability is substantial.

A lack of specificity for VEP abnormalities often makes localization difficult. Demyelinating lesions, as occur in multiple sclerosis, often produce increased latencies. Other optic neuritides decrease amplitude, whereas neurotransmitter abnormalities, glaucoma, refractive error, and normal aging alter latency. Optic atrophy, amblyopia, and refractive error also may affect amplitude.

33. What specific populations and industries have been associated with VEP abnormalities?

Printing press workers and rotogravure printing workers exposed to toluene, adhesive bandage and vegetable oil extract manufacturing workers exposed to *n*-hexane, workers in the manufacturing of lead-containing items, and chloralkali workers exposed to inorganic mercury have been found to have subclinical deficits in visual evoked response latency.

34. What is critical flicker fusion?

Critical flicker fusion (CFF) is the threshold frequency at which a flickering light is perceived as constant. CFF is sensitive to changes in central nervous system activity. Thus, CFF threshold has been argued to be a measure of cortical arousal, but it is just as likely to reflect retinal or intermediate visual pathway function.

35. What populations have been associated with CFF abnormalities?

CFF detected abnormalities in lead smelters, workers in a battery production plant, and others in the lead industry in Australia.

36. What is contrast sensitivity?

Contrast sensitivity is the ability to perceive slight changes in luminance between regions that are not separated by definite borders. Assessment of contrast sensitivity involves a presentation of vertical bars on a panel or television screen. The number of cycles of light to dark per degree of visual angle is termed the spatial frequency and is expressed in cycles per degree.

Contrast visual testing is a psychophysical visual test of undetermined diagnostic capability in many neurovisual disorders. A decrement in contrast sensitivity in the presence of normal visual acuity is thought to reflect neurologic dysfunction, because this pattern has been noted in multiple sclerosis and cerebral lesions. It is not, however, specific to any particular neurovisual disease or neural locus of damage; deficits have been noted with many diverse conditions.

A selective deficiency in intermediate spatial frequencies is characteristic of multiple sclerosis. A more general spatial frequency loss observed among patients with compressive lesions of the anterior visual pathways seems to reflect more diffuse disturbance of the optic nerve.

37. Which populations and agents have been associated with abnormalities in contrast sensitivity?

Abnormalities in contrast sensitivity have been observed in microelectronics workers exposed to mixed solvent solutions, volunteers exposed to perchloroethylene, and patients receiving ethambutal therapy for pulmonary tuberculosis.

BIBLIOGRAPHY

Brain cancer
1. Thomas TL: Primary brain tumors associated with chemical exposure. In Bleeker M (ed): Occupational Neurology and Clinical Neurotoxicology. Baltimore, Williams & Wilkins, 1994.
2. Thomas TL, et al: Risk of astrocytic brain tumors associated with occupational chemical exposures: A case referent study. Scand J Work Environ Health 13:417–423, 1987.
3. Wu W, et al: Cohort and case control analyses of workers exposed to vinyl chloride: An update. J Occup Med 31:518–523, 1989.

Cerebellar syndromes
4. Bleeker ML: Clinical presentations of selected neurotoxic compounds. In Bleeker ML (ed): Occupational Neurology and Clinical Neurotoxicology. Baltimore, Williams & Wilkins, 1994.
5. Feldman RG: Recognizing the chemically exposed person. In Feldman RG (ed): Occupational and Environmental Neurotoxicology. Philadelphia, Lippincott-Raven, 1999.
6. Rosenberg NL, Spitz MC, Filey CM, et al: Central nervous system effects of chronic toluene abuse—Clinical brainstem evoked responses and magnetic resonance imaging studies. Neurotoxicol Teratol 23: 611–614, 1988.
7. Yokoyama K, Araki F, Murata K, et al: Subclinical vestibulocerebellar anterior cerebellar lobe and spinocerebellar effects in lead workers in relation to current and past exposure. Neurotoxicology 18:371–380, 1997.

Cranial nerve disorders
8. Ashford NA, Miller CS: Chemical Exposures: Low Levels and High Stakes. New York, Van Nostrand Reinhold, 1998.
9. Bell IR: Neuropsychiatric aspects of sensitivity to low levels chemicals: A neural sensitization model. Toxicol Indust Health 10:277–312, 1994.
10. Bleeker ML: Occupational Neurotoxicology and Clinical Neurotoxicology. Baltimore, Williams & Wilkins, 1994.
11. Feldman RG: Occupational and Environmental Neurotoxicology. Philadelphia, Lippincott-Raven, 1999.
12. Feldman RG,White RF: Role of neurologist in hazard identification and risk assessment. Environ Health Perspect 104:227–237, 1996.
13. Rosenberg NL (ed): Occupational and Environmental Neurology. Boston, Butterworth-Heinemann, 1995.
14. Rosenberg NL: Neurotoxicity of organic solvents. In Rosenberg NL (ed): Occupational and Environmental Neurology. Boston, Butterworth-Heinemann, 1995.

Visual toxicology
15. Altmann L, Bottger A, Wiegand H: Neurophysiologic and psychological measurements reveal effects of acute low level organic solvent exposure in humans. Int Arch Occup Environ Health 62:493–499, 1990.
16. Anger K: Neurobehavioral tests used in NIOSH supported worksite studies, 1973–1983. Neurobehav Toxicol Teratol 7:359–368, 1985.
17. Bakir F, Damluji SF, Aminz Aki L, et al: Methyl mercury poisoning in Iraq. Science 181:230–240, 1973.
18. Baloh RW, Langhofer L, Brown CP, Spivey GH: Quantitative eye tracking tests in lead workers. Am J Indust Med 1:109–113, 1980.
19. Broadwell DK, Darcey DJ, Hudnell HK, et al: Work site clinical and neurobehavioral assessment of solvent exposed microelectronics workers. Am J Indust Med 27:677–698, 1995.
20. Cavallieri A, Belotti L, Gobba F, et al: Colour vision loss in workers exposed to elemental mercury vapour. Toxicol Lett 77:351–356, 1995.
21. Chang YC: Neurotoxic effects of N-hexane on the human central nervous system: Evoked potential abnormalities in n-hexane polyneuropathy. J Neurol Neurosurg Psychiatry 50:269–274, 1987.
22. Chia SE, Jeyaratnam J, Ong CN, et al: Impairment of color vision among workers exposed to low concentrations of styrene. Am J Indust Med 26:481–488, 1994.
23. Ellingsen DG, Morland T, Andersen A, Kjuus H: Relation between exposure related indices and neurological and neurophysiologic effects in workers previously exposed to mercury vapor. Br J Indust Med 50:736–744, 1993.
24. Fallas C, Fallas J, Maslard P, Dally S: Subclinical impairment of color vision among workers exposed to styrene. Br J Indust Med 49:679–682, 1992.

25. Feldman RG, White RF: Role of neurologist in hazard identification and risk assessment. Environ Health Perspect 104(S2):227–237, 1996.
26. Galloway N: Electrodiagnosis. In Walsh TJ (ed): Neuro-ophthalmology. Philadelphia, Lea & Febiger, 1992, pp 353–390.
27. Grant WM: Toxicology of the Eye, 3rd ed. Springfield, IL, Charles C. Thomas, 1986.
28. Hart WM: Acquired dyschromatopsias. Surv Ophthalmol 32:10–31, 1987.
29. Karai I, Sugimoto K, Goto S: A case comparison study of carbon disulfide retinopathy and diabetic retinopathy using flourescein fundus angiography. Acta Ophthalmol 61:1074–1086, 1983.
30. Lilienthal H, Winneke G, Ewert T: Effects of lead on neurophysiologic and performance measure: Animal and human data. Environ Health Perspect 89:21–25, 1990.
31. Lorance RW, Kaufman D, Wray SH, Mao C: Contrast visual testing in neurovisual diagnosis. Neurology 37:923–929, 1987.
32. Marsh DO: Organic mercury: Clinical and neurotoxicological aspects. In Wolff FA (ed): Handbook of Clinical Neurology. Elsevier Science, 1994, pp 413–429.
33. Mergler D, Huel G, Bowler R, et al: Visual dysfunction among former microelectronics assembly workers. Arch Environ Health 46:326–334, 1991.
34. Moller C, Odkvist L, Larsby B, et al: Otoneurological findings in workers exposed to styrene. Scand J Work Environ Health 16:189–194, 1990.
35. Nakatsuka H, Watanabe T, Takeichi Y, et al: Absence of blue-yellow color vision loss among workers exposed to toluene or tetrachloroethylene mostly at levels below occupational exposure limits. Int Arch Occup Environ Health 64:113–117, 1992.
36. Otto D, Hudnell K, Boyes R, et al: Electrophysiological measures of visual and auditory function as indices of neurotoxicity. Toxicology 49:205–218, 1988.
37. Raitta C, Teir H, Tolonen M, et al: Impaired color discrimination among viscose rayon workers exposed to carbon disulfide. J Occup Med 233:189–192, 1981.
38. Rosenman KD, Valcuikas JA, Glickman L, et al: Sensitive indicators of inorganic mercury toxicity. Arch Environ Health 41:208–215, 1986.
39. Ruitjen MW, Salle HJ, Verberk MM, Muiijser H: Special nerve functions and colour discrimination in workers with long term low level exposure to carbon disulphide. Br J Indust Med 47:589–595, 1991.
40. Rustam H, Hamdi T: Methyl mercury poisoning in Iraq. A neurological study. Brain 97:500–510, 1974.
41. Seppalainen AM, Raitta C, Huuskonen MS: N-hexane induced changes in visual evoked potentials and electroretinograms of industrial workers. Electroencephalogr Clin Neurophysiol 47:492–498, 1979.
42. Sugimoto K, Goto S, Kanda S, et al: Studies on angiography due to carbon disulphide. Retinopathy and index of exposure dosages. Scand J Work Environ Health 4:151–158, 1978.
43. Urban P, Lukas E: Visual evoked potentials in rotogravure printers exposed to toluene. Br J Indust Med 47:819–823, 1990.
44. Xintaras C, Johnson BL, Ulrich CE, et al: Application of the evoked response technique in air pollution toxicology. Toxicol Appl Pharmacol 8:77–87, 1966.

36. PERIPHERAL NERVOUS SYSTEM DISEASE

Gary M. Liss, M.D., M.S., FRCPC, Gyl Midroni, M.D., FRCP(C), and Ronald A. House, M.D., M.Sc., FRCPC

1. What is the extent of occupational peripheral neuropathy?

Symptomatic occupationally induced toxic neuropathy is rare in North America, but asymptomatic toxic neuropathy may be more common among certain exposed groups. A number of chemicals, principally some solvents, heavy metals, and pesticides, have been found to cause toxic neuropathy; specific examples are described below. The potential for exposure in numerous industries and the relative rarity of reports of clinically apparent toxic neuropathy suggest that underrecognition and underreporting are likely. Between 1980 and 1994, the Workers' Compensation Board in the Province of Ontario (which has a population of over 10 million) allowed 19 claims for toxic peripheral neuropathy (excluding those associated with repetitive strain and trauma) and rejected 12 claims. Of the accepted claims, 8 were associated with *n*-hexane.

The clinical syndromes of peripheral nervous system disease may be divided into **polyneuropathies** and **focal or multifocal neuropathies**. In polyneuropathies the involvement is diffuse and therefore symmetric, whereas in focal or multifocal syndromes lesions may be localized to specific site(s) in individual nerve trunks. Occupational toxin exposure is generally associated with polyneuropathy, whereas acute or chronic trauma and compression are important occupational causes of focal neuropathies.

2. What are the two basic forms of peripheral nerve damage due to neurotoxins?

Most toxic polyneuropathies result from metabolic upset of the neuron with subsequent **axonal degeneration**. Often the most distal parts of the axon are affected first, with increasingly proximal involvement as the disease worsens. This pattern has led to the term **dying-back neuropathy**, although the term **central-peripheral distal axonopathy** is perhaps more accurate, reflecting the fact that central nervous system axons also may be affected. A much less common mechanism in toxic polyneuropathies is demyelination, which affects Schwann cells or their myelin independently of the axon. Confusion sometimes arises because axonal degeneration may cause a mild degree of secondary demyelination. The most important means of distinguishing between axonal and demyelinating polyneuropathies is nerve conduction studies. Prominent slowing signals the presence of demyelination, whereas muscle denervation identifies a loss of axons. The distinction is important in that recovery from demyelination is usually faster and more complete than recovery from axonal degeneration.

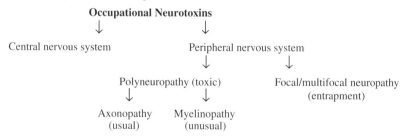

3. Why is the peripheral nervous system so vulnerable to toxin-induced or entrapment neuropathies?

The length of the axon is an important determinant of susceptibility; longer nerves and larger-diameter myelinated fibers are more vulnerable. In many cases, the pathophysiologic mechanisms resulting in distal axonopathy are not known. The nerve damage appears to involve interference with the transport of nutritional and metabolic materials toward the end of the axon; consequently, the distal portion is more at risk.

4. What are the main peripheral neurotoxins in the workplace? In the environment?

Various neurotoxins in industry induce a symmetric sensorimotor polyneuropathy, including the classic neurotoxic agents *n*-hexane and methyl-*n*-butyl ketone as well as carbon disulfide, acrylamide, mercury, and some organophosphates. *n*-Hexane and methyl-*n*-butyl ketone are hexacarbon solvents; the neurotoxicity of both may be exacerbated by concurrent exposure to methyl ethyl ketone and is thought to be mediated by 2,5-hexanedione, which is formed during metabolism. Arsenic has been associated with predominantly sensory neuropathy, whereas lead induces a predominantly motor polyneuropathy with weakness of the wrist and finger extensors (e.g., the "wrist drop" emphasized in older descriptions). Two outbreaks of autonomic neuropathy resulting in bladder dysfunction were caused by the catalyst, dimethylaminopropionitrile (DMAPN), which is used in the production of polyurethane foam. Trichloroethylene has induced trigeminal neuropathy.

Environmental organic mercury poisoning has induced episodes of distal limb paresthesias as well as central nervous system disturbances (e.g., Minamata, Japan). Although lead is also frequently encountered in the environment, in children the main concern is effects on the central nervous system (including neurobehavioral changes) rather than the peripheral nervous system.

5. What are the main symptoms and signs of chemically induced peripheral neuropathy?

Most toxic neuropathies have a subacute onset with gradual progression. The initial manifestations are usually sensory and may include intermittent paresthesias such as numbness, burning, tingling, pain, and/or anesthesia. Symptoms usually appear initially in a stocking distribution (feet), followed later by a glove distribution (hands), based on the relationship to fiber length. Motor manifestations often follow, such as cramps, stiffness, weakness in feet and hands, and atrophy. If only the hands are affected, the clinician should consider the possibility of another diagnosis. The ankle reflexes are first to be reduced or absent, but other tendon reflexes also should be tested. Most toxins do not cause focal damage. As a classic example, the hexacarbon neuropathies are characterized by the insidious development of progressive distal weakness and sensory loss more marked in the lower extremities. A slapping gait and difficulty with finger movements and grasping of heavy objects also occurred in more severe cases.

As a general rule, toxic neuropathies are subacute to chronically progressive, relatively mild, predominantly sensory, symmetric, and length-dependent; they show axonal features on conduction studies. However, this pattern is common and nonspecific and usually cannot be distinguished clinically from neuropathy due to such relatively frequent etiologies as diabetes, renal failure, vitamin deficiency, or paraproteinemic neuropathy. Rapid progression, a significant degree of asymmetry, motor predominance, and demyelinating features on conduction studies are atypical and suggest a nontoxic etiology, such as acute or chronic inflammatory demyelinating neuropathy, vasculitic neuropathy, or a genetically determined process. Careful questioning about family history is required to avoid overlooking an inherited neuropathy.

6. What types of clinical tools are recommended for the evaluation of a patient with potential peripheral neuropathy due to occupational or environmental exposure?

For the clinical evaluation of individual patients, electrophysiologic testing with nerve conduction studies (NCS) (both motor and sensory studies) and electromyography (EMG) are the principal diagnostic tools for confirmation of neuropathy. NCS may help to identify the site of nerve compression in focal neuropathies. In diffuse polyneuropathies, NCS may help to differentiate axonal and demyelinating subtypes.

Usually it is not possible to distinguish between toxic and nontoxic etiologies on clinical grounds. Once the existence of neuropathy is verified by NCS, a diagnostic work-up is required to exclude the common nontoxic etiologies. At a minimum, the work-up should include a fasting glucose, complete blood count, erythrocyte sedimentation rate, vitamin B_{12}, creatinine, thyroid-stimulating hormone, serum and urine immunoelectrophoresis, and chest radiograph. HIV testing and cerebrospinal fluid examination also may form important parts of the diagnostic work-up, and nerve biopsy may be indicated if no diagnosis can be made otherwise. In outbreaks of toxic neuropathies extensive work-up may be required only for the first index cases; more limited testing may be performed in patients who have a known toxin exposure and a typical clinical presentation.

7. In an epidemiologic study of manufacturing workers exposed to methyl-*n*-butyl ketone, nerve conduction velocities were measured to diagnose cases of peripheral neuropathy. When are NCS or other ancillary tests indicated for diagnosis and case definition in an epidemiologic study? What confounders need to be considered?

Although NCS are critical for clinical diagnosis, on some occasions they have been incorporated as part of group screening. NCS are subject to a number of limitations. Most importantly, the wide range of normal values limits the ability to detect mild abnormalities. Because conduction study results depend on age, sex, and body habitus, appropriately matched control data are required for studying subtle changes in a group of patients with a toxic exposure. In general, reduction and loss of sensory amplitudes and prolongation of sensory distal latencies are the earliest NCS abnormalities in toxic neuropathies. However, these parameters are highly dependent on limb temperature, which should be rigorously controlled. Another limitation is that only large myelinated fibers are assessed by NCS; thus significant disease of small myelinated and unmyelinated fibers may pass undetected. The major advantage of NCS is that they are completely uninfluenced by patient cooperation and thus provide an unbiased measure of nerve function.

Quantitative sensory testing (QST) is a helpful adjunct to NCS. QST assesses the patient's ability to perceive various stimuli, including vibration, touch/pressure, and thermal sensations. Its main advantage is the ability to test specific sensory modalities, including those mediated by fiber types that are not amenable to NCS (e.g., small fiber-mediated thermal sensations). However, QST is subject to the same limitations as NCS; unless it is performed rigorously, the results may be unreliable. QST results are also highly dependent on cooperation and accurate reporting by the patient (its major limitation). Berger and Schaumburg note that QST is recommended for "rapid screening of large populations (e.g., workers at risk for toxic neuropathy)" and that in diffuse peripheral neuropathies abnormalities on QST may precede abnormalities in NCS. Generally, QST and NCS provide complementary information; hence, both should be used in epidemiologic studies if possible.

In all epidemiologic studies of peripheral neuropathy, one must consider other causes of peripheral nerve damage, including nerve compression, dietary factors (malnutrition, alcohol), and diabetes. In an outbreak investigation involving many cases of possible toxic neuropathy, one can exclude uncertain cases with confounding exposures from the analysis. However, if fewer cases are available, one may analyze the associations between the exposure under study and cases of neuropathy, both including and excluding cases with nonoccupational risk factors. If differences between the two analyses are found, they may permit assessment of the interaction between risk factors.

8. When should you recommend nerve biopsy, if ever?

Nerve biopsy is generally not indicated in the investigation of toxic neuropathy; the diagnosis should be suggested by a carefully taken history and confirmed by clinical improvement after withdrawal from the offending material. The great majority of occupational toxin neuropathies reveal nonspecific histologic features of axonal degeneration and/or regeneration, occasionally with mild degrees of secondary demyelination. Such findings cannot be distinguished from the findings in most acquired axonopathies. A unique exception involves the hexacarbon neuropathies, in which axonal swellings filled with massive neurofilament accumulations are a prominent feature. Biopsy may be helpful for patients in whom some other acquired or genetically determined cause of neuropathy is a diagnostic option and also should be considered when a novel cause of toxic neuropathy is suspected.

9. What other, less frequently reported agents are possible causes of chemically induced peripheral neuropathy?

In addition to the classic agents described above, peripheral neuropathy also has been associated in the past with the solvent styrene, mixed organic solvents, polychlorinated biphenyls, and the gases methyl bromide, ethylene oxide, and carbon monoxide (neuropathy due to carbon monoxide may occur only after severe acute exposure). Recently cases of peripheral neuropathy have been reported in Canada in association with exposure to 1,1,1-trichloroethane after skin immersion. The cases involved the potential for both cutaneous and inhalation routes of exposure, and the neuropathy appeared to be primarily sensory. In addition, recent cases of neuropathy have been reported after exposure to multiple solvents (roofers and painters), heating tar epoxy resin paint, and n-heptane (in a shoemaker in whom n-hexane was not detected). Confirmation is required to establish the causal nature of these associations. Peripheral neuropathy also may be encountered among workers exposed to hand-arm vibration; this subject is addressed in chapter 28.

10. What is the prognosis of chemically induced peripheral neuropathy?

Some degree of recovery after removal from exposure is the rule, although a period of months may be required. Recovery has usually been complete in mild and moderate cases of neuropathy. Recovery from axonopathy tends to be slower and more likely to be incomplete than recovery from myelinopathy. Occasionally patients continue to deteriorate for some weeks after removal from toxin exposure (the "coasting" phenomenon).

11. What are the characteristic findings in a patient with acrylamide toxicity?

The vinyl monomer acrylamide ($CH_2=CHCONH_2$), a white crystalline solid, was introduced in the 1950s as a chemical grouting agent and has been used in soil waterproofing, during mining and tunneling operations, and in the production of polymers, surface coatings, and adhesives. In cases of intoxication, exposure has occurred during tunneling operations, mixing of dry acrylamide powder, and polymerization of monomer. The neuropathy is characterized by the gradual, progressive development of sensory and motor findings with numbness and weakness in the feet and hands, muscle aching, decreased ankle reflexes, and decreased vibration sensation. Concomitant findings may include nystagmus, unsteadiness of the legs, ataxia, and tremor, which may reflect central (cerebellar involvement). Skin irritation manifested by redness, peeling, and even blistering of palmar skin may precede neuropathy. Excessive sweating of the palms and feet also has been reported. Recovery after cessation of exposure was not complete in severely poisoned workers.

12. Which entrapment syndromes are commonly associated with occupational exposures or traumas?

Peripheral nerves are vulnerable to focal injury through compression, traction, or other mechanisms in a variety of occupational settings. Carpal tunnel syndrome, probably the most common example, is discussed in chapter 36. The table below lists specific occupational settings that can lead directly to focal peripheral nerve injury.

NERVE	SYMPTOMS/SIGNS	SETTING
Long thoracic	Shoulder pain, winging of scapula	Carrying heavy shoulder pack
Lower trunk brachial plexus (TOS)	Arm pain, tingling of inner arm and/or little finger, wasting/weakness of hand muscles	Musicians
Suprascapular	Shoulder pain, weakness of arm abduction	Baseball pitchers
Ulnar (at elbow)	Forearm pain, tingling of fifth finger, weakness/wasting of hand/forearm muscles	Musicians
Ulnar (at wrist)	Hand pain, weakness/wasting of hand muscles	Manual workers
Peroneal (at fibula)	Foot drop, numbness/tingling of foot	Prolonged squatting
Femoral	Buckling of knee, numbness/pain along anterior thigh/inner leg	Dancers, gymnasts
Saphenous	Numbness/pain along inner aspect of leg	Prolonged kneeling

TOS = thoracic outlet syndrome.

13. What methods best prevent toxic peripheral neuropathy in the workplace?

In general, premarket screening by animal testing for detection of potential neurotoxic effects has too low a yield and is too expensive to be recommended for all chemicals before introduction into industry. However, a case can be made for premarket animal testing for some substances with chemical structures or mechanisms of action similar to those of known neurotoxic agents. The most effective means of prevention is reduction or elimination of exposure by engineering controls such as process enclosure and local exhaust ventilation. When possible, a less toxic chemical should be substituted for a neurotoxic agent. Workers should be informed of the neurotoxic effects of chemicals and advised of the importance of proper safety procedures, including the use of personal protective equipment such as gloves and respirators. Safety procedures are especially important during clean-ups of leaks and spills. Biologic monitoring (measurement of the substance or its metabolites in blood, urine, or other biologic media) is used routinely for some neurotoxic chemicals such as lead and also may be used on a periodic or ad hoc basis for other chemicals to determine the level of exposure and effectiveness of personal protective equipment.

BIBLIOGRAPHY

1. Allen N, Mendell JR, Billmaier DJ, et al: Toxic polyneuropathy due to methyl-n-butyl ketone: An industrial outbreak. Arch Neurol 32:209–218, 1975.
2. Baker EL: Neurologic disorders. In Rom WN (ed): Environmental and Occupational Medicine, 2nd ed. Toronto, Little, Brown, 1992, pp 561–572.
3. Berger AR, Schaumburg HH: Disorders of the peripheral nervous system. In Rosenstock L, Cullen MR (eds): Textbook of Clinical Occupational and Environmental Medicine, 2nd ed. Toronto, W.B. Saunders, 1994, pp 482–503.
4. Billmaier D, Yee HT, Allen N, et al: Peripheral neuropathy in a coated-fabrics plant. J Occup Med 16:665–671, 1974.
5. Cherry N, Gautrin D: Neurotoxic effects of styrene: Further evidence. Br J Indust Med 47:29–37, 1990.
6. Cone JE, Bowler R, So Y: Medical surveillance for neurologic endpoints. Occup Med State Art Rev 5:547–562, 1990.
7. Demers RY, Markell BL, Wabeke R: Peripheral vibratory sense deficits in solvent-exposed painters. J Occup Med 33:1051–1054, 1991.
8. Guirguis S: Acrylamide and acrylonitrile. In Rom WN (ed): Environmental and Occupational Medicine, 2nd ed. Toronto, Little, Brown, 1992, pp 947–953.
9. Gruenner G, Dyck PJ: Quantitative sensory testing: Methodology, applications, and future directions. J Clin Neurophysiol 11:568–583, 1994.
10. Herbert R, Gerr F, Luo J, et al: Peripheral neurologic abnormalities among roofing workers: Sentinel case and clinical screening. Arch Environ Health 50:349–354, 1995.
11. House RA, Liss GM, Wills MC: Peripheral sensory neuropathy associated with 1,1,1-trichloroethane. Arch Environ Health 49:196–199, 1994.
12. Landrigan PJ: Occupational Neurological Disease: Teaching Epidemiology in Occupational Health. National Institute for Occupational Safety and Health, 1987 [DHHS (NIOSH) Publication Nol 87-112].
13. Lederman RJ: Neurologic disorders in performing artists. In Rosenberg NL (ed): Occupational and Environmental Neurology. Stoneham, MA, Butterworth-Heinemann, 1995, pp 309–339.
14. Liss GM: Peripheral neuropathy in two workers exposed to 1,1,1-tricohloroethane [letter]. JAMA 260:2217, 1988.
15. Midroni G, Bilbao JM: Biopsy Diagnosis of Peripheral Neuropathy. Stoneham, MA, Butterworth-Heniemann, 1995, pp 331–351.
16. Murata K, Araki S, Yokoyama K: Assessment of the peripheral, central, and autonomic nervous system function in styrene workers. Am J Indust Med 20:775–784, 1991.
17. Murata K, Araki S, Yokoyama K, Maeda K: Autonomic and peripheral nervous system dysfunction in workers exposed to organic solvents. Int Arch Occup Environ Health 63:335–340, 1991.
18. Sakai T, Araki S, Sata F, Araki T: Analysis of toxic gas produced by heating tar epoxy resin paint to assess work atmosphere. Sangyo Igaku—Jpn J Indust Health 36:412–419, 1994.
19. Spencer PS, Schaumburg HH: Central-peripheral distal axonopathy: The pathology of dying-back polyneuropathies. Prog Neuropathol 3:253–295, 1976.
20. Schaumburg HH, Spencer PS: The neurology and neuropathology of the occupational neuropathies. J Occup Med 18:739–742, 1976.
21. Stewart JD: Focal Peripheral Neuropathies, 2nd ed. New York, Raven Press, 1993.
22. Valentini F, Agnesi R, Dal Vecchio L, et al: Does n-heptane cause peripheral neurotoxicity? A case report in a shoemaker. Occup Med 44:102–104, 1994.

37. OCCUPATIONAL AND ENVIRONMENTAL NEUROPSYCHOLOGY

Rosemarie M. Bowler, Ph.D., M.P.H.

1. What is neuropsychology?

Neuropsychology is the scientific study and application of principles of brain-behavior relationships using assessment strategies involving both quantitative (systematic research) and qualitative (clinical) approaches. Neuropsychological methods use standardized tests that permit comparison of a patient's functional abilities with normative data obtained from comparable populations. The principal assessment method consists of an extensive clinical history and an individualized test battery administered and interpreted by a specially trained neuropsychologist who is knowledgeable about brain injuries and diseases.

2. What do neuropsychologists do?

Neuropsychologists are trained in the measurement and interpretation of brain function by use of neuropsychological tests. Clinical psychologists are trained in brain pathology, neuroanatomy, and physiology to perform neuropsychological evaluations. They are trained to administer psychometric tests developed during the First and Second World Wars to screen U.S. military recruits and to diagnose brain-injured and/or behaviorally disordered U.S. military personnel. At present, neuropsychologists not only assess central nervous system dysfunction but also serve as an interface between general medicine and neurology. They can document impairment associated with and resulting from traumatic injuries and toxic exposures. Although most of the neuropsychological tests in use are normed across different age levels, many are insufficiently normed against different cultures and socioeconomic groups. Caution needs to be applied in the interpretation of test results for such groups. For this reason, it is desirable to include similar control groups in epidemiologic research to eliminate bias.

3. How is neuropsychology used in occupational and environmental medicine?

Occupational medicine. Neuropsychologists quantify behavioral effects of accidents, toxic exposures, and repetitive disorders, such as carpal tunnel syndrome, in terms of functional limitations and disabilities. The rehabilitative potential of an injured worker can be assessed and appropriate treatment and rehabilitation programs prescribed. The neuropsychologist also determines the effects of stress-related illnesses on work function. A neuropsychologist with background in toxic exposures can (1) determine the likelihood of association between exposure and dysfunction, (2) rule out other contributing factors, (3) make recommendations to the physician about psychiatric medication and additional medical evaluations, and (4) in cases of large-scale work exposure, propose a screening test battery that can be used before and after implementation of workplace improvements. Although low-level chemical exposures and their effects on function are controversial, hysterical formation of symptoms is rather rare in educated and industrial workers.

Environmental medicine. Neuropsychologists are asked to evaluate the functional effects of environmental contaminants such as toxicants and neurotoxicants. Examples include organic solvents, heavy metals, gases, and pesticides. Exposures may occur in accidental injuries to groups of workers (e.g., sick buildings or accidents) or spills of solvents or pesticides that contaminate the environment and become human health hazards.

4. What type of neuropsychological tests are available?

Although an attempt was made to create complete and comprehensive assessment test batteries, such as the Halstead-Reitan Neuropsychological Test Battery and the Luria-Nebraska

Neuropsychological Test, most neuropsychologists use a flexible battery of individual tests, chosen specifically for each evaluation. The two main tests in use for psychometric and neuropsychological assessments are the Wechsler Adult Intelligence Scale-III (WAIS-III) and the Wechsler Memory Scale-III (WMS-III), which were revised and improved by using greater age and education ranges, broader ethnic composition, and four different geographic regions.

5. Describe the domains of brain function and the tests frequently used to measure them in a thorough evaluation.

1. **Verbal ability and cognition.** Tests of learning achievement, such as the Wide Range Achievement Test (WRAT), yield school-grade equivalents. Word knowledge is measured by vocabulary tests. Abstract verbal reasoning is measured by the Similarities Test from the WAIS-III. Verbal fluency is typically measured with Benton's Controlled Oral Word Association Test.

2. **Learning.** Verbal learning is measured by word list and spatial reasoning tests. Word learning lists are included in the Memory Assessment Scale (MAS) and the California Verbal Learning Test (CVLT). The Category Test of the Halstead-Reitan Battery measures the ability to learn nonverbal sets, and both the Symbol Digit Modalities Test (SDMT) and the Digit Symbol Test of the WAIS-III measure speed of learning geometric symbols.

3. **Information processing and cognitive flexibility** (both verbal and nonverbal tests). Processing of information is measured by tests of cognitive flexibility and processing speed. The ability to shift from verbal to nonverbal stimuli, to sequence, and to scan and track a sequence visually is measured by the SMDT, Stroop Color Word Test, Short Category Test from the Halstead-Reitan Battery, and Trail Making Test B. In addition, the WAIS-III has an index score for Processing Speed composed of visuospatial tasks.

4. **Attention and memory.** Memory is measured over a range of modalities. The two most frequently used memory batteries are the WMS-III and the Memory Assessment Scale (MAS). The recently revised WMS-III also includes an index score for Working Memory, a construct assessing capacity to remember and manipulate information presented both visually and orally in short-term memory. In addition, it has separate primary indices for Immediate Memory and General (delayed) Memory. It also separates single-trial learning from retention and retrieval. Memory index scores are similar to IQ scores; a mean of 100 equals the 50th percentile and the standard deviation is 15.

5. **Executive function.** Executive function involves complex purposive behavior, such as planning and organizing. A patient with frontal lobe dysfunction scores poorly on these and on other tests of social competence, such as the Comprehension Subtest of the WAIS-III or the Proverbs Test.

6. **Concept formation** (visual and verbal). Visual concept formation is measured by the Category Test from the Halstead-Reitan Battery, and the Wisconsin Card Sorting Test and the Raven's Progressive Matrices Test measure the ability to abstract from visually presented tasks. The WAIS-III Picture Completion and Picture Arrangement Subtests also measure visual reasoning and perception. Verbal abstraction is measured by the Similarities Subtest from the WAIS-III.

7. **Psychomotor speed, gross motor strength, tactile function, and reaction time** (tested bilaterally). Psychomotor speed is assessed with a fingertapper; gross motor strength by the dynamometer; tactile function by either the Purdue Pegboard Test, the Grooved Pegboard Test, or the Santa Ana Test; and reaction time by a number of different electronic or computerized tests of simple and/or complex reaction.

8. **Visual and visuospatial ability.** Visual ability is tested by the Snellen Near Visual Acuity Test; contrast sensitivity (the ability to differentiate between shades of gray) by tests such as the Vistech Test of Contrast Sensitivity; and color vision sensitivity by tests such as the Lanthony D15 Color Vision Test (desaturated panel). Visuospatial functions are tested by Symbol Digits Modalities Test and the Digit Symbol and Block Design Subtests from the WAIS-III. Visuoperceptual function can be tested by the Picture Completion and Picture Arrangement Subtests of the WAIS-III and visuospatial construction ability by the Block Design Subtest of the WAIS-III.

9. **Emotionality.** Tests of affect and mood are essential in cases of both functional and possible organic (limbic system) causes. The most widely used objective test of personality and mood is the Minnesota Multiphasic Personality Inventory (MMPI-2), a true-false test of 564 items. Summary scores are plotted graphically for 10 clinical and 3 validity scores. Other tests of personality are the Beck Depression Inventory (BDI), the Profile of Mood States (POMS), and The Symptom Checklist 90-Revised (SCL 90-R) or its shorter version, the Brief Symptom Inventory (BSI). To obtain additional information about personality and to assist the psychologist in screening for psychotic processes, projective personality tests are useful, such as the Rorschach Ink Blot Test and the Thematic Apperception Test (TAT). Projective tests ask the patient to project onto ambiguous or unstructured stimuli their own needs, experiences, and unique ways of experiencing the world. Brain-injured patients frequently show evidence of constriction, stimulus boundedness, response rigidity, fragmentation, simplification, conceptual confusion and disorientation, hesitancy and doubt, and psychotic processes.

6. How does the neuropsychologist test for malingering?

The trained neuropsychologist is able to evaluate the overall test results and clinical observations (during the history taking and test administration) to rule out a conscious effort to produce poor responses. The neuropsychologist may give several tests measuring the same domain of function; valid test protocols show a consistency of performance. Several specific tests of malingering are available, such as the Rey 15-Item Visual Memory Test and the Portland Digit Substitution Test. The validity scales of the MMPI-2 also may be used to rule out consciously produced deficits.

7. When should a patient be referred to a neuropsychologist?

Referrals can be made for a number of presentations. Patients may report early potential changes in brain function, such as not feeling like the same person as before, or family members or friends may notice that their personality has changed. Patients may report forgetfulness (getting lost, forgetting whether they locked the house, forgetting work tasks that they were required to do, or, in more severe cases, familiar work tasks have become too difficult), problems with memory for recent events but not with long-term memory or overlearned events, excessive fatigue, changes in sleep patterns, behavioral changes, word-finding difficulties, irritability, or sudden, unprovoked changes in mood. Some patients may engage in increased drug or alcohol use, whereas some neurotoxicant-exposed patients may suddenly become intolerant of alcohol.

8. When you refer, what should you provide for the neuropsychologist? What can you expect from a neuropsychological evaluation?

All relevant summaries of medical records and a specific referral question should be provided before the patient's first appointment with a neuropsychologist. If an injured worker is off work, the neuropsychologist can be asked whether the worker will be able to return to his or her prior job or whether the worker needs retraining in another job or other rehabilitative training. In neurotoxicant-induced disorders, the neuropsychologist can be asked whether the dysfunction is specific to the particular exposure. If the neuropsychologist is not familiar with the effects of particular chemicals to which the worker was exposed, it is desirable to provide material safety data sheets (if available) or to include brief statements about known health effects associated with such exposures.

9. What typical patterns of abnormalities may be found in neurotoxicant-exposed patients?

The typical patterns are well described by the World Health Organization (WHO), which has defined three types of disorders due to organic solvent exposure. Similar patterns are found in patients exposed to neurotoxicants, such as pesticides, heavy metals, and gases. Type 1 includes the usual symptoms of neurotoxicity, such as dizziness and nausea, confusion, disorientation, headache, weakness and fatigue, and concentration problems. Type 2a includes adverse mood problems, and type 2b includes both adverse mood problems and neuropsychological deficits in attention and concentration, memory, cognitive flexibility, information processing, and motor functions. Word knowledge is generally resistant to deterioration. Type 3 includes the more serious toxic encephalopathies with impairment in both cognitive and mood function, as well as neurologically detectable findings.

10. How do mood changes cause dysfunction? Why are they often reported after neurotoxicant exposure?

Workers who suffer moderate-to-severe levels of depression and anxiety after a chemical exposure are unable to apply the same level of concentration, vigilance, and accuracy to their work. Such changes may impair the worker's ability to deal with the public and coworkers, as well as family and social life. Neurotoxicants have been shown to cause mood changes (WHO type 1 and 2 impairment). The mood changes may be reactive (functional) to impairment and illness but also may involve changes in neurotransmitter release or actual changes in the limbic system of the central nervous system.

11. What are the typical functional effects of neurotoxicant exposure or minimal brain injury?

Workers who have suffered toxic exposure or minimal brain injury are likely to show diffuse deficits in attention, sustained concentration, and memory, as well as alterations in mood. Such changes may be reflected by impaired speed in performing work tasks. They also may result in excessive fatigue and problems in relating to others at the work site, resulting in work inefficiency, forgetfulness, and an increase in the potential for accidents.

12. What are the organic effects of neurotoxicant exposure or minimal brain injury?

Organic brain effect from neurotoxicant exposure may be difficult to diagnose for the inexperienced neuropsychologist. In part this difficulty is due to the presence of both cognitive and mood dysfunctions, which may mimic symptoms of functional disorders such as depression or anxiety. However, in the types of diffuse minimal brain dysfunction associated with neurotoxicant disorders, patients frequently show deficits in sustaining concentration, visuospatial function, and cognitive flexibility and information processing. In general, such deficits are consistent across various tests.

13. What are the typical diagnoses after neurotoxicant exposure or injury?

Common diagnostic categories include an organic disturbance, such as a mental disorder not otherwise specified due to a toxic exposure or personality change due to a toxic exposure. The diagnosis also may be coded as a cognitive disorder not otherwise specified in patients with mild impairment in cognitive functioning. Although toxic encephalopathy may be used descriptively, it is not a formal DMS-IV diagnosis. Severe memory disturbance may diagnosed as amnestic disorder not otherwise specified. If the precipitating accident or event was outside usual and ordinary human experience, the patient may develop posttraumatic stress disorder (PTSD). PTSD may be accompanied by loss of the ability to concentrate and by mood changes, particularly anxiety. Patients with PTSD characteristically may either avoid thinking about the stressful stimuli or be flooded with unwanted stimulation and flashbacks.

14. What is the controversy surrounding hysteria and conversion disorder? Can conversion disorder develop after chemical exposures?

The controversy is due largely to the fact that, with the exception of lead, no biologic markers are available for neurotoxicant exposure. Although styrene can be measured in the urine of active workers by checking the levels of mandelic acid and cholinesterase testing may show organophosphate poisoning, such analyses must take place within hours or days of exposure—too short a period to be feasible in most cases. The literature describes some workers who have been intoxicated by either solvents or other neurotoxic substances as having hysterical and/or conversion reactions. Although rare, on occasion workers develop true hysteria or conversion disorder, which is serious and disabling.

15. What treatments are available for conversion disorder?

Treatment for conversion disorder is lengthy and of doubtful outcome, particularly in older patients or patients who have no predisposition toward developing psychological insight. In such cases, biofeedback may help the patient to cope with disabling symptoms.

16. What should a neuropsychological report address?

A neuropsychological report should address (1) the referral question; (2) prior occupational and educational history (often school transcripts or prior test scores are helpful adjuncts in determining premorbid level of functions); (3) prior medical and psychiatric history, including psychiatric medication, alcohol, and recreational drug use; (4) childhood history; (5) family and marital history; (6) prior injuries; and (7) a detailed work history. The neuropsychological report also should include a section about behavioral/clinical observations, a list of the scores and percentile standing on each test administered, and a detailed interpretation of each functional brain area. The report should conclude with a summary statement about possible relationships between specific impairments and the exposure or accident. It also should include detailed recommendations for treatment and specify any further assessments that may be required.

17. What treatments are available for neuropsychological injury?

Treatment recommendations by the neuropsychologist may include individual psychotherapy to treat new mood or anxiety disorders; evaluation for psychiatric medication, if indicated; biofeedback for anxiety problems; or, if the deficits are primarily in cognitive function and memory, cognitive retraining, which helps patients to compensate for loss by retraining in memory and visual tasks through rehearsal on computer models.

18. When should a patient be referred for such treatments?

The above treatments should be prescribed as soon as possible—the longer the patient does not receive treatment, the more difficult it is to treat the illness.

19. When should a patient be retested?

After the patient has had the appropriate treatment and after at least 6 months to 1 year have elapsed. Retesting also assists in releasing an injured worker for return to work.

20. Are computer-administered neuropsychological tests available?

Several computer-administered test batteries have been developed, such as the Neurobehavioral Test Battery and NES. They are used primarily in large-scale epidemiologic studies rather than in individual clinical evaluations. They are less sensitive than traditional assessment methods, patients may have visual problems that compound test findings, and workers may be unfamiliar and uncomfortable with computer screens and handicapped by lack of typing skills. Computer-generated interpretive profiles of mood tests are available, but the Ethics Guidelines of the American Psychological Association clearly indicate that they should not be used to diagnose a patient or to interpret the patient's level of performance.

21. If a group of workers are injured, what screening test batteries are available? What can be expected from these batteries?

Whenever possible, it is desirable to have collaborating data in accidents or toxic exposures in which several workers may be injured. In such situations it may not be feasible to conduct comprehensive individual evaluations immediately after the incident. For such occasions or in large-scale epidemiologic investigations, test batteries can be used to screen function in large groups. Typically, screening test batteries should address the specific problem under study with brief tests chosen for their relevance to the health effect under investigation. It is desirable to combine specific and sensitive but brief clinical tests suitable for large-scale screening. Screening batteries do not yield the type of information that permits individual diagnoses but give useful information about overall group effects. Screening test batteries may be as brief as 20–30 minutes per patient, but they require the direction of an experienced neuropsychologist. Medical/psychological staff can be trained to administer some screening tests under supervision.

BIBLIOGRAPHY

1. Delis DC, Kramer JH, Kaplan E, Ober BA: California Verbal Learning Test: Adult Version. San Antonio, TX, Psychological Corporation, 1987.
2. Golden CJ, Purisch AD, Hammeke TA: Luria-Nebraska Neuropsychological Battery: Forms I and II. Los Angeles, Western Psychological Services, 1985.
3. Golden CJ: Stroop Color and Word Tests. Chicago, Stoelting Company, 1978.
4. Gorham DR: Clinical Manual for the Proverbs Test. Missoula, MT, Psychological Test Specialists, 1956.
5. Halstead WC: Brain and Intelligence. Chicago, University of Chicago Press, 1947.
6. Jastak S, Wilkinson GS: Wide Range Achievement Test–Revised. Wilmington, DE, Jastak Achievement Services, 1984.
7. Lezak MD: Neuropsychological Assessment, 3rd ed. New York, Oxford University Press, 1995.
8. Reitan RM, Wolfson D: The Halstead-Reitan Neuropsychological Test Battery: Theory and Clinical Interpretation. Tucson, AZ, Neuropsychology Press, 1993.
9. Smith A: Symbol Digit Modalities Test (SDMT): Manual (Revised). Los Angeles, Western Psychological Services, 1988.
10. Spreen O, Strauss E: A Compendium of Neuropsychological Tests. New York, Oxford University Press, 1991.
11. Wechsler D: WAIS-III and WMS-III Technical Manual. San Antonio, TX, Psychological Corporation, 1997.
12. Williams JM: Memory Assessment Scales Manual. Odessa, FL, Psychological Assessment Resources, 1991.

38. FEVER AT WORK

Ware G. Kuschner, M.D.

1. What are the most common infectious causes of fever at work? Which occupations are most affected?

Infections may be acquired on the job from infected persons, animals, or point sources. Person-to-person transmission of infection is an occupational hazard particularly associated with the health care profession. Important infections transmitted in this setting that may result in a febrile illness include viral hepatitis, infection with the human immunodeficiency virus, tuberculosis, and, in susceptible workers, measles and rubella. Other occupations at increased risk of person-to-person transmission of infectious diseases at work include transportation workers (e.g., flight attendants who may be at increased risk of acquiring tuberculosis), military recruits and day-care workers (febrile upper respiratory tract illnesses), and commercial sex workers (HIV, hepatitis, syphilis).

Zoonoses are an important group of infectious diseases caused by organisms transmitted from either living or dead animals to humans. Workers at risk of contracting zoonotic infection include agricultural workers, veterinarians, animal handlers, slaughterhouse workers, and farmers. Over 100 zoonoses have been described worldwide. Some of the more common occupational zoonoses occur in the agricultural industry: anthrax from beef cattle, Q fever from sheep and dairy cattle, histoplasmosis from poultry, tularemia from sheep, and brucellosis from swine.

Point sources of infection also may be important causes of occupational febrile syndromes. Examples include building-related *Legionella* spp. infection, fungal infection in construction workers or archaeologists, and infections with waterborne pathogens in sewage workers.

2. What preventive measures should be taken against infectious causes of fever?

Vigilant adherence to preventive measures, including vaccination, blood and body fluid universal precautions, respiratory protection, and routine surveillance skin testing for tuberculosis, can reduce morbidity and mortality in high-risk groups. Childhood immunization should be completed and documented in all workers. Current adult immunization recommendations from the Centers for Disease Control and Prevention include booster vaccination with tetanus and diphtheria toxoid (TD) every 10 years throughout adulthood.

The hepatitis B three-dose series is recommended for children and should be considered absolutely mandatory for health care workers and other persons at high risk. Three intramuscular injections of recombinant hepatitis B vaccine induce adequate antibody response in 80–95% of persons. Postvaccination testing for adequate antibody response is recommended for high-risk groups, including health care workers. Deltoid intramuscular injection is preferred in adults. Subcutaneous or buttock administration should not be utilized.

Yearly vaccination against influenza A and B should be available to all adults and should be mandatory among health care workers when no contraindication is present. Additional comprehensive up-to-date vaccination information is available from the Centers for Disease Control and Prevention through an automated information service that can be reached at 1-800-CDC-SHOT.

3. What are the most common noninfectious causes of fever at work? Which occupations are most affected?

Many noninfectious causes of work-related fever result from various inhalational exposures; not all inhalational exposures, however, result in clinically relevant pulmonary sequelae.

Acute hypersensitivity pneumonitis, also known as extrinsic allergic alveolitis outside the United States, is an important immunologically mediated occupational febrile syndrome. It is caused by inhalational exposure to organic dusts or proteins in a sensitized worker. In addition to fever, chills, and malaise, hypersensitivity pneumonitis is characterized by pulmonary findings that typically include cough, dyspnea, arterial oxygen desaturation, alveolar and interstitial infiltrates on chest radiograph, and reduced lung volumes on pulmonary function tests. Farmer's lung, caused by exposure to moldy hay harboring thermophilic *Actinomyces* species, is a classic example. Many other causes of hypersensitivity pneumonitis also have been described. The diverse occupations at risk include those involving exposure to contaminants or byproducts of sugar cane, mushrooms, maple bark, cork, cheese, wood pulp, malt, turkeys, and pigeons. The specific antigens that have the potential to induce hypersensitivity pneumonitis have not been characterized in all settings. Nevertheless, *Actinomyces* species, a type of bacteria with the morphology of fungi, and various plant and animal proteins have been identified as likely causes in many cases.

Various inhalational exposures, collectively known as **inhalation fever**, are clinically and pathophysiologically distinct from hypersensitivity pneumonitis but also may cause work-related fever. Three important subtypes of inhalation fever are metal fume fever, polymer fume fever, and bioaerosol inhalation fever, which includes, most notably, organic dust toxic syndrome. These different forms of inhalation fever are linked by the similar short-lived, generally benign, flulike syndrome that characterizes each, as well as by shared pathophysiology. The specific noxious agents that cause inhalation fever are apparently completely unrelated except for their etiologic roles. Pulmonary findings are generally not impressive in inhalation fever.

Metal fume fever is caused by inhalation of certain metal oxide fumes, including zinc oxide and possibly magnesium oxide. Occupations at risk include welders who work with zinc-containing metals such as galvanized steel and brass foundry workers.

Polymer fume fever is caused by exposure to the combustion products of fluoropolymers, including polytetrafluoroethylene (Teflon). Exposure may occur in industrial settings where polymers are applied for their nonstick properties, including production of home cookware and lime conveyor parts.

Inhalation of bioaerosols, including woodchip dust and moldy grain, may cause **organic dust toxic syndrome** (ODTS). Typically, heavy-to-massive dust exposures are required, whereas lower exposure burdens may cause hypersensitivity pneumonitis. Inhaled endotoxins (lipopolysaccharides) are thought to be among the noxious agents that precipitate ODTS. ODTS has been described in farming, forestry, paper pulp industry, grain elevator operation, and loading and unloading grain from ships. Other bioaerosols, including mists originating from contaminated water, may cause inhalation fever. The most important variant of inhalation fever caused by contaminated mist is commonly known as humidifier fever.

Finally, fever can be associated with acute lung injury resulting from inhalation of irritant gases (such as phosgene or nitrogen dioxide) or certain toxic metals (such as cadmium and mercury). This syndrome should not be confused with either hypersensitivity pneumonitis or inhalation fever.

4. What is Monday morning fever?

Monday morning fever is an informal term used in occupational settings where inhalation fever (e.g., metal fume fever, polymer fume fever, ODTS, humidifier fever) occurs. The term highlights the clinical feature of tachyphylaxis that characterizes inhalation fever. Tachyphylaxis refers to the attenuation in clinical response to multiday exposure to an inhalant that causes inhalation fever. After an extended exposure-free period, however, such as a vacation or perhaps a weekend, reexposure may result in a fulminant clinical response; hence the term Monday morning fever.

5. What are the most important differences between hypersensitivity pneumonitis and inhalation fever?

Both inhalation fever and hypersensitivity pneumonitis, also known as extrinsic allergic alveolitis, are occupational febrile syndromes caused by inhalation of noninfectious agents. These work-related febrile syndromes cause short-lived flulike syndromes that can be similar in clinical presentation. To make matters even more confusing, a form of inhalation fever, ODTS, may occur in the same occupational setting in which hypersensitivity pneumonitis occurs (i.e., agricultural exposure to grains and hay). There are, however, important differences, both pathophysiologically and prognostically, between the syndromes.

Hypersensitivity pneumonitis is immunologically mediated. IgG antibodies against the offending antigen should be present. Low-dose antigen exposure is sufficient to precipitate an episode of acute hypersensitivity pneumonitis or to perpetuate disease in a sensitized worker. Pulmonary findings include dyspnea, rales, hypoxia, and radiographic infiltrates. Bronchoalveolar lavage reveals lymphocytosis. Chronic exposure to the offending antigen may result in irreversible chronic interstitial lung disease characterized by pulmonary fibrosis and reduced lung volumes.

In contrast with hypersensitivity pneumonitis, the inhalation fevers, including ODTS, do not require sensitization. Pulmonary findings may be minimal or absent in inhalation fever. Bronchoalveolar lavage findings in ODTS and metal fume fever include increased concentrations of neutrophils, not lymphocytes. In ODTS, high-dose exposure to organic dust, usually contaminated with endotoxin, is necessary. Repeated exposure to inhalants that cause inhalation fever results in downregulation of the febrile response (i.e., tachyphylaxis) rather than induction of the magnified (amnestic) response of hypersensitivity pneumonitis. Long-term sequelae are not associated with the various inhalation fevers.

Hypersensitivity Pneumonitis vs. Inhalation Fever

FEATURES	HYPERSENSITIVITY PNEUMONITIS	INHALATION FEVER
Example	Farmer's lung	Metal fume fever
Etiologic exposure	Thermoactinomyces	Zinc oxide fume
Pathophysiology	Hypersensitivity reaction	Probably cytokine-mediated
Exposure dose	Low dose sufficient	High dose required
Sensitization required	Yes	No
Fever	Yes	Yes
Flulike symptoms	Yes	Yes
Cough	Expected	Not necessary
Dyspnea	Typically yes	Typically no
Chest exam	Rales	Typically normal
Radiographic findings	Diffuse interstitial and alveolar infiltrates	Typically no abnormalities
Pulmonary function tests	Decreased volumes and diffusing capacity	Typically minimal changes
Bronchoalveolar lavage	Lymphocytosis	Neutrophil increase
Chronic sequelae	Potentially yes	None

6. What is the pathophysiology of metal fume fever?

Metal fume fever is one of the better understood occupational febrile syndromes. Cytokines, biochemical regulators of inflammation, appear to play an important role. Animal and human experimental data have shown that exposure to zinc oxide fumes produces an impressive inflammatory cellular response in the lungs, beginning a few hours after exposure. This response is characterized by dose- and time-dependent increases in neutrophils and proinflammatory cytokines. In controlled experimental human exposures, increases in pulmonary tumor necrosis factor-alpha, as quantified in bronchoalveolar lavage fluid, have been demonstrated 3 hours after zinc oxide fume inhalation, followed by increases in interleukin 8 and an associated influx of neutrophils. The mechanistic links between these pulmonary inflammatory responses and the constitutional symptoms that characterize metal fume fever need to be elucidated more clearly. The extent to which cytokine networking plays a role in mediating other inhalational febrile syndromes is unclear.

7. What elements of the clinical history are important to the evaluation of patients reporting fever at work?

The occupational medical history is likely to be the most important part of the evaluation of a patient with suspected occupational febrile syndrome. The physical examination and laboratory data are frequently nonspecific and in some circumstances only support rather than not confirm the diagnosis suggested by the history. The notable exceptions are occupationally acquired infections, which may be demonstrated by culture of body fluids and tissue or serology studies.

In all evaluations of suspected occupational fever, arguably the most important question to ask the patient is, "What do you think is the cause of your illness?" The answer may be particularly useful if the patient suspects a link between work and the febrile syndrome. Other important information to obtain and questions to ask include:

1. Describe in as much detail as possible exactly what you do at work (a job title without other descriptive information is insufficient).

2. What is new at work?

3. Is the febrile syndrome associated with work? Does it resolve during periods away from work, such as vacation?

4. What symptoms are you experiencing now or have you experienced in the past with episodes of fever?

5. Are you exposed to fumes or dusts?

6. Are particulate matter or other air pollutants visible in the air you breathe at work?

7. What protective equipment do you use at work, including respiratory protective appliances?

8. Are you aware of other workers, currently or previously employed, who have experienced similar symptoms?

8. What treatment strategies are available for fever at work?

Treatment for infectious causes of fever at work is the same as for infectious diseases in general and includes antimicrobial therapy directed at the likely etiologic agent. In addition, important measures to prevent reinfection include hand-washing and, when appropriate, precautions against contact with contaminated aerosols and fluids.

There are few well-established strategies to treat noninfectious causes of fever at work. Of historical interest, milk has been used by workers as far back as the early 19th century to treat and prevent metal fume fever. The value of milk as a therapeutic agent in this or other forms of inhalation fever, however, has not been satisfactorily scrutinized in clinical studies. Corticosteroids are often used in hypersensitivity pneumonitis (extrinsic allergic alveolitis); however, removal from the exposure is the most important therapeutic intervention.

In general, the acute febrile inhalational syndromes resolve spontaneously. Symptomatic relief, including antipyretics and analgesics, may be offered. Long-term strategies should focus on prevention, including reducing the risk of repeated toxic exposures at work.

BIBLIOGRAPHY

1. Blanc P, Boushey HA: The lung in metal fume fever. Sem Respir Med 14:212–225, 1993.
2. Kligman EW, Peate WF, Cordes DH: Occupational infections in farm workers. Occup Med State Art Rev 6:429–443, 1991.
3. Kuschner WG, D'Alessandro A, Wintermeyer SF, et al: Pulmonary responses to purified zinc oxide fume inhalation. J Investig Med 43:371–378, 1995.
4. Lewis CE, Kerby GR: An epidemic of polymer fume fever. JAMA 191:103–106, 1965.
5. Patterson WB, Craver DE, Schwartz DA, et al: Occupational hazards to hospital personnel. Ann Intern Med 102:658–680, 1985.
6. Rask-Andersen A: Organic dust toxic syndrome among farmers. Br J Indust Med 46:233–238, 1989.
7. Salvaggio JE: Hypersensitivity pneumonitis. J Allergy Clin Immunol 79:558–571, 1987.
8. Schenker M, Ferguson T, Gamsley T: Respiratory risks associated with agriculture. Occup Med State Art Rev 6:415–428, 1991.

39. WORK-RELATED LOW BACK PAIN

Bradley Evanoff, M.D., M.P.H.

1. What is low back pain?

One of the difficulties in studying low back pain is the plethora of definitions and the different ways in which patients can be identified—by symptoms, by medical treatment, or by disability. Most people with symptoms of low back pain do not come to medical attention; most episodes of low back pain that come to medical attention result in no change in work status; most alterations of work status due to low back pain are temporary. Thus, very different profiles of low back pain emerge from differing definitions.

Low back pain may be a symptom of a serious spinal or systemic condition. After such a condition is excluded, low back pain can be classified as **sciatica**, lower limb symptoms suggesting lumbosacral nerve root compromise, or **nonspecific low back pain**, with symptoms confined primarily to the back without symptoms or signs of sciatica or a serious underlying condition.

2. How common is low back pain?

Low back pain is a very common disorder and is among the most frequent reasons for seeking medical attention. In a given year, up to 50% of the population has an episode of low back pain; 50–70% of people will experience in their lifetimes an episode of low back pain severe enough to limit activity. In persons < age 45, low back problems are the most common cause of disability.

3. How serious is the problem of work-related low back pain?

Low back pain attributed to work is a major cause of cost and time lost from work. Fifteen to 24% of all compensable claims in workers' compensation are for low back pain; these claims account for about one-third of workers' compensation costs. Considerable variability in rates of claims for low back pain between workers is found in different industries and between workers in different countries.

4. What are the causes of work-related low back pain?

NIOSH has recently conducted a comprehensive review of the scientific literature in low back pain. The evidence strongly suggests that low back pain disorders are associated with work-related lifting, forceful movements, and whole-body vibration. Working in awkward postures (bending and twisting) and heavy physical work also may be associated with increased risk for low back pain disorders. The NIOSH review also noted that psychosocial factors. such as job satisfaction, personality traits, perception of intensified workload, and job control are associated with low back pain. It is unclear whether these factors affect the development of low back pain or whether they primarily affect the reporting of low back pain; in most studies, psychosocial factors may account for a small fraction of work-related low back disorders.

5. What are nonoccupational causes of low back pain?

A number of non-work factors have been associated with low back pain. These include age, gender, overall level of physical fitness, lumbar mobility, lumbar strength, tobacco use, non-work physical activities, past history of low back disorders, and congenital structural abnormalities such as spondylolisthesis.

6. Can low back pain be caused by work and non-work factors simultaneously?

Low back pain is clearly multifactorial in origin and, in a given patient, the onset, severity, reporting, and prognosis of low back pain may be influenced by a variety of work and non-work factors. The presence of personal risk factors in a patient does not rule out work-relatedness, just as work may not be the sole cause of an individual patient's symptoms.

7. How is low back pain diagnosed?

The diagnosis of low back pain relies primarily on the patient history. Physical examination and diagnostic testing are of limited diagnostic utility, particularly in acute low back pain.

8. What elements should be included in the history of patients with low back pain?

It is important to determine if a patient has pain related to a serious condition such as a fracture, a systemic disorder such as malignancy or infection, or cauda equina syndrome. The history should focus on "red flags" that indicate the possible presence of a disorder more serious than nonspecific low back pain. Red flags include a history of trauma, age > 50 years or < 20 years, history of malignancy or immune compromise, pain that worsens when supine, recent onset bowel or bladder dysfunction, saddle anesthesia, and severe or progressive neurologic deficit of the lower extremities. Past history of low back disorders also should be sought, as should information on the onset and time course of symptoms and any functional limitations due to symptoms. Location of symptoms should be determined, specifically radiation of pain or paresthesias to the distal lower extremity.

9. What are the physical examination findings in low back pain?

The physical examination is important for the evaluation of radiculopathy, and evidence of sensory deficit, motor deficit, and altered deep tendon reflexes should be sought on examination. Evidence of prior low back pathology, such as surgical scars and differences in muscle bulk, should be noted. Other findings, such as restricted range of motion and muscle spasm, have limited prognostic or diagnostic utility but are often useful in tracking the clinical course in individual patients.

10. What diagnostic tests should be performed in patients with low back pain?

Diagnostic tests play a very limited role in the initial management of acute low back pain. In the absence of red flags in the history as discussed in question 8, plain radiographs of the lumbosacral spine are unlikely to change diagnosis or therapy and are widely overused. Radiographs are appropriate in cases of chronic or recurrent low back pain, and should be ordered to rule out fracture or systemic disorder only if suggested by the history. The use of magnetic resonance imaging (MRI) is problematic because a substantial proportion of persons without back pain have disc abnormalities revealed by MRI; anatomic abnormalities seen on MRI must be evaluated critically for their importance in individual patients. In some settings, electromyography may be useful in the diagnosis of radiculopathy. The usefulness of other diagnostic modalities for chronic pain, including discography, remains controversial.

11. What specific questions should be asked about the patient's workplace in evaluating the possibility of work-related low back pain?

Work exposures such as lifting, bending, twisting, whole body vibration, and prolonged, awkward postures should be assessed. Exacerbation of symptoms by specific activities should be noted. The physician should explore possibilities for temporary modification of work duties to reduce physical stresses on the back.

12. How is low back pain treated?

A large literature reviews the treatment of both acute and chronic low back pain disorders. Unfortunately, the literature is full of contradictory evidence, and many studies are of low quality. Expert panels in several countries have produced evidence-based guidelines for the treatment of low back pain.

The chance for natural resolution of acute low back pain is good even in the absence of any treatment; treatment should thus focus on symptom relief, reassurance, and rapid return to function.

Acetaminophen, nonsteroidal antiinflammatory drugs (NSAIDs), muscle relaxants, and active exercise are appropriate treatments for acute low back pain. Spinal manipulation also is an acceptable treatment. Evidence suggests that various NSAIDs and muscle relaxants are equally effective in the treatment of low back pain. Exercise therapy has little benefit in the treatment of acute low back pain. Epidural steroid injections may be of use in the treatment of acute sciatica.

The difficulty of treating chronic low back pain effectively is demonstrated by the wide variety of therapeutic modalities that have been tried for the disorder. As with acute low back pain, a major goal of treatment should be return to work and usual activities. Evidence supports the use of back schools (in an occupational setting), exercise therapy, spinal manipulation, and multidisciplinary treatment programs. Evidence also suggests that NSAIDs are effective in symptomatic pain relief, but does not support the use of physical modalities such as transcutaneous electrical nerve stimulation (TENS), biofeedback, orthoses, and acupuncture. In the setting of work-related lower back pain, surgical interventions such as lumbar fusion have not been shown to improve patient outcomes. Even among patients with radiculopathy it is not clear that surgery improves long-term patient outcomes, although discectomy brings faster resolution of symptoms in patients suffering from sciatica secondary to disc herniation.

13. What are effective strategies for preventing low back pain in working populations?
Strategies to prevent low back pain may focus on changing the workplace or on changing the worker. As noted above, work activities are clearly associated with low back pain. A growing body of evidence indicates that workplace changes that decrease low back stresses from lifting, bending, and vibration result in lower rates of low back pain. Such ergonomic interventions may reduce lost time even more than injury rates, because workers with activity restrictions due to low back pain can return to jobs with lower physical demands.

Back pain may be prevented by changing the characteristics of individual workers through education, aerobic exercise, back specific exercise, and the use of back supports (corsets or back belts). Some evidence supports the effectiveness of exercise programs in preventing back pain. Studies of educational programs and back supports have not provided convincing evidence of the effectiveness of these interventions in preventing back pain among asymptomatic workers.

BIBLIOGRAPHY

1. Bernard B (ed): Musculoskeletal Disorders and Workplace Factors. NIOSH Publication no. 97-141. Cincinnati, OH, National Institute for Occupational Safety and Health, U.S. Department of Health and Human Services, 1997.
2. Bigos S, Bowyer O, Graen G, et al: Acute low back pain problems in adults. Clinical Practice Guideline no. 14. AHCPR Publication no. 95-0642. Rockville, MD, Agency for Health Care Policy and Research, Public Health Service, U.S. Department of Health and Human Services, 1994.
3. Cherkin DC, Deyo RA, Battie M, et al: A comparison of physical therapy, chiropractic manipulation, and provision of an educational booklet for the treatment of patients with low back pain. N Engl J Med 8:1021–1029, 1998.
4. Deyo RA, Rainville J, Kent DL: What can the history and physical examination tell us about low back pain? JAMA 268:760–765, 1992.
5. Pope MH, Andersson GBJ, Frymoyer JW, Chaffin DB: Occupational low back pain: Assessment, treatment, and prevention. St. Louis, Mosby Year Book, 1991.
6. Spitzer WO, LeBlanc F, Dupuis M (eds): Scientific approach to the assessment and management of activity-related spinal disorders. Spine 7(Suppl):1–59, 1987.
7. Van Tulder MW, Koes BW, Bouter LM: Conservative treatment of acute and chronic nonspecific low back pain. Spine 18:2128–2156, 1997.

40. KNEE PAIN

Franklin T. Hoaglund, M.D.

1. When a patient complains of knee pain spontaneously or after an injury, what are the possible causes?

After a thorough examination of the knee joint, one must look proximally for other causes of knee pain. The segmental innervation of the knee is from lumbar the 3rd and 4th roots. A ruptured lumbar disc, infection, or tumor may be causing a radiculopathy of L3 or L4. These nerve roots are part of the femoral nerve that also may be irritated by tumor or infection as the nerve passes retroperitoneally and beneath the inguinal ligament into the proximal thigh. The possibility of radiculopathy or neuropathy requires medical history related to the back genitourinary (GU), gastrointestinal (GI), and gynecologic systems. Neurologic examination, including motor power, reflexes, and sensory deficit in the lower extremity is indicated.

Hip disease that causes referred pain to the distal thigh or knee without other hip complaints is more common than an L3 or L4 radiculopathy. The anatomic basis for the pain is the overlapping nerve supply for sensory innervation of the hip and the subsartorial plexus. Hip disease can usually be excluded by looking for pain when putting the hip through a range of motion while keeping the knee immobile.

2. Describe a thorough examination of the knee.

Observe the patient as he or she arises from a chair and walks. Ask him or her to walk on the heels or toes and observe for signs of pain or limp. Compare configuration of the knee with the opposite side, observing for atrophy of vastus medialis. Kellgren's bulge test is used to test for a synovial effusion. Ligamentous stability is tested by stressing the knee in varus and valgus and determining anteroposterior (AP) stability. Range of motion is tested from full extension to full flexion. The joint lines are palpated for signs of tenderness and the patellar grind tests are performed to look for chondromalacia or patellar femoral osteoarthritis. The examination is not complete without including a brief lower extremity neurologic examination and a test of hip joint range of motion.

3. A 30-year-old man presents with a painful and swollen knee after being struck by a moving car, which caused him to twist his knee and then to fall directly on the same knee. What kind of imaging is necessary?

AP and lateral plain film x-rays should be sufficient to rule out a fracture. However, if a tibial plateau fracture is suspected, plain or oblique x-rays are helpful. If the patient does not have a fracture and does not improve with conservative treatment, magnetic resonance imaging (MRI) may be subsequently necessary to look for internal derangements (menisci tears or cruciate insufficiency).

4. A 45-year-old man has pain along the medial knee joint line associated with activity, but no catching, locking, or giving way. What kind of imaging should be requested in the initial work-up?

An AP x-ray of both knees standing should be requested to determine joint space narrowing from cartilage loss compared with the normal side. Whenever x-rays of the knee are obtained, weight-bearing films should be done to gather information about cartilage loss. Early joint space loss may be missed with non–weight-bearing x-rays. Skyline and lateral views for the patellar femoral relationships are done on the painful side. A tunnel view is done to further delineate the posterior femoral condyles for lesions such as early osteonecrosis.

5. What surgical treatment should be considered in a patient with early-to-moderate medial compartment degenerative arthritis of the knee that has not responded to conservative treatment?

The number one consideration for a younger patient (i.e., < 55 years of age) is a valgus tibial osteotomy in which the upper tibia is realigned so that the varus deformity from joint space loss is corrected by realignment of the proximal tibia into the valgus. This allows weight transfer during stance phase of gait to occur in the lateral compartment and minimizes or eliminates pain from medial compartment loads. The rehabilitation for osteotomy requires waiting for the bone to heal (3–4 months). After healing, there are no protective restrictions on activity; the patient may engage in any activities that he or she is comfortable with.

Total knee replacement should be avoided in the younger patient, because the implant and its relation to host tissue has a finite life. For older patients with more severe pain, a total knee replacement may be done. After experiencing night pain, the patient usually elects to have surgery. Because it is the operation for early or late disease, no penalty exists for delaying total knee replacement. The final decision rests with the patient.

6. Compare hip and knee osteoarthritis with respect to the severity of symptomology.

For most patients with hip disease who have night pain and significant mechanical pain with walking, total hip replacement is usually necessary because the symptoms are expected to continue. In comparison, patients with knee osteoarthritis may have no significant mechanical pain and night pain may resolve spontaneously to a tolerable level. In the early-to-moderate stages of osteoarthritis of the knee, symptoms are episodic. Intraarticular steroids injected into the knee may provide temporary relief.

7. Is there any urgency to diagnose torn menisci in order to remove it in the early stages following a knee injury?

No! MRI or arthroscopy is necessary to diagnose meniscal pathology. However, because some small tears or degenerative lesions of the meniscus either may heal or become asymptomatic, they can be watched expectantly. If the patient does not improve in a few weeks, definitive studies with an MRI and arthroscopic evaluation may be done. There is no penalty for leaving a torn meniscus in place if the patient is asymptomatic, because it does not cause degenerative arthritis. For persistently symptomatic patients, arthroscopic surgical repair of the torn menisci or partial meniscotomy may be undertaken.

8. What would be the most likely diagnosis in a 25-year-old female worker who has had previous episodes of anterior knee pain, and developed recurrent symptoms after starting a new job in which she is frequently required to carry small loads up and down the stairs?

In a young woman with anterior knee pain, the most common diagnosis is chondromalacia patellae (i.e., abnormal or bad cartilage). Such patients have pain while getting out of a chair or walking. Descending stairs is worse than ascending, because descending requires a greater range of motion. On physical examination patients have crepitus with passive patellar femoral motion. Symptoms are reproduced with passive depression of the patella in the groove and the patient actively contracts the quadriceps. A small synovial effusion is extremely rare. Plain x-rays are usually not helpful. The condition seems to occur in patients who have 3–5° hyperextension of the knees.

9. A 40-year-old nurse struck the medial aspect of her proximal tibia knee region on a low metal cart in the operating room. She had immediate pain that resolved. Swelling did not occur, and within a few days she experienced extreme pain in the anterior lateral aspect of the proximal tibial region. She walks without a limp, has no effusion, and no evidence of chondromalacia. However, the patient has extreme sensitivity to light touch over the upper anterior and lateral aspects of the tibial region. What is the diagnosis?

The key physical finding is the hyperesthesia over the skin supplied by the infrapatellar branch of this saphenous nerve. The patient has a traumatic injury or neuroma on this nerve branch that supplies sensation to the skin of this part of the knee. Diagnosis is made by tapping carefully with a fingertip over the area of the suspected neuroma. A Tinel's sign is elicited when pain is reproduced. Although this injury is rare, it may occur from a direct blow or be seen after arthroscopic surgery or total knee replacement in which the nerve has been directly injured.

10. A 55-year-old office worker is seen for the gradual onset of pain and swelling of the posterior aspect of the knee. No recent injury has occurred, and she is otherwise healthy. Physical examination reveals slight restriction of full flexion and a 20 cc effusion. Diffuse swelling is present in the popliteal fossa without evidence of tenderness or redness. What is the cause of the popliteal swelling?

This patient has a history of low-grade symptoms and findings of restricted knee motion and synovial affusion. She has developed a Baker's or synovial cyst. Synovial fluid from the knee joint is forced back through a ball valve gap in the semimembranous bursae from which it cannot return. Baker's cyst occurs in older patients with torn menisci or degenerative arthritis. Treatment needs to to address the primary problem. Excision of the cyst is rarely indicated.

11. A 35-year-old office worker gets up from her desk, turns, and strikes the anterior aspect of her knee on an open file drawer. She suffers acute severe pain, and over the next 2–3 days develops gradual swelling over the anterior aspect of the patella. When seen 3 days later, diffuse swelling and a baggy thickening of the tissue is observed anterior to the patella beneath the skin. No redness or abrasion is found. What is the most likely diagnosis and appropriate treatment?

The patient most likely has traumatic prepatellar bursitis. Depending on the severity of the local findings, plain x-rays may be necessary to rule out a patellar fracture. Treatment includes instructions to the patient to avoid knee flexion, application of a knee immobilizer in extension, and antiinflammatory medication for pain. One can expect resolution of symptoms in 7–10 days.

12. What techniques are available for repairing articular cartilage defects?

Full-thickness articular cartilage losses do not heal with normal hyaline articular cartilage. In the past, attempts at local drilling of the subchondral bone by microfracture or even abrasion arthroplasty have been performed. These techniques result in the development of fibrocartilage that does not have the mechanical strength of hyaline articular cartilage and does not yield long-term solutions. The technique of implementing autogenous osteochondral grafts (mosaicplasty) involves harvesting small cylindrical graphs from the non–weight-bearing periphery of the patellar femur area and implanting them into a small defect. The defect must be small because the protection of this grafted area requires the architectural support of the surrounding normal cartilage. This technique will not help an osteoarthritic joint.

Another technique is to culture autologous chondrocytes that are removed arthroscopically and subsequently implanted into a small cartilage defect under a periosteal flap. The defect must be small and the surrounding articular cartilage normal for biomechanical support of the grafted area. This technique is not useful if the surrounding cartilage is osteoarthritic, nor is it applicable to broad areas of osteoarthritic cartilage. No recent clinical reports have followed the successful original work in Sweden. When this technique was studied in a canine model, repair was unsuccessful. It is uncertain whether either of these techniques will prove valuable in the future.

13. A 63-year-old female worker falls at work with a direct blow onto her knee. By the time she is seen at the hospital, she has an abrasion over the anterior aspect over the knee, a diffusely swollen knee, and severe pain with any motion of the knee. What diagnosis should be considered?

The patient has a hemarthrosis due to soft tissue or bone injury. The patient may have any fracture about the knee, patella, distal femur, proximal tibia, or damage to articular surfaces. Injury to any of the soft tissues of the knee from the menisci to the collateral cruciate patellar ligaments and quadriceps mechanisms should be considered.

With any trauma it is possible to overlook a second lesion because of the severity of pain from the primary injury. In an elderly woman with this type of fall, a knee injury may coexist with a hip fracture producing referred pain to the knee.

14. What are the indications to repair a torn anterior cruciate ligament (ACL) ?

Considerations include the level of symptoms experienced by the patient, the occupational or athletic demands of the patient, and the age of the patient.

The classic mechanism of injury of an ACL is a decelerating twisting injury associated with a feeling of giving way or an audible "pop" and the subsequent development of a bloody effusion that arises slowly over the next 24 hours. The injury may occur with internal or external rotation.

Many isolated ACLs with normal or nonathletic activity are asymptomatic. If a torn cruciate ligament is associated with torn menisci or associated collateral ligament injury, the patient may have recurrent episodes of catching, locking, or giving way of the knee such that cruciate repair, augmentation, or substitution is indicated.

Many patients may be quite asymptomatic in terms of activities of daily living, but can become symptomatic with athletic endeavors. For the rare torn ACL of a low-demand patient > 50 years of age, cruciate surgery is usually not necessary.

Various surgical procedures are tailored to the functional demands of the patient. Surgical options include intraarticular autogenous ACL reconstruction with a mid-third patellar tendon graft or allograft, or extraarticular techniques, such as an iliotibial band transfer.

BIBLIOGRAPHY

1. Breinan HA, Minas T, Hsu HP, et al: Effect of cultured autologous chondrocytes defects on repair of chondral defects in a canine model. J Bone Joint Surg 79A:1439–1451, 1997.
2. Brittberg M, Lindahl A, Nillson A, et al: Treatment of deep cartilage defects in the knee with autologous chondrocyte transplantation. N Engl J Med 331:889–895, 1994.
3. Feagin JA (ed): The Cruciate Ligaments, 2nd ed. New York, Churchill Livingstone, 1994.
4. Font R, Scuderie GR, Insall JN: Survivorship of cemented total knee arthroplasty. Clinl Orthop Rel Res 345:79–86, 1997.
5. Fulkerson JP, Hungerford DS: Disorders of the Patellofemoral Joint, 2nd ed. Baltimore, Williams & Wilkins, 1990.
6. Hoppenfeld S: Physical examination of the knee. In Physical Examination of the Spine and Extremities. New York, Appleton Century Cross, 1976, pp 171–196
7. Insall JN (ed): Sugery of the Knee, 2nd ed. New York, Churchill Livingstone, 1993.

41. NERVE ENTRAPMENTS

Margit L. Bleecker, M.D., Ph.D., and Thomas C. Bruff, M.D., M.P.H.

Entrapment of the median nerve in the carpal canal, the widely publicized carpal tunnel syndrome, is discussed in chapter 36. The following discussion focuses on other nerve entrapment syndromes in the upper extremities that may be related to occupational ergonomic stressors. The figure below illustrates the most common sites of nerve entrapment in the upper extremity combined with their ergonomic risk factors and associated occupations.

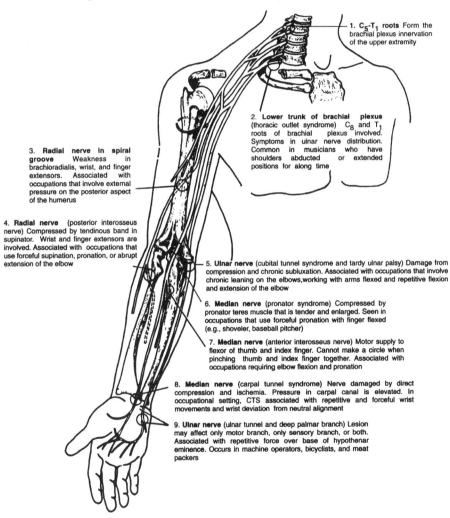

1. **C_5-T_1 roots** Form the brachial plexus innervation of the upper extremity

2. **Lower trunk of brachial plexus** (thoracic outlet syndrome) C_8 and T_1 roots of brachial plexus involved. Symptoms in ulnar nerve distribution. Common in musicians who have shoulders abducted or extended positions for along time

3. **Radial nerve in spiral groove** Weakness in brachioradialis, wrist, and finger extensors. Associated with occupations that involve external pressure on the posterior aspect of the humerus

4. **Radial nerve** (posterior interosseus nerve) Compressed by tendinous band in supinator. Wrist and finger extensors are involved. Associated with occupations that use forceful supination, pronation, or abrupt extension of the elbow

5. **Ulnar nerve** (cubital tunnel syndrome and tardy ulnar palsy) Damage from compression and chronic subluxation. Associated with occupations that involve chronic leaning on the elbows,working with arms flexed and repetitive flexion and extension of the elbow

6. **Median nerve** (pronator syndrome) Compressed by pronator teres muscle that is tender and enlarged. Seen in occupations that use forceful pronation with finger flexed (e.g., shoveler, baseball pitcher)

7. **Median nerve** (anterior interosseus nerve) Motor supply to flexor of thumb and index finger. Cannot make a circle when pinching thumb and index finger together. Associated with occupations requiring elbow flexion and pronation

8. **Median nerve** (carpal tunnel syndrome) Nerve damaged by direct compression and ischemia. Pressure in carpal canal is elevated. In occupational setting, CTS associated with repetitive and forceful wrist movements and wrist deviation from neutral alignment

9. **Ulnar nerve** (ulnar tunnel and deep palmar branch) Lesion may affect only motor branch, only sensory branch, or both. Associated with repetitive force over base of hypothenar eminence. Occurs in machine operators, bicyclists, and meat packers

Anatomic sites of nerve entrapments in the upper extremity and their associated ergonomic stressors (From Bleecker ML: Clinical presentation and treatment of nerve entrapment occurring in the workplace. In Bleecker ML (ed): Occupational Neurology and Clinical Neurotoxicology. Baltimore, Williams & Wilkins, 1994, pp 269–282, with permission.)

ULNAR NERVE

1. Where does the ulnar nerve become entrapped?

The ulnar nerve, formed from the roots of C7, C8, and T1, runs down the medial aspect of the upper arm, passes behind the medial epicondyle in the condylar groove, and then enters the cubital tunnel. The elbow is the most common site of ulnar nerve entrapment. The ulnar nerve continues down the medial aspect of the forearm and enters Guyon's canal, a less common site of entrapment. Guyon's canal is next to the carpal tunnel, the roof of which is formed by the transverse carpal ligament. The sides are formed by the pisiform bone and hook of the hamate bone. The contents of Guyon's canal include the ulnar vessels but, unlike the carpal tunnel, no tendons.

2. What causes the impingement at the cubital tunnel and Guyon's canal?

Direct trauma as well as prolonged leaning on the elbows may damage the ulnar nerve. In the cubital tunnel repeated flexion and extension, prolonged flexion, or an abnormally fibrous aponeurosis of the flexor carpi ulnaris may cause irritation and stretch or compress the nerve. At Guyon's canal, external pressure from hand-held tools, bicycle handlebars, or canes may increase pressure on the nerve. Internally, ganglions, cysts, lipomas, and anomalous muscles may cause ulnar nerve compression at the wrist.

3. What occupations are most at risk for ulnar nerve entrapment at the elbow? At the wrist?

At the elbow: carpenters, painters, glass cutters, switchboard operators, seamstresses, musicians, clerical workers, jewelers, and students.

At the wrist: pipe cutters, metal polishers, mechanics, and professional cyclists.

Any occupation that requires prolonged forceful grasp of a hand tool, such as a knife in meat cutting, is at risk for compressive neuropathy at the palm.

4. What are the clinical manifestations of ulnar neuropathy?

If impingement occurs **at the elbow**, numbness and tingling are present in the little finger and, to a variable extent, the ring finger. Pain in the forearm may awaken the patient from sleep. Tinel's sign may be positive but is not highly specific because of the superficial location of the ulnar nerve at the elbow. Motor symptoms may or may not be present. However, an important early motor sign is weakness of the third palmar interosseous muscle, which manifests as an abducted posture of the little finger.

When the ulnar nerve is compressed **at the wrist**, the symptoms are usually weakness or poor coordination of the ulnar-innervated intrinsic muscles of the hand. Pain may be present; characteristically, it is worse at night. A callus may be present on the involved palm. Also possible, but uncommon, is a pure sensory deficit that may cause lack of sensation in the ulnar distribution.

5. If the site of ulnar nerve compression is not obvious from the history, what can help to differentiate compression at the elbow from compression at the wrist?

Weakness of the flexor carpi ulnaris or the flexor digitorum profundus results from compression at the elbow, which also may produce sensory changes in the dorsal ulnar aspect of the hand.

6. What are the treatments for entrapment of the ulnar nerve?

In patients with significant muscle weakness or muscle atrophy, surgery is indicated. Otherwise, conservative measures should be used. For entrapment **at the elbow**, the patient should be shown the course of the ulnar nerve and instructed to avoid leaning on the elbows. Elbow pads may help if avoidance is not possible. Ice and a trial of nonsteroidal antiinflammatory drugs (NSAIDs) may be beneficial. An ergonomic evaluation of the patient's occupational duties may be indicated. Avoidance of forceful and repeated flexion-extension decreases tension on the nerve. Extensor splints or a pillow fastened together in the shape of a doughnut with the arm in the middle may be effective during sleep.

With compression **at the wrist**, instructing the patient to avoid forceful grasping with the involved hand may be all that is needed. Occasionally, a volar hand splint may be helpful. The above measures should be used for 8 weeks or longer before considering surgery, unless the clinical situation worsens.

7. If conservative measures have failed, what are the surgical options?

With compression **at the elbow**, release of the aponeurotic cover of the cubital tunnel, transposition of the ulnar nerve from the condylar groove to the medial forearm, or medial epicondylectomy are most commonly used. Release of the transverse carpal ligament with exploration of the ulnar nerve is the surgical treatment for compression **at the wrist**.

8. What is the role of nerve conduction studies?

Nerve conduction studies are not used initially unless the patient shows evidence of significant muscle weakness or muscle atrophy. The test is used after conservative measures have failed and surgery is contemplated. Nerve conduction studies may be useful in the few cases in which the site of compression is not evident after a thorough history and physical examination.

RADIAL NERVE

9. Where does radial nerve entrapment occur?

In the proximal forearm the posterior interosseous nerve, a branch of the radial nerve, may be compressed. The radial nerve also may be compressed in the radial groove of the humerus in association with fractures, and the superficial branch of the radial nerve may be compressed at the wrist by tight bracelets, watchbands, or handcuffs. Some cases of injury to the superficial branch of the radial nerve may result in symptoms of complex regional pain syndrome, formerly known as reflex sympathetic dystrophy.

10. What compresses the posterior interosseous nerve?

The arcade of Frohse near the origin of the supinator, a tendinous band in the supinator muscle or at its distal edge, may impinge on the posterior interosseous nerve. The vascular leash of Henry, an arcade of vessels arising from the radial artery, also may compress the nerve.

11. What is resistant tennis elbow?

Resistant tennis elbow, also called radial tunnel syndrome, is a pain syndrome in the extensor muscle mass distal to the lateral epicondyle. The pain is exacerbated by extension; other symptoms are uncommon. Patients may have had multiple treatments for lateral epicondylitis, including a trial of NSAIDs, steroid injections, and possibly surgery.

12. How does one distinguish radial tunnel syndrome from lateral epicondylitis?

Passive flexion of the wrist causes discomfort with lateral epicondylitis, with tenderness primarily over the lateral epicondyle. Patients with radial tunnel syndrome have exquisite tenderness over the extensor muscle mass distal to the lateral epicondyle. The middle finger test is positive and causes pain in the radial tunnel syndrome. The test is performed with the patient's elbow extended and the wrist in neutral position; the middle finger is extended against resistance, causing pain over the radial tunnel. A trigger point in the area of the radial tunnel may cause pain in the forearm that radiates both proximally and distally. If no neurologic deficit is found, presence of an active trigger point causing the pain becomes more likely.

13. What occupations are associated with radial tunnel syndrome?

Mechanics, factory workers, clerical workers, athletes, food workers, farmers, musicians, or housekeepers. Some workers report an episode of trauma to the forearm.

14. What is the posterior interosseous nerve syndrome?

The posterior interosseous nerve syndrome consists primarily of motor findings at the same location as the radial tunnel syndrome. Radial deviation may result from weakness of the extensor carpi ulnaris in mild cases; severe cases may involve wrist drop and inability to extend the fingers. The cause for this different constellation of findings is not precisely known, but lipomas, bursae, cysts, or ganglia are more likely than work-related factors.

15. What is the treatment of radial tunnel and posterior interosseous syndromes?

The conservative measures are similar and include relative rest, splinting of the wrist and possibly the fingers in extension, and avoidance of forceful supination. Modification of the ergonomic stressors must be included in the treatment protocol. A trial of NSAIDs may be more effective in radial tunnel syndrome. Conservative measures should be continued for at least 12 weeks before considering surgery.

MEDIAN NERVE

16. Where may the median nerve become entrapped in the forearm?

Pronator syndrome, as the name implies, refers to entrapment of the median nerve as it passes between the superficial and deep heads of a hypertrophied pronator teres. However, other structures in the forearm also may entrap the median nerve: a thickened lacertus fibrosus (a fascial band between the biceps tendon and forearm fascia), a fibrous band within the pronator teres, and a tight fibrous arch of the flexor digitorum superficialis (sublimis bridge). The ligament of Struthers (a fibrous band extending from a humeral supracondylar spur to the medial epicondyle), if present, courses over the median nerve and may result in compression and symptoms that mimic pronator syndrome.

17. What clinical features suggest median nerve compression in the forearm?

Pronator syndrome occurs predominantly in men, whereas median nerve compression at the wrist (carpal tunnel syndrome) has an increased prevalence in women. Symptoms in the dominant arm include paresthesias in the hand accompanied by pain and tenderness in the forearm. Weakness in the hand is not a frequent complaint. There is no nocturnal exacerbation of symptoms, a classic feature of carpal tunnel syndrome. Examination finds muscle weakness most commonly in the flexor pollicis longus with less involvement of the abductor pollicis brevis, flexor digitorum profundus, and opponens pollicis. Diminished sensation in the median nerve distribution is subtle but usually present. Virtually all cases have tenderness over the pronator teres muscle and a positive Tinel's sign when the median nerve is percussed at this location.

18. Entrapment of which other branch of the median nerve mimics pronator syndrome?

The anterior interosseous nerve arises from the median nerve approximately 6 cm below the lateral epicondyle. It is a pure motor branch of the median nerve and innervates the flexor pollicis longus, flexor digitorum profundus to the index finger, and pronator quadratus. Weakness in these muscles prevents the patient from pinching the tip of the index finger and thumb to form a circle. The tendinous origin of the pronator teres or flexor digitorum superficialis may compress the anterior interosseous nerve. However, many cases have resulted from direct trauma to the forearm; occupations that require repetitive elbow flexion and pronation, such as butchers, carpenters, and weightlifters, also have been implicated.

19. Are nerve conduction studies helpful?

Because the clinical presentation of pronator syndrome may be confused with carpal tunnel syndrome, nerve conduction studies help to make the diagnosis. Normal median motor and sensory distal latencies, with slowed motor conduction velocity in the forearm and forearm flexor weakness, are compatible with pronator teres syndrome but not with carpal tunnel syndrome.

20. Which occupational ergonomic stressors are associated with pronator teres syndrome?

Occupations that demand forearm muscular activity, especially the combination of pronation with finger flexion, including shovelers, woodworkers, mechanics, baseball pitchers (fast ball), fiddlers, and barbers.

21. Is surgery the treatment of choice?

Surgery should be considered the last resort. Most cases respond to modification of the ergonomic stressor, such as power tools to prevent forceful pronation of the forearm. Sometimes immobilization is required. Corticosteroid infiltration of the pronator teres may need to be repeated for complete relief but should be part of the treatment protocol.

THORACIC OUTLET SYNDROME (TOS)

22. Describe the anatomic structures responsible for the symptoms of TOS.

TOS is the compression or irritation of the brachial plexus and subclavian vessels as they pass between the anterior and middle scalene muscles, behind the clavicle, over the first rib, and beneath the coracoid process of the scapulae, where the pectoralis minor muscle is inserted. Depending on which structures of the neurovascular bundle are compromised, the clinical presentation may be neurogenic, vasogenic, or both.

Neurogenic symptoms most commonly result from involvement of the lower trunk of the brachial plexus because it is in contact with the first rib. The lower trunk contains ulnar motor and sensory fibers of the hypothenar muscles and fifth digit as well as median motor fibers of the thenar muscles. True neurogenic TOS is rare, estimated at one per million people.

The more common vascular symptoms of TOS result from compromise of the subclavian artery or vein. The subclavian artery travels with the lower trunk of the brachial plexus behind the anterior scalene muscle and over the first rib. The subclavian vein crosses in front of the anterior scalene muscle and behind the clavicle to enter the axilla.

23. What are the potential causes of TOS?

The known anatomic abnormalities that may cause TOS include cervical ribs, fibrous bands extending either from incomplete cervical ribs or from the transverse process of C7, anomalies of the clavicle, and anomalies of the scalene muscles. The prevalence of cervical ribs in the general population is 0.5%, but symptoms of TOS occur in only 10% of this group. The controversy over the etiologic role of these anatomical structures in TOS results from the fact that corrective surgery does not necessarily result in resolution of symptoms.

Functional TOS is more common and implies that the compromise of the neurovascular bundle may be corrected by altering postural alignment or usage of the upper extremities. For example, people with low-set shoulders and long necks ("droopy shoulder syndrome") or shoulder dysfunction, middle-aged women with rounded shoulders, and heavy-breasted women are more prone to functional TOS. Occupations that require arm use at shoulder height, repeated lifting of heavy items, and hyperabduction of the arms have an increased prevalence of TOS symptoms. Static work that stresses the upper extremities may transfer the stress load to the costotransverse joint of the first rib; alteration in the movement of this joint in turn causes the scalene muscles to tense and to compress the lower roots of the brachial plexus and subclavian artery. Work that places the shoulder in abduction results in tightening of the pectoralis minor with narrowing of the subcoracoid space, where the neurovascular bundle is located. Occupations at risk for TOS include industrial workers who perform repetitive manual tasks, secretaries, cashiers, hairdressers, nursing staff, painters, and construction workers.

24. What are the symptoms of TOS?

The largest group of patients presents with varying features of brachial plexus and vascular compromise. Neurogenic features frequently include pain in the distribution of the lower roots, namely the medial aspect of the arm, forearm, and hand. In other cases the pain is diffuse.

Intermittent paresthesias and aching along the inner side of the upper extremity is eventually accompanied by weakness in the small muscles of the lateral thenar eminence with less involvement of muscles of the hypothenar eminence or the forearm. A common complaint is arm fatigue with use.

The symptoms of intermittent subclavian artery compression are diffuse arm pain, fatigue and aching with use, coldness, and weakness. Fewer patients have axillary/subclavian vein involvement with edema, discoloration of the arm, and achiness and tenderness over the axillary vein.

25. Which clinical signs help to support the diagnosis of TOS?

Stress tests are performed to increase compression or traction of the neurovascular bundle at the thoracic outlet. However, because of the high false-positive rate, the patient must have the appropriate symptoms; if the stress test is positive, it should reproduce the original symptoms.

Ninety-degree abduction-external rotation test. The thoracic outlet is narrowed by abducting the arm to shoulder height with the elbow flexed to 90°. The shoulder is externally rotated while the head is turned to the opposite side. If no symptoms develop, the patient is asked to open and close the fist slowly for 3 minutes. Resolution of symptoms when the arm is lowered also helps to confirm the diagnosis.

Adson test. The radial pulse is monitored for obliteration while the patient takes in a long breath with the neck extended and turned to the affected side. Because of contraction of the scalene muscles and elevation of the first rib, many normal people may show pulse obliteration.

The **chest radiograph** demonstrates cervical ribs, an elongated C7 transverse process, and abnormalities of the clavicle.

Nerve conduction studies may show features of chronic axon loss with diminished amplitudes in the motor response of the median and ulnar nerves and the sensory action potential of the ulnar nerve but normal conduction velocities. Chronic partial denervation of the small intrinsic hand muscles is also present. Obviously the studies are positive only if neurogenic involvement is present. Somatosensory-evoked potentials are not as sensitive as nerve conduction studies for the detection of neurogenic abnormalities.

Arteriography or venography of the subclavian vessels may be needed to assess the extent of obstruction. MRI of the brachial plexus is useful for tumors but otherwise contributes little to identifying the responsible lesion.

26. Is conservative management the treatment of choice?

Stretching exercises, strengthening exercises to correct the alignment of the shoulders and poor posture, and weight reduction are frequently adequate. When symptomatic patients have supernumerary bony or fibrotic abnormalities, surgery is required, but in the absence of such structures resection of the first rib remains controversial. Before surgery is contemplated, other clinical conditions should be excluded and conservative medical management deemed a failure. Remember that conservative medical management includes modification of the ergonomic stressors.

BIBLIOGRAPHY

1. Bleecker ML: Clinical presentation and treatment of nerve entrapment occurring in the workplace. In Bleecker ML (ed): Occupational Neurology and Clinical Neurotoxicology. Baltimore, Williams & Wilkins, 1994, pp 269–282.
2. Bozenthe DJ: Cubital tunnel syndrome pathophysiology. Clin Orthop Rel Res 351:90–94, 1998.
3. Cuetter AC, Bartisek DM: The thoracic outlet syndrome: Controversies, overdiagnosis, overtreatment, and recommendations for management. Muscle Nerve 12:410–419, 1989.
4. Dawson DM, Hallett M, Wilbourn AJ: Entrapment Neuropathies, 3rd ed. Philadelphia, Lippincott-Raven, 1998.
5. Kleinert JM, Mehta S: Radial nerve entrapment. Orthop Clin North Am 27:305–315, 1996.
6. Leffert RD, Gumley G: The relationship between dead arm syndrome and thoracic outlet syndrome. Clin Orthop Rel Res 223:20–31, 1987.
7. LeForestier N, Moulonguet A, Maisonobe T, et al: True neurogenic thoracic outlet syndrome: Electrophysiological diagnosis in six cases. Muscle Nerve 15:390–395, 1998.

8. Lindgren KA, Manninen H, Rytkonen H: Thoracic outlet syndrome: A functional disturbance of the thoracic upper aperture? Muscle Nerve 18:526–530, 1995.
9. Millender LH, Louis DS, Simmons BP (eds): Occupational Disorders of the Upper Extremity. New York, Churchill Livingstone, 1992.
10. Morris HH, Peters BH: Pronator syndrome: Clinical and electrophysiological features in seven cases. J Neuro Neurosurg Psychiatry 39:461–464, 1976.
11. Netscher DT, Cohen V: Ulnar nerve entrapment at the wrist: Cases from a hand surgery practice. South Med J 91:451–456, 1998.
12. Pang D, Wessel HB: Thoracic outlet syndrome. Neurosurgery 22:105–121, 1988.
13. Ritts GD, Wood MB, Linscheid RL: Radial tunnel syndrome: A ten-year surgical experience. Clin Orthop Rel Res 219:201–205, 1987.

42. SLEEP DISORDERS CAUSING DAYTIME SLEEPINESS

Richard B. Berry, M.D.

1. What are sleep stages? Why are they important?

Sleep is composed of different stages characterized by typical electroencephalographic (EEG), electrooculographic (EOG), and electromyographic (EMG) patterns. EEG reflects brain-wave patterns; EOG, eye movement; and EMG, muscle tone. Sleep is divided into non–rapid-eye-movement (NREM) and rapid-eye-movement (REM) cycles. During the night there are usually 4–5 cycles (episodes) of NREM sleep, each followed by REM sleep. The episodes of REM sleep increase in duration toward the end of the sleep period. NREM sleep is further divided into stages 1 and 2 (light sleep) and stages 3 and 4 (deep or slow-wave sleep). Sleep stages affect respiration and other bodily functions differently. For example, patients with breathing disorders such as sleep apnea typically have the lowest oxygen levels during REM sleep, which is associated with skeletal muscle hypotonia. Disorders that interrupt sleep frequently, such as sleep apnea, may decrease the amounts of stages 3 and 4 NREM as well as REM sleep.

2. What are possible causes of workers falling asleep during work?

- Obstructive sleep apnea
- Upper airway resistance syndrome
- Narcolepsy
- Periodic leg movements in sleep
- Idiopathic hypersomnia
- Depression
- Withdrawal from stimulants
- Rotating shifts/nightshift work
- Poor sleep environment (e.g., noise, crying child)
- Medications (some tricyclic antidepressants, clonidine)
- Insufficient sleep syndrome

3. When is sleep monitoring (polysomnography) indicated?

Sleep monitoring is indicated to determine the cause of excessive daytime sleepiness when no obvious problems, such as inadequate sleep or medications, are apparent. Some patients have more than one sleep disorder (e.g., narcolepsy and obstructive sleep apnea). Sleep monitoring is less useful for evaluation of insomnia.

4. What is commonly measured during complete polysomnography?

MEASUREMENT	PURPOSE
EEG: central and occipital positions	Detect presence and stage of sleep
EOG	Detect eye movements (associated with REM sleep and wake)
Chin EMG	Detect reduction in muscle tone associated with REM sleep
Electrocardiogram	Cardiac rate and rhythm
Airflow	Detect apnea (absent airflow for $\geq$ 10 sec) or hypopnea (reduced airflow for $\geq$ 10 sec)
Chest and abdominal movement	Detect presence or absence of respiratory effort during apnea
Pulse oximetry	Detect arterial oxygen desaturation
Anterior tibialis (leg) EMG	Detect periodic leg movements (PLMs) in sleep

5. How is obstructive sleep apnea (OSA) diagnosed?

Airflow is monitored to detect periods of apnea (absence of airflow for $\geq$ 10 sec) or hypopnea (reduction in airflow). Bands around the chest and abdomen detect movement associated with respiration. **Obstructive apnea** is an absence of airflow despite continued respiratory effort. **Central apnea** is characterized by an absence of inspiratory effort (chest and abdominal movement). **Mixed apnea** is composed of an initial central portion followed by an obstructive portion. **Hypopnea** is a reduction in airflow (usually to less than 50% of baseline) for 10 seconds or longer. Hypopneas also may be classified as central (reduced ventilatory effort) or obstructive (upper airway narrowing). However, distinction between the two types is not always possible with routine monitoring methods. Obstructive hypopneas are often associated with paradoxical chest and abdominal movement (one moves inward while the other moves outward). Patients with OSA typically have a combination of obstructive and mixed apneas and hypopneas, although a few central apneas also may be present. A fall in arterial oxygen saturation (desaturation) is commonly associated with apneas and hypopnea; the nadir in saturation follows termination of these events.

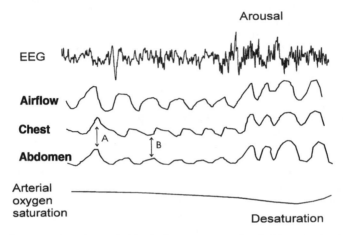

Obstructive hypopnea. A = chest and abdominal movement associated with respiration. B = paradoxical chest and abdominal movement.

6. Why are patients with OSA sleepy during the day?

Patients with OSA have repetitive episodes of upper airway narrowing or closure during sleep. When upper airway muscle activity fails to maintain upper airway patency, the result is obstructive apnea (no airflow—airway closed) or hypopnea (reduced airflow—airway narrowed) despite continued respiratory effort. These events are terminated by arousals (partial brief awakenings) characterized by speeding of the EEG and typically lasting 3–5 seconds. Frequent arousals prevent sleep from being restorative, even if the total amount of sleep is normal. The brief awakenings are too short to be recalled by patients with OSA. In patients with moderate-to-severe OSA, the amounts of stages 3 and 4 NREM and REM sleep are also usually reduced.

7. When should OSA be suspected?

Heavy snoring, periods of apnea or gasping observed by the bedmate, and a large neck circumference are the three best predictors of OSA. Men are about twice as likely as women to have OSA. Obesity and the regular, heavy use of ethanol also predispose to OSA. Patients with sleep apnea tend to underestimate the severity of their sleepiness. Other symptoms of OSA include morning headache or grogginess, decreased intellectual performance, or personality change.

8. How is the severity of OSA quantified?

The most commonly used index of severity is the apnea + hypopnea index (AHI), which is also called the respiratory disturbance index (RDI). The AHI is the mean number of episodes of apnea and hypopnea per hour of sleep. The total number of events is divided by the hours of any stages of sleep that were recorded. In general, an AHI of 5 or less is considered normal; < 20 indicates mild, 20–40 moderate, and > 40 severe apnea. However, other findings of polysomnography must be considered in assessing severity, including severity of arterial oxygen desaturation, frequency of arousals from sleep, and presence of apnea-associated cardiac arrhythmias.

9. Are effective treatments available for OSA?

Modest weight loss of 10–15% may improve sleep apnea and should be attempted in all obese patients. Unfortunately, weight loss is difficult to maintain. Some patients have much less apnea when sleeping on their sides (position therapy). Tracheostomy is effective but rarely performed today. Nasal continuous positive airway pressure (CPAP) is the treatment of choice for most patients with moderate-to-severe OSA. Oral appliances are effective for mild-to-moderate cases and an occasional patient with severe OSA. Most are mandibular-advancing devices that move the jaw (and hence the tongue) forward. Uvulopalatopharyngoplasty (UPPP) is an effective procedure for snoring. A portion of the palate and redundant pharyngeal tissue is removed. However, this procedure has only a 40–50% chance of reducing the AHI by 50% to below 15/hour. Therefore, UPPP is not the procedure of choice for severe disease. Laser-assisted palatoplasty is used for snoring and perhaps mild OSA.

Treatment Options for Obstructive Sleep Apnea

MILD OSA	MODERATE OSA	SEVERE OSA
Weight loss	Weight loss—adjunctive	Weight loss—adjunctive
Position therapy	Nasal CPAP	Nasal CPAP
Oral appliances	Oral appliances	Tracheostomy
UPPP	UPPP	± UPPP
± Nasal CPAP	Maxillofacial surgery	± Oral appliances
		Maxillofacial surgery

10. How does nasal CPAP prevent obstructive apnea?

Nasal CPAP maintains upper airway patency via a pneumatic splint. Patients wear a nasal mask connected to a source of pressurized airflow. The level of pressure required to keep the airway open is determined by a nasal CPAP titration study. The pressure is incrementally increased until apnea, hypopnea, and snoring are prevented. This treatment is highly effective, but the compliance rate is only around 60%. Partial night sleep studies consisting of an initial diagnostic portion followed by nasal CPAP titration are commonly used in many sleep laboratories for economic reasons.

11. When should upper airway resistance syndrome be suspected?

Upper airway resistance syndrome (UARS) consists of repeated arousals from sleep related to respiratory effort. Like traditional OSA, UARS results in daytime sleepiness. The sleep study shows repeated arousals with little or no frank apnea or hypopnea. Breathing through a narrowed upper airway results in increased respiratory effort, which causes patients to arouse from sleep before frank apnea or hypopnea develops. Routine airflow monitoring using thermistors to measure temperature changes induced by airflow may not detect the pattern of breathing diagnostic for UARS. In the figure (top of next page) only subtle changes in thermistor airflow are noted despite a flattened airflow profile measure accurately by a pneumotachograph (a) and increased respiratory effort (esophageal pressure deflections). Frequent unexplained arousals should trigger the suspicion of UARS. UARS is treated in the same way as mild OSA, and most experts consider it simply one end of the spectrum of OSA.

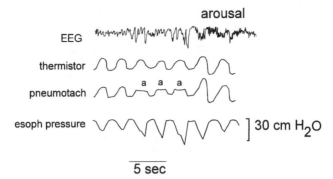

Respiratory effort-related arousal (RERA) event.

12. What historical elements suggest a diagnosis of narcolepsy?

Narcolepsy is a disorder of unknown etiology that is frequently not recognized until many years after onset of symptoms. The classic symptom tetrad of narcolepsy consists of (1) sleep attacks, (2) cataplexy, (3) hypnogogic hallucinations, and (4) sleep paralysis. Only a minority of patients with narcolepsy have all four symptoms. Cataplexy is the only symptom specific for narcolepsy. Unfortunately, some patients with narcolepsy have onset of sleep attacks several or many years before cataplexy begins. Narcolepsy usually begins in adolescence or early adulthood.

Classic Tetrad of Narcolepsy Symptoms

Sleep attacks	Episodes of irresistible sleepiness
Cataplexy	Loss of muscle tone triggered by high emotion (laughter, embarrassment, surprise)
Sleep paralysis	Inability to move while conscious at sleep onset or after awakening
Hypnogogic hallucinations	Vivid visual imagery at sleep onset (e.g., stranger in the room)

13. How does sleep monitoring support a diagnosis of narcolepsy?

Polysomnography is performed to rule out disorders such as sleep apnea and PLMs during sleep as a cause of daytime sleepiness. A very **short REM latency** (time from sleep onset until the first episode of REM sleep) is characteristic of narcolepsy. The normal REM latency is around 70–120 minutes, but patients with narcolepsy may have a REM latency < 15 minutes. However, the presence of a short REM latency on nocturnal polysomnography is neither sensitive nor specific for narcolepsy. Less than 50% of patients with narcolepsy have a short REM latency on a given night. Other causes of short nocturnal REM latency include sleep apnea, depression, and withdrawal from REM-suppressing medications. If narcolepsy is suspected, polysomnography is followed the next day by a multiple sleep latency test (MSLT).

14. What is the MSLT?

The MSLT is a series of 4 or 5 naps scheduled every 2 hours over the day. The patient is given 20 minutes from lights-out to fall asleep. The time from lights-out to first sleep is called the **sleep latency**. If sleep occurs, the patient is given another 15 minutes to reach REM sleep. If no sleep or REM sleep occurs within the allotted time (or after unequivocal REM sleep is noted), the test is stopped and the patient gets out of bed until the next nap. A short sleep latency during the day documents excessive daytime sleepiness. The presence of two or more REM periods is noted in patients with narcolepsy, sleep apnea, prior REM deprivation, or withdrawal of REM-suppressing medications.

Interpretation of MSLT Data

MEAN SLEEP LATENCY	SEVERITY OF SLEEPINESS	NUMBER OF REM PERIODS IN 5 NAPS	
		0–1	2 OR MORE
< 5 min	Severe	Normal	Abnormal
5–10 min	Moderate		
10–15 min	Mild sleepiness (some normal subjects)		
> 15 min	Normal		

15. What findings on the MSLT support a diagnosis of narcolepsy?

The classic criteria for narcolepsy are shown below. A positive MSLT may occur with sleep apnea or prior REM sleep deprivation; for this reason, polysomnography is performed before MSLT. Recent withdrawal of drugs suppressing REM sleep also may increase the probability of REM periods during the MSLT. The results of the MSLT must be interpreted with the clinical history and polysomnography findings in mind. If OSA is present on nocturnal polysomnography, the MSLT must be repeated after adequate treatment of OSA. For example, patients treated with nasal CPAP undergo a repeat sleep study on CPAP to document successful treatment of OSA. This test is followed by an MSLT on CPAP. If the MSLT still meets criteria for narcolepsy despite adequate OSA treatment, the findings support a diagnosis of narcolepsy.

MSLT FINDINGS SUPPORTING A DIAGNOSIS OF NARCOLEPSY	OTHER DISORDERS GIVING 2 OR MORE REM PERIODS IN 5 NAPS
Mean sleep latency < 5 min	Sleep apnea
2 or more REM periods in 5 naps	REM deprivation from any cause
	Withdrawal of REM-suppressing medication

16. Does a negative MSLT rule out narcolepsy?

Only about 80% of patients with narcolepsy have a positive MSLT on any given day. If a patient with daytime sleepiness has unequivocal cataplexy, a clinical diagnosis of narcolepsy may be made. In the absence of cataplexy, however, laboratory confirmation is needed. If the patient has no obvious cause for daytime sleepiness (no sleep apnea) on the polysomnogram and has a short sleep latency on the MSLT without REM periods, one must consider four diagnoses: narcolepsy (false-negative MSLT), idiopathic hypersomnia, UARS, and prior insufficient sleep. Idiopathic hypersomnia is a diagnosis of exclusion. Daytime sleepiness in this disorder is treated with stimulants, as in narcolepsy. Insufficient sleep syndrome is ruled out by having patients keep a sleep diary for 2 weeks before the MSLT.

17. How is narcolepsy treated?

The excessive daytime sleepiness of narcolepsy is treated with stimulant medications such as methylphenidate (Ritalin) or dextroamphetamine. Fair control of symptoms can be obtained in most patients. Some patients also find short naps during periods of sleepiness very refreshing. The symptoms of cataplexy may not require treatment in all patients. If necessary, good control is possible with tricyclic antidepressants (protriptyline, imipramine) or selective serotonin reuptake inhibitors.

18. Do PLMs during sleep always result in daytime sleepiness?

No. Patients with PLMs more commonly present with complaints of insomnia (frequent awakenings) than daytime sleepiness. Many older patients also have PLMs but are asymptomatic. The cause of the leg movements is unknown. PLMs are associated with uremia, treatment with tricyclic antidepressants, and withdrawal of seizure medications. The leg movements are harmless but result in arousal and sleep disturbance that may cause either insomnia (difficulty in maintaining sleep) or nonrestorative sleep resulting in excessive daytime sleepiness.

19. Do patients with PLMs during sleep report the leg movements?

No. Patients with PLMs during sleep may recall frequent awakenings during the night, but they usually do not recall the leg movements. The patient's bed partner usually reports that the patient kicks the covers or jerks during sleep. PLMs should not be confused with a brief whole body jerk at sleep onset (hypnic jerk or sleep start). PLMs consist of dorsiflexion of the toes, flexion at the ankle, and flexion at the knee (much like the Babinski response).

20. What does sleep monitoring show in patients with PLMs?

Monitoring of the EMG of the anterior tibialis muscle reveals periodic activity. Leg movement bursts are seen in groups of 4 or more; the intermovement interval usually lasts from 20–90 seconds. The **periodic movement index** is usually reported as the number of leg movements per hour of sleep. The **periodic leg movement arousal index** is the number of leg movements associated with arousal per hour of sleep. Significant daytime sleepiness is usually with a PLM arousal index of 20–25/hr or greater.

21. How does restless leg syndrome (RLS) differ from PLM syndrome?

RLS consists of sensations of creeping/crawling in the legs that are temporarily terminated by movement of the legs. These sensations usually occur at bedtime while the patient is awake. Most patients with RLS also have PLMs. However, most patients with PLMs do not have RLS. A history of RLS is important because it usually means that a sleep study is not indicated unless other disorders, such as sleep apnea, are suspected.

22. What treatments are available for RLS and PLMs during sleep?

Clonazepam (0.5–2 mg at bedtime) or other benzodiazepines may improve sleep in patients with PLMs by decreasing the number of arousals. In general, there is no decrease in the number of PLMs. Clonazepam has a long half-life and may cause morning grogginess. Starting with a low dose several hours before bedtime may minimize this side effect. Shorter-acting benzodiazepines, such as temazepam or triazolam, also have been used successfully. Most clinicians consider the combination of carbidopa and levodopa the treatment of choice for PLMs. This medication decreases the frequency of PLMs. Carbidopa/levodopa, 25/100 mg, is started at $\frac{1}{2}$ pill at bedtime with a repeat $\frac{1}{2}$ pill during the night if needed. The dose can be titrated upward slowly until a response is noted (maximal dose = 3 pills nightly). At low doses the main side effect is nausea.

RLS is often more difficult to treat than PLMs. Although clonazepam and carbidopa/levodopa may work in mild cases, moderate-to-severe RLS may require dopamine agonists such as pergolide and/or narcotics. Treatment of RLS with carbidopa/levodopa at doses > 200 mg of levodopa nightly may result in augmentation, in which symptoms spread to earlier parts of the day and involve the arms. Switching to pergolide or other agents may help.

23. When should insufficient sleep syndrome be suspected?

The amount of sleep required for a given person to function optimally is probably genetically determined. The average amount of required sleep is around 7.5–8 hours. Many people in modern society arrange their schedules to sleep less during the work week. They tend to sleep longer on the weekends, thereby repaying their "sleep debt." People may compensate for less than optimal sleep by taking stimulants (caffeine) or maintaining activity. In one study of normal people, a reduction in sleep time from 8 to 6 hours reduced the sleep latency on an MSLT from 12 to 8 minutes.

24. Can sleeping pills cause daytime sleepiness?

Hypnotics with a long duration of action (flurazepam) have the potential to cause drug hangover the next day. Temazepam (intermediate half-life) and triazolam (short half-life) usually avoid this problem but may reduce the amount of stages 3 and 4 NREM sleep. Problems with memory or coordination may occur, especially in elderly patients. The nonbenzodiazepine zolpidem (short half-life) does not appear to reduce the amount of stages 3 and 4 sleep, but it is much more expensive than temazepam and triazolam. In general, all hypnotics should be used in the lowest effective dose for limited periods. Slowly weaning the dose avoids rebound insomnia when the drugs are discontinued.

25. Is depression more commonly associated with insomnia or excessive daytime sleepiness?

Affective disorders most commonly are associated with complaints of insomnia. Sleep maintenance insomnia and early morning awakening are common complaints. Depression also may be associated with a short REM latency (although usually not as short as narcolepsy). Fatigue and malaise rather than daytime sleepiness are common daytime manifestations. However, excessive daytime sleepiness may be associated with the depressive phase of bipolar disease, seasonal depression, and atypical depression. Atypical depression is characterized by weight gain, rejection hypersensitivity, and hypersomnia.

26. What is the shiftwork maladaptation syndrome?

The shiftwork maladaptation syndrome consists of (1) chronic sleep disturbance and waking fatigue, (2) gastrointestinal symptoms (constipation, diarrhea), (3) alcohol or drug abuse, (4) higher accident or near-miss rates, (5) depression and malaise, and (6) difficult interpersonal relationships. Some or all of these symptoms are common in patients who work nightshifts, especially those on rotating shifts. In one study 40–80% of industrial night workers reported disturbed sleep compared with 10–15% of day workers.

27. Why is adaptation to the nightshift so difficult?

Alertness and sleep propensity are closely tied to 24-hour (circadian) biologic rhythms. The major internal clock is believed to be the suprachiasmic nucleus (SCN) of the hypothalamus. The SCN receives important input from the retina (retinohypothalamic tract) that enables body rhythms to adapt to the cycles of light (day) and night (dark). Light is the strongest stimulus that resets the SCN. Abrupt attempts to alter the timing of activity (work) and sleep are opposed by strong biologic rhythms. Workers on the nightshift find it difficult to stay awake at night and have trouble sleeping during the day. With time some adaptation may occur. However, most nightshift workers revert to the normal night sleeping pattern on weekends for societal reasons and thus never truly adapt. Rotating shifts are the most difficult because the body never fully adapts to the new schedule.

28. What measures can maintain alertness during nightshift work?

Measures that delay the phase of the internal body clock, such as bright light (equivalent in intensity to outdoor light) or vigorous exercise in the evenings or first part of the night in the work environment, may induce phase delays (delay in the nadir in body temperature that normally occurs at night). Sleep maintenance is easier during periods of low and falling body temperature. Thus, a phase delay may improve daytime sleep. Conversely, avoidance of bright light in the morning (dark glasses, minimal exposure to outdoor light) minimizes the phase-advancing properties of morning daylight. Stimulants such as caffeine also may help to maintain alertness during the night but may make sleep during the following day more difficult. A quiet bedroom with black-out window shades or eye masks also may help workers to sleep during the day. Although short-acting hypnotics may increase daytime sleep, chronic use is not recommended. Some preliminary studies have found melatonin to improve daytime sleep; however, the long-term safety and efficacy of melatonin have not been proved. In general, nightshift work or rotating shifts should be avoided if at all possible in patients with other sleep disorders.

BIBLIOGRAPHY

1. Aldrich MS, Chervin RD, Malow BA: Value of the multiple sleep latency test for the diagnosis of narcolepsy. Sleep 20:620–629, 1997.
2. American Sleep Disorders Association: International Classification of Sleep Disorders: Diagnostic and Coding Manual. Rochester, MN, American Sleep Disorders Association, 1997.

3. American Sleep Disorders Association: The clinical use of the multiple sleep latency test. Sleep 15:268–276, 1992.
4. Bassetti C, Aldrich MS: Narcolepsy. Neurol Clin 14:545–569, 1996.
5. Bonnet MH: Performance and sleepiness as a function of frequency and placement of sleep disruption. Psychophysiology 23:263–271, 1986.
6. Carskadon MA, Rechtschaffen A: Monitoring and staging human sleep. In Kryger MH, Roth T, Dement WC (eds): Principles and Practice of Sleep Medicine. Philadelphia, W.B. Saunders, 1994, pp 943–960.
7. Flemons WW, Whitelaw WA, Brant R, et al: Likelihood ratios for a sleep apnea clinical prediction rule. Am J Respir Crit Care Med 150:1279–1285, 1994.
8. Guilleminault C: Narcolepsy syndrome. In Kryger MH, Roth T, Dement WC (eds): Principles and Practice of Sleep Medicine. Philadelphia, W.B. Saunders, 1994, pp 549–561.
9. Guilleminault C, Stoohs R, Clerk A, et al: A cause of excessive daytime sleepiness: The upper airway resistance syndrome. Chest 104:781–787, 1993.
10. Monteplaisir J, Lapierre O, Warnes H, et al: The treatment of restless leg syndrome with or without periodic leg movements in sleep. Sleep 15:391–395, 1992.
11. Strollo PJ, Rodgers RM: Obstructive sleep apnea. N Engl J Med 334:99–104, 1996.
12. Van Reeth O: Sleep and circadian disturbances in shift work: Strategies for their management. Horm Res 49:158–161, 1998.

43. PSYCHOLOGY AND WORKER HEALTH

Robert Smither, Ph.D.

1. What is an employee assistance program (EAP)?

Employee assistance programs (EAPs) were developed to address issues, usually related to psychology, that affect worker performance. Although such programs existed before World War II, during the 1970s and 1980s employers increasingly took an interest in how problems with alcohol, stress, drugs, and other areas affected productivity. Employers also recognized that often such problems can be treated effectively in the workplace. Recent estimates suggest that about 25% of a company's workforce will use an EAP over a 5-year period.

2. Who typically uses an EAP?

Men and women typically use an EAP in proportion to their numbers in the workforce, but men tend to use more counseling time than women. Married white or Hispanic men who hold premanagerial positions are most likely to use an EAP. In addition, EAP clients tend to have been with the company for a number of years before they use the EAP's services.

3. What are the concerns of employees about EAP usage?

Employees will not use an EAP if they have concerns about confidentiality. They are also typically concerned about the hours of the EAP, convenience of appointments, and costs associated with treatment.

4. What are the five basic models of employee assistance programs?

1. The **hot-line model** is a telephone service that allows employees to talk about their problems and to get a referral to other services if necessary. The hot-line model preserves confidentiality, but diagnoses made over the telephone are questionable. In addition, hot-line models offer no way of follow-up to see whether a caller received proper treatment.

2. In the **consortium model**, several organizations form an EAP that serves all employees. This model usually requires some payment from the patient, based on income, and is housed at a site away from the workplace.

3. The **outside contractor model** refers employees to an outside organization that specializes in the treatment of problems related to job performance. This is probably the most common type of EAP.

4. In the **in-house EAP**, companies provide facilities and staff to treat employees on site. This model allows easy accessibility to counselors but engenders the most concerns about confidentiality. Other considerations are employer liability and the problem of providing qualified staff.

5. In the **union-based EAP**, union members volunteer their services to other members.

5. How does psychological counseling affect medical center usage?

EAPs arose in part as a way of containing medical costs. In a landmark study at the Kaiser-Permanente Medical Center in San Francisco, researchers demonstrated how providing counseling to employees reduced the number of visits to the medical center over time. Because it is much less expensive to provide psychological counseling than medical treatment, many employers moved to cut medical costs by making counseling available for employees. Another important factor in the rise of the EAP is the number of young people who entered the workforce during the 1970s and 1980s. Because this group is particularly at risk for drug and alcohol problems, many employers have found it necessary to expand counseling programs.

6. How prevalent is alcoholism in the workplace?

Alcoholism in the workplace has been a problem for decades and was the initial reason for establishing counseling programs at work. There are at least 13 million problem drinkers in the U.S., and the cost to employers is over $60 billion annually. Obvious costs include absenteeism, sick leave, accidents, and insurance claims. Hidden costs include poor quality work, early retirements, poor decisions, and higher worker compensation claims. Typical health problems of alcoholics are cirrhosis, gastritis, pancreatitis, hypertension, and cancer of the mouth, tongue, throat, and liver.

7. What is the profile of a typical alcoholic employee?

Although the stereotypical alcoholic employee is a blue-collar worker, alcoholism is actually more common among white-collar workers and professionals. White males, aged 35–50 years, appear to be the group at greatest risk for alcoholism. Of all working alcoholics, probably less than 15% receive some kind of treatment.

8. Discuss gender differences in alcoholism.

Stress and emotional isolation appear to be the factors most likely to cause onset of alcohol abuse among men. In contrast, women typically start drinking in response to specific life crises. Men are more likely to drink socially; women begin their alcoholism by drinking alone or with an alcoholic partner. Although alcoholism occurs more frequently among men, women are more likely to abuse other drugs at the same time. Overall, prognoses for female alcoholics are poorer than for male alcoholics.

9. What are the success rates of treatment for alcoholism?

Early treatment programs for alcoholism consisted largely of moral appeals to stop drinking. Not surprisingly, such appeals rarely worked, particularly when an employee was in an advanced stage of alcoholism. Currently the typical program consists of 28 days of inpatient treatment. A newer treatment, pioneered by health maintenance organizations, is provided on an outpatient basis outside working hours. This new approach is less costly, but its effectiveness has not been fully demonstrated. Although recovery rates for alcoholics are now at 50% or higher, experts recognize that most alcoholics recover without seeing a professional—they just stop drinking.

10. What is the relationship between drug use and job performance?

Research indicates that drug use has a negative effect on performance. One study found that employees who used drugs have a 60% higher absence rate than nonusers and a 47% rate of involuntary termination. Another study found that people who had been arrested for a drug offense were far more likely to be discharged than those who had not been arrested, even if the arrest did not result in conviction. Drug use is usually a more serious problem for employers than alcoholism. In contrast with the alcoholic, who tries to keep his or her drinking secret, drug users are likely to try to support their habit by selling to other employees. A high percentage of drug users are attracted to the retail industry, where shoplifting helps to support their habit.

11. What is the prevalence of drugs in the workplace?

In a given year, approximately 10% of the workforce has used illicit drugs. About two-thirds of drug abusers are employed. Whereas the use of illegal drugs is concentrated among younger employee groups, older workers and women in particular are likely to abuse prescription drugs.

12. What factors are related to use of illicit drugs?

Factors related to the use of illicit drugs include youth, gender (male), lack of involvement in religious organizations, low self-esteem, and family or friends who use drugs. Other correlates of drug use include stress at work, job dissatisfaction, lack of faith in management, lack of job involvement, and lack of commitment to the organization.

13. What is the prevalence of drug testing?

Historically, employers have taken little interest in rehabilitating drug users and typically terminated them as soon as their drug use was discovered. Because of the need for workers, however, many employers have modified their policies. Currently testing occurs after an accident or suspicious behavior rather than randomly.

14. How can drug users be identified?

Drug use is often difficult to identify because different drugs cause different behavioral changes. Typical problems associated with drug use include absenteeism, unexplained absences from the work area, falling asleep on the job, lengthy trips to the restroom, and serious financial problems. One of the best ways to identify drug users is urinalysis. Although no one disputes the right of an employer to require a drug test of applicants, incumbent employees may object to drug testing. Typical objections include concerns about privacy or the possibility of error. Overall, employees are more accepting of drug testing when their job carries substantial safety risk, such as airline pilots and physicians.

15. What is the effect of employee gambling on the workplace?

In recent years, some people have come to regard gambling as a disease that affects job performance. Gambling is a major cause of white-collar crime. Of the approximately 90 million gamblers in the U.S., 85% steal from their employers. Of interest, because gamblers need a constant cash flow, they may be hard workers who earn substantial bonuses and raises for their efforts on the job. Compulsive gamblers tend to be above average in intelligence and have a high need for achievement and a reputation for enjoying gambling.

16. What characteristics are associated with stress?

Stress is a physiologic or psychological response to demands made on an individual. Typical physiologic responses to stress include elevated heart rate, high blood pressure, increased respiration, hypertension, heart disease, or ulcer. Psychological symptoms include headaches, insomnia, and anxiety.

17. What stressors are typically found in the work environment?

Stress is a complex phenomenon that has different effects on different people. Stress may occur when a job does not meet the expectations of the employee or when job requirements are demanding. Researchers also know that job scope affects stress—employees who have too few or too many duties are likely to report feelings of stress. Role ambiguity, or uncertainty about job-related expectations, is another source of stress. Of interest, both pleasant and unpleasant situations may cause stress. For example, being promoted can be as stressful as being fired.

18. What personality characteristics are related to stress?

Workers with negative affectivity (negative self-concept and attitude toward life in general) are more likely to experience stress. In addition, people who have physical ailments typically express more stressful feelings than healthy people.

Other factors that affect stress levels include uncertainties about the management or future direction of an organization, lack of support from a supervisor, or the requirement to adhere to an inflexible schedule. According to the National Institute of Occupational Safety and Health (NIOSH), the 12 most stressful jobs are laborer, secretary, inspector, clinical laboratory technician, office manager, supervisor, manager/administrator, waitress/waiter, machine operator, farm owner, miner, and painter.

19. What is type A behavior?

Type A refers to a syndrome of behaviors associated with higher levels of stress. People who experience type A behavior tend to have a chronic sense of time urgency, impatience, hostility, and competitiveness. Typically, type A personalities have heightened arousal of the autonomic nervous system and muscle tension. They often use rapid speech patterns, tend to be extroverted, and have a strong need for power. Type B personalities, on the other hand, are more easygoing, relaxed, satisfied, and unhurried. Type A syndrome has been associated with greater risk for heart attack and stroke.

Often the success of an organization depends on type A behavior in certain employees. Ways of managing type A behavior include redesigning jobs, eliminating work overloads, and allowing more employee participation in decision making. Other approaches to managing stress include classes in goal setting, time management, exercise, and meditation.

20. How common is violence in the workplace?

In recent years, violence has become a serious workplace problem. In 1994, for example, almost 1100 people were murdered on the job. Although transportation accidents are the number one cause of death at work, homicide is now second. Less serious forms of violence are much more common than murder. During an 18-month period, for example, the U. S. Postal Service recorded 700 cases of employee-supervisor violence. Violence is most prevalent in the health care and social service industries.

Violence has a terrible effect on both employees who experience the violence and employers who witness it. Typical employee responses to violence include stress and lower productivity. In terms of legal costs, a workplace death typically results in a jury verdict of $2.2 million; a rape on the job averages $1.8 million.

21. What are the federal guidelines for prevention of violence in the workplace?

In 1996 OSHA introduced the following guidelines for preventing violence in the workplace: (1) analysis of the worksite to identify high-risk situations; (2) prevention and control through engineering and administrative processes; (3) training and education of workers about risks associated with violence; and (4) management commitment to avoiding violence.

22. Which people are most likely to become violent?

Researchers have yet to identify the factors that make a person become violent. Nonetheless, some characteristics of people who commit violent acts have emerged. Many are younger men with a history of violence. In addition, they tend to be loners who are often angry, depressed, or paranoid. Finally, they often have a fascination with weapons.

Behavioral indications of possible violent behavior include lateness and absence from work, taking up a great deal of a supervisor's time with complaints, low productivity, poor relations with other workers, frequent accidents, deteriorating hygiene or appearance, inappropriate comments, and evidence of a personal crisis outside work.

23. What is the effect of AIDS on the workplace?

One of every 300 workers in the United States has acquired immune deficiency syndrome (AIDS); 90% of people with AIDS are working. The majority of AIDS cases occur in health care, pharmaceutical, broadcasting, communications, recreation, and food-service industries. Current estimates of the treatment cost for an AIDS patient from infection to death is about $125,000. Another problem related to AIDS is the concern of other workers that they may contract the disease. Employers often deal with fears about AIDS through education programs that discuss how the virus is transmitted and dispel incorrect beliefs about the illness.

AIDS is covered under the Americans with Disabilities Act (ADA), and organizations are required to protect the rights of people with HIV/AIDS by making reasonable accommodations to meet their job-related needs.

24. What are health promotion programs?

Health promotion programs are designed to improve worker health and longevity by changing behavior. In other words, they attempt to prevent problems before they occur. Health promotion typically occurs at three levels. At the simplest level, managers try to raise employee awareness of health issues by providing newsletters, holding health fairs, and offering health-related classes. At the second level, companies provide specific programs to employees on an ongoing basis, such as fitness classes or memberships at health clubs. At the third level, the company may provide an in-house fitness facility, offer health foods in the company cafeteria, and keep workers informed about advances in health care.

Although health promotion programs appear to have an obvious benefit to employers and employees, certain factors need to be taken into consideration before introducing such a program. Examples include needs analysis, estimation of cost, and procedures for evaluating the program's effectiveness. Four qualities associated with successful health promotion programs include specific and quantifiable goals developed through consultation with management, employees, and fitness specialists; a long-term commitment from management and the providing of high quality staff; a strategy for evaluation; and a program of outreach to employees.

BIBLIOGRAPHY

1. Axel H: Corporate Experiences with Drug Testing Programs. New York, Conference Board, 1990.
2. Breuer NL: Emerging trends for managing AIDS in the workplace. Personnel J 74:125–134, 1995.
3. Brief AP, Burke MJ, George JM, et al: Should negative affectivity remain an unmeasured variable in the study of job stress? J Appl Psychol 73:193–198, 1988.
4. Chen PY, Spector PE: Negative affectivity as the underlying cause of correlations between stressors and strains. J Appl Psychol 76:398–407, 1991.
5. Cummings NA, Follette WT: Brief psychotherapy and medical utilization: An eight-year follow-up. In Dorken H Dorken and Associates (eds): Handbook of Organizational Communication: An Interdisciplinary Perspective. Newbury Park, CA, SAGE, 1976.
6. Delaney WP, Ames G: Work team attitudes, drinking norms, and workplace drinking. J Drug Issues 25:275–290, 1995.
7. French MT, Zarkin GA, Bray JW: A methodology for evaluating the costs and benefits of employee assistance programs. J Drug Issues 25:451–470, 1995.
8. Gebhardt DL, Crump CE: Employee fitness and wellness programs in the workplace. Am Psychol 45:262–272, 1990.
9. Harris MM, Heft LL: Alcohol and drug use in the workplace: Issues, controversies, and directions for future research. J Manage 18:239–266, 1992.
10. Johnson PR, Indvik J: Workplace violence: An issue of the nineties. Public Personnel Manage 23:515–523, 1994.
11. Lehman WEK, Farabee DJ, Holcom ML, Simpson DD: Prediction of substance use in the workplace: Unique contributions of personal background and work environment variables. J Drug Issues 25:253–274, 1995.
12. McDaniel MA: Does pre-employment drug use predict on-the-job suitability? Personnel Psychol 41:717–729, 1988.
13. McShulskis E: Less is less when it comes to substance abuse treatment. HR Mag Dec:24–25, 1996.
14. Micco L: Debate flares over OSHA's night retail guidelines. HR News Jan:3, 1997.
15. Normand J, Salyards S, Mahoney J: An evaluation of preemployment drug testing. J Appl Psychol 75:629–639, 1990.
16. O'Donnell MP: Design of workplace health promotion programs. Royal Oak, MI, American Journal of Health Promotion, 1986.
17. Waxman HS: Putting workplace violence in perspective. Security Manage Sept:123–126, 1995.
18. Woo J: Businesses find suits on security hard to defend. Wall Street J September 1, 1993, section B1.

44. ORGANIZATIONAL DYNAMICS IN THE WORKPLACE

Len Sperry, M.D., Ph.D.

1. Why should occupational physicians be concerned about organizational dynamics?

Because occupational physicians spend several hours a day contending with the organizational behavior of employees and management, a knowledge of organizational dynamics is as useful and necessary as training in injury prevention, industrial hygiene, toxicology, and ergonomics. A working knowledge of organizational dynamics greatly increases the occupational physician's effectiveness in day-to-day transactions in the workplace.

2. What mnemonic is useful for conceptualizing and recalling organizational dynamics?

A useful mnemonic for conceptualizing and recalling the dynamics of organizations and organizational behavior involves anatomic and physiologic terminology. An organization can be thought of as having

1. Five anatomic subsystems: strategy, structure, culture, leadership, and workers
2. Six physiologic processes or developmental stages: birth, expansion, professionalization, consolidation, early bureaucratization, and late bureaucratization.

Physicians find it relatively painless to learn about organizational dynamics if the subject is approached from a systems perspective in the way that anatomy and physiology are usually taught. Whereas anatomy and physiology focus largely on the cellular and organ system level, organizational dynamics emphasizes the more complex system levels: employee, work team, and organizational systems. The physician can understand these complex systems as living organisms that have a recognizable anatomy and physiology.

3. How is a work organization similar to a living organism or system?

Organizations have much in common with living systems or organisms whose organs are linked. The image of an organization as a living system can be quite useful for the occupational physician. Although organizations are less unified than organisms, they form complex, evolving systems of mutually supported elements organized around stable central themes. Essential properties of a system include its subsystems, boundaries, level or degree of homeostasis (**fit**), and its rules of communication and feedback patterns. Critical events for a system are its developmental crises, the transition of members in and out of the system, and changes that occur within its suprasystem or environmental context.

4. What are the anatomic components of a work organization?

The anatomy of an organizational system can be thought of as a set of five overlapping, concentric circles representing the subsystems of structure, culture, strategy, leaders, and workers within a larger circle representing the suprasystem or external environment. (See figure at top of next page.)

5. What is the structural subsystem of an organization?

Structure refers to mechanisms that help an organization to achieve its intended task and goals. The task is divided into smaller person-sized jobs or roles and clustered into larger sets labeled teams, departments, or divisions. It specifies the reporting relationship of all roles, their span of control and scope of authority, and their location in a hierarchy of roles, called an organizational chart. An organization's structural system specifies the ways in which the person within a role performs. It is the means of measuring job performance, which is called performance appraisal.

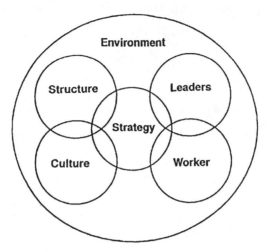

The anatomy of an organization: Five subsystems. From Sperry L: Corporate Therapy and Consulting. New York, Brunner/Mazel, 1996.

6. What are roles and norms?

Roles are expectations that prescribe the boundaries of acceptable behavior for a particular job and the individual or individuals holding that job. Norms, on the other hand, define group behavior. Norms are shared group expectations about what constitutes appropriate behavior. They are not written expectations as are policies but nevertheless are known by all.

7. What is the cultural subsystem of an organization?

Culture refers to the constellation of shared experiences, beliefs, assumptions, stories, customs, and actions that characterize an organization. The major determinants of culture are the values held by senior executives, the history of the corporation, and the chief executive's vision of the organization. These determinants translate into culture through the shared experiences, memories, stories, and actions of employees. The corporate culture provides a guide to action for new situations and new employees. Culture is to the organization what personality and temperament are to the individual. Thus, culture defines an organization's identity both to those inside and outside the organization. The culture of a corporation may be difficult to describe in words, but everyone senses it. It gives an organization its unique flavor; essentially it is "just the way we do things around here." Culture subtly controls the behavior of its members. Accordingly, management can influence its workers by effectively managing the organization's culture.

8. What is the leader subsystem of an organization?

The leader subsystem involves both the leadership and management functions of an organization. Leadership refers to a process of influence whereby a leader persuades, enables, or empowers others to pursue and achieve the intended goals of the organization. Leadership and management were used synonymously until recently.

9. What is the difference between leadership and management?

Many authors contend that management involves the five functions of planning, organizing, staffing, directing, and controlling, whereas leadership involves only one component of the directing function. Thus, an effective leader creates a vision that tells members where the corporation is going and how it will get there. The leader then galvanizes members' commitment to the vision by being ethical, open, empowering, and inspiring.

10. What are the common styles of leadership?

There are at least three ways of conceptualizing the leadership process. The first is to assume that effective leaders have the flexibility to shift their style from boss-centered (autocratic) to employee-centered (participative) to accommodate the needs of specific situations. A second concept is to think of leadership as combining two styles simultaneously but in different proportions. One style is task-centered, whereas the other is employee- or person-centered. Blake and Mouton plotted the two styles on a 2×2 chart, which they call the "managerial grid." The third concept, called **situational leadership**, is the best form of leadership. It is based on situational needs: personal characteristics of the leaders, nature of the organization, and worker characteristics.

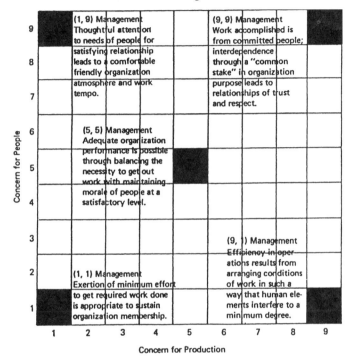

The managerial grid. From Blake R, Mouton J: The Managerial Grid. Houston, Gulf, 1964.

11. What is the worker subsystem of an organization?

The worker subsystem involves the way in which employees relate to each other, their leaders, and the organization's mission and specific goals. Also called **followership style**, this subsystem is an important key to the leader's and organization's success. Research shows that workers in a given organization have a preference for the autocratic, democratic, or participative leadership style. Workers function best with leadership that corresponds with their followership style. For example, a subordinate with an affinity for the autocratic approach responds favorably to autocratic leadership. The lack of match between leadership and followership styles probably accounts for conflict, stress, and decreased worker productivity and performance.

12. What is an informal organization? How does it affect the overall organization?

People do not work in isolation but form memberships in small groups as a way to increase their adaptability within the organizational system. These groups may be a formal part of the structural subsystem, such as work teams, or they may be informal. The informal organization is a group of workers that forms around a workplace issue or an outside activity. Such groups accomplish much of the organization's work. Chance meetings at the coffee machine, impromptu lunch meetings, and informal telephone calls go a long way toward defining and achieving the organization's intended goals. Needless to say, the presence of a disaffiliative or hostile informal organization can seriously undermine the organization's objective.

13. What is the strategy subsystem of an organization? How does strategy differ from mission and vision?

Strategy refers to the organization's overall plan or course of action for achieving its identified goals. Corporate strategy is based on the organization's vision and mission statements. The **vision statement** answers the question, "What can the organization become, and why?" The **mission statement** answers the question, "What business are we in, and who is our customer?" **Strategy** answers the question, "How do we do it?" There are three levels of strategy: (1) the corporate strategy, which charts the course for the entire organization; (2) the business strategy, which is charted for each individual business or division within the corporation; and (3) the functional strategy, which deals with basic functional areas, such as marketing, finance, and personnel.

14. What is strategic planning?

Strategy takes the form of a strategic plan, and the process of developing and implementing the strategy is called strategic planning and management. An important consideration in strategic planning is to achieve a good fit between the strategic and structural subsystems, because a given strategy can best be carried out by a given structure. An effective, integrative corporate strategy should affect positively all of the other subsystems and probably will require changes in the structural subsystem.

15. What is the environmental subsystem of an organization?

The five subsystems interact and mutually influence one another. The configuration of these subsystems is also greatly affected by its suprasystem, the environment, especially during times of major changes, such as economic recessions, war, or other natural disaster. The environmental suprasystem refers to factors outside an organizational system that influence and interact with it. The environment includes economic, legal, political, and sociocultural factors. It also includes technologic factors, such as competitors, shareholders, customer demands, and standard industrial practices.

16. What is organizational design?

The design of an organization can be likened to the skeletal subsystem of a person, which provides a framework that supports the other subsystems. Organizational design refers to the overall configuration and interrelationships, particularly among the roles and positions in the structural subsystem, but it also reflects the configuration of all of the subsystems and suprasystem. An organizational chart illustrates these positions and relationships.

17. What are the most common organizational designs?

The continuum of organizational designs ranges from the hierarchical or bureaucratic at one end to the adaptive at the other end. The **hierarchical design** takes a pyramidal shape with a clear chain of command, strict division of specialized jobs, and a comprehensive set of rational rules and rigid guidelines. Communication and decision-sending proceed from the top—the senior executive level—of the pyramid downward through middle management and then to the worker at the bottom of the pyramid. Hierarchical organizations are designed for stable times and conditions and seem particularly suited for a manufacturing or industrial economy. The **adaptive design**, on the other hand, emphasizes flexibility, horizontal communication, a low level of specialization and standardization, and high levels of cooperation. It may be likened to a network in which managers function much as switchboard operators, coordinating the activities of employees, suppliers, customers, and other stockholders.

18. How can the physiology of an organization be described?

Describing how organizations work is no small undertaking. Organizational behavior is the field of study devoted to describing organizational physiology or how work organizations function.

Two physiologic processes are related to organizations: homeostasis (**fit**) and adaptation, or stages of development and decline.

19. What is person-organization fit?

Achieving and maintaining a sense of balance and harmony is central to organizational well-being. Balance is usually described by the concept of **person-organization fit**. Achieving balance and a good fit between person and organization is a challenge to corporate leadership and the consultants whom they engage. A good fit results in higher job performance, higher job satisfaction, increased self-esteem, and less stress. Similarly, dysfunctional responses to poor fit include increased level of stress, burnout (defined as a syndrome of emotional exhaustion and cynicism among employees who engage in people work), role ambiguity, and role conflict. Poor fit does not necessarily reflect deficits within either the person or the organization. Rather, problems usually are functions of the lack of fit between the needs and resources of the person and those of the setting. Person-organization fit can be improved or enhanced by altering the person (i.e., by coaching or training), by altering the organization (i.e., by job redesign), or by some combination of the two.

20. What are the six stages of an organizational system?

The six stages of organizational growth and decline are new venture, expansion, professionalization, consolidation, early bureaucratization, and late bureaucratization.

21. Describe the new venture stage.

The first stage of an organization involves the conception of a new venture. The critical tasks at this stage include defining a target clientele and developing a service that targets such a group. Accomplishing these tasks requires the ability to extend or create a market need, the willingness to make a risky investment of time, energy, and money to create an organization that satisfies the unmet need, and the ability to create a basic organizational structure that can support the service and clientele. These abilities are characteristic of the entrepreneurial leader, the leadership style most compatible with this stage. At first, the organization is likely to be quite small in terms of members and clientele; thus its structure can be flexible and informal. This stage involves developing a basic system for day-to-day operations and finding individuals to staff the organization. Often there is little role differentiation between leaders and followers.

22. Describe the expansion stage.

Expansion is the stage of rapid growth. It may begin quickly or after the organization has been in the first stage for a number of years. The major problems in the expansion stage involve growth rather than survival. Organizational resources are stretched to their limits as a new wave of members joins the organization, as demands for services increase, and as the organization's rather primitive day-to-day operating system becomes overwhelmed. Organizational growing pains are painfully present. Growing pains signal that changes are needed and cannot be ignored; they imply that the organization has not been fully successful in developing the internal system it needs at a given stage of growth. If the founder of the organization is unable to cope with the management problems that arise, the organization is likely to flounder and even fail. Not surprisingly, the critical task at this stage is to develop an infrastructure of operating systems that result in efficiency and effectiveness. As this more complex operating system develops, the organizational structure becomes more differentiated. Basic human management training becomes a necessity. Whereas little formal management structure was needed in the first stage, more managerial structure is needed here, particularly with delegation of authority.

23. Describe the professionalization stage.

When a critical size has been achieved, the structure and operating system of the organization must be further formalized. A new generation of employees who were not involved on the ground floor requires more formal planning, defined roles and responsibilities, performance standards, and control systems. Developing a strategic planning and management system becomes the critical task in the professionalization stage. This, in turn, requires some sort of organizational development effort that provides the concurrent level of skill training needed to implement the management system. Optimal leadership involves a mixture of administrative and integrative styles. Not surprisingly, an organizational climate that encourages consultative and participative management matches well employees who are able to function relatively interdependently.

24. Describe the consolidation stage.

After transitioning to a professionally managed system, the organization can focus its efforts on consolidation. Consolidation means maintaining a reasonable increase in growth while developing organizational culture. In the first three stages the organization's culture was transmitted by the founder(s) to the first—and possibly the second—generation. But this informal mode of socialization becomes much less effective and less adequate with subsequent waves of members. Culture becomes a critical concern in the consolidation stage, as does structure. The organizational structure is a further enhancement and articulation of the organizational structure of the previous stage. Knowledge of and commitment to the organization's mission statement and implementation strategies must be widespread throughout the organization. The mission statement must be reflected in both orientation for new workers and newsletters to existing members. Employees are respected and prized; thus, human resources development and employee assistance programs (EAPs) become integrated parts of the organization. Members' horizons, knowledge base, and skills must be regularly upgraded. Leadership that combines entrepreneurship and integration is most compatible with the consolidation stage. Self-renewal must become the organization's basic strategy. Failure to plan strategically and to manage the corporation may result in the organization's decline.

25. Describe the early bureaucratization stage.

As the organization transitions to the early bureaucratization stage, there is a subtle but clear shift from substance to form. Status seeking, business as usual, and appearances characterize the behavior of members. The organization is usually well endowed and may be cash-rich for the first time in its history. Later the focus shifts to internal turf wars. Backbiting, coalition building, and paranoia are common. Growing pains are particularly intense as members' dissatisfaction mounts. In some organizations, negativity threatens to poison the organization's climate. Leadership at first was content to rest on the organization's laurels but now shifts to a self-protective mode. Cliques become the usual mode of communication. The best and brightest employees start to leave the organization. The emphasis has clearly shifted from growth and maintenance to decline. The structures and the planning and development functions are much less responsive than in previous stages. Leadership is marked first by administration and by inefficient administration. Decentralization and delegation become increasingly threatening to leadership, and efforts to recentralize power are expected behaviors.

26. How can the late bureaucratization stage be described?

Many of the subunits and subsystems of the organization become clearly dysfunctional during the late bureaucratization stage. Miscommunication is commonplace, and two-way communication is limited or nonexistent. Coordination and follow-through are the exception rather than the rule. New employees are no longer socialized in the mission statement and strategy, and for all members the organizational culture reflects a sense of helplessness and a lack of common direction. The critical function is to forestall and avoid extinction, as the organization is figuratively in intensive care and is maintained by external life-support systems. The organization's subsystems are conflictual and nonresponsive to the needs of both employees and clientele. Little if any training and development occur. Administrators struggle to buy time and prolong the organization's life. But inefficiency and ineffectiveness are to be expected. Clients find that access to responsive subsystems is the exception rather than the rule. Not surprisingly, the reemergence of dependency among members complements the autocratic style of leaders. The eventual demise of the organization seems inevitable, unless draconian measures are taken.

BIBLIOGRAPHY

1. Bennis W, Nanus B: Leaders: The Strategies for Taking Charge. New York, Harper & Row, 1985.
2. Blake R, Mouton J: The Managerial Grid. Houston, Gulf, 1964.
3. Deal J, Kennedy A: Corporate Cultures: The Rites and Rituals of Corporate Life. Reading, MA, Addison-Wesley, 1982.
4. Sperry L: Corporate Therapy and Consulting. New York, Brunner/Mazel, 1996.

45. SPECIAL SENSORY FUNCTIONS OF SMELL, TASTE, AND HEARING

Thomas J. Callender, M.D.

OLFACTION

1. Why is olfactory testing relevant to occupational medicine?

1. It is a basic component of the general physical examination.

2. It is important to determine a worker's ability to detect odors for avoidance of dangerous environments.

3. It provides a nonspecific measure of overexposure to certain toxic agents.

4. Olfactory dysfunction may be associated with significant distress, impairment, and adverse effect on quality of life.

5. Olfactory impairments suggest damage to the nasosinuses or central nervous system, providing an indication for definitive work-up and treatment.

6. The Occupational Safety and Health Administration (OSHA) requires that users of air-purifying respirators be able to detect the hazardous compound at levels below toxicity in case the compound penetrates the filter system.

2. What areas of the central nervous system (CNS) are involved in olfaction?

Neural projections from the olfactory bulb to the olfactory cortex have interconnections to the hippocampus, thalamus, hypothalamus, and frontal lobes.

3. What peripheral nerves are involved in the process of perception of inhaled substances?

The olfactory nerve (cranial nerve [CN] I) senses odors. Some inhaled substances are irritants sensed by CN V (e.g., acetone, ammonia, menthol).

4. How many simultaneous odors can a person perceive?

Most people cannot perceive more than four odors at a time; therefore, complex mixtures may result in the inability to perceive dangerous substances.

5. How do genetic factors affect olfaction and worker safety?

Congenital defects in olfaction may make it difficult for workers to avoid dangerous environments. For example, about 40–45% of the general population cannot detect the bitter almond smell of cyanide. This defect may be a sex-linked recessive trait.

6. Give examples of industrial chemicals for which olfactory perception is influenced by genetics.

Hydrogen cyanide, n-butyl mercaptan, trimethylamine, and isovaleric acid.

7. How should olfactory acuity be quantitatively tested?

1. Each nostril should be tested separately for olfactory acuity because tremendous asymmetries may result from various factors.

2. Qualitative testing is performed by using a collection of common odors in glass tubes. The University of Pennsylvania Smells Test (UPST) provides a quantitative, standardized, and well-documented odor identification method.

8. **What are the clinical indications for olfactory testing?**
   1. History of inhalation of smoke or irritant chemicals
   2. Possible injury of the olfactory nerve or temporal lobes of the brain via trauma, tumors, CNS infections, or toxic encephalopathy
   3. Screening workers who must use their sense of smell to avoid dangerous situations
   4. Serial olfactory testing to measure progression of disease as well as response to therapy
   5. Investigating loss of smell or taste as an adverse response to overexposure to toxic chemicals.

9. **Define the general categories of odor dysfunction.**
   Anosmia: absence of the sense of smell.
   Dysosmia or parosmia: distorted perception of smell.
   Cacosmia: a type of dysosmia characterized by the perception of a foul smell when none exists.
   Phantosmia: a type of dysosmia whereby the person experiences a sensation of smell without stimulus.
   Torqosmia: a type of dysosmia in which a burnt or metallic smell is perceived without an actual stimulus.

10. **What nonoccupational diseases need to be considered in evaluating a patient with dysosmia?**
   Addison's disease, hypothyroidism, temporal lobe epilepsy, psychosis, pregnancy, and head injuries. Dysosmia from peripheral causes involves any abnormality of the nose, sinuses, or upper respiratory tract.

11. **What toxins are commonly associated with an impaired sense of smell with chronic or high levels of exposure?**
   Hydrogen sulfide, volatile hydrocarbons, cadmium, carbon disulfide, hydrazine, acrylic acid, methyl bromide, sulfur dioxide, formaldehyde, or inhalation of any mucous membrane irritant. For such agents the sense of smell is a poor method of protection.

TASTE

12. **Describe the pathophysiology of taste dysfunction.**
   1. Rapidly reproducing taste bud cells on the tongue, palate, throat, and upper third of the esophagus are frequently renewed and highly susceptible to toxins that adversely affect cell reproduction.
   2. Autonomic neurotoxins may affect innervation of any of the following:
      - Anterior two-thirds of the tongue and palate facial nerve (CN VII)
      - Posterior one-third of the tongue (glossopharyngeal nerve [CN IX])
      - Laryngeal and epiglottal areas (CN X)
   3. Toxins that adversely affect protein production or zinc metabolism may adversely affect zinc-containing salivary proteins (e.g., gustins) that are necessary to identify ingested flavors.
   4. Taste is also greatly affected by simultaneous odor and taste receptor stimulation.
   5. Excessive or abnormal mucous production or the presence of atypical substances in the mouth (e.g., sinusitis or gingival disease) may block contact of ingested substances with the taste buds.

13. **Define the general categories of taste dysfunction.**
   Ageusia: lack of perception of taste.
   Hypogeusia: decreased sensitivity.
   Dysgeusia: distortion of normal taste.
   Cacogeusia: a type of dysgeusia in which a foul or perverted taste is perceived; metallic taste.

14. Give examples of toxins that may cause dysgeusia.

Acetaldehyde, arsenicals, cadmium, copper, ferrous salts, lead, mercuric chloride, and mercury. A sweet metallic taste or absence of taste is often associated with lead, selenium, tellurium.

HEARING

15. What factors other than noise levels need to be considered in evaluating a patient for hearing protection measures?

Ototoxic industrial chemicals or medications as well as familial tendencies can synergize or potentiate noise-induced hearing loss and need to be considered in evaluating workers.

16. What industrial and environmental ototoxic agents are usually associated with hearing loss?

Carbon monoxide, bromates, arsenic, mercury, nitrogen mustard, lead, 2,4-dinitrophenol, methyl mercury, toluene, xylene, and styrene.

17. What toxins usually cause tinnitus?

Heavy metals, bromates, and aromatic hydrocarbons.

BIBLIOGRAPHY

1. Doty RL, Gregor T, Monroe C: Quantitative assessment of olfactory function in an industrial setting. J Occup Med 28:6:457–460, 1986.
2. Goldfrank LR (ed): Toxicological Emergencies, 5th ed. Norwalk, CT, Appleton & Lange, 1994, pp 350–394.
3. Keeve JP: Ototoxic drugs and the workplace. Am Fam Physician 38:177–181, 1988.
4. Kimbrough RD, Mahaffey KR, Grandjean P, et al: Clinical Effects of Environmental Chemicals: A Software Approach to Etiological Diagnosis. New York, Hemisphere Publishing Corporation, 1989. pp 33–34.
5. Kisiel DL, Bobbin RP: Miscellaneous ototoxic agents. In Brown RD, Daigneault EA (eds): Pharmacology of Hearing: Experimental and Clinical Basis. New York, Wiley, 1981, pp 231–269.
6. Ryan CM, Morrow LA, Hodgson M: Cacosmia and neuro-behavioral dysfunction associated with occupational exposure to mixtures of organic solvents. Am J Psychiatry 145:1442–1445, 1989.
7. Sandmark B, Broms I, Lofgren L, Ohlson CG: Olfactory function in painters exposed to organic solvents. Scand J Work Environ Health 15:60–63, 1989.

46. OCCUPATIONAL EYE INJURIES AND EXPOSURES

Eric J. Poulsen, M.D., and Gordon K. Klintworth, M.D., Ph.D.

1. Name the parts of the eye indicated in the figure below.

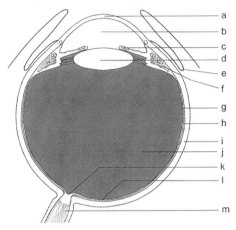

a. Cornea	f. Ciliary body	j. Vitreous
b. Anterior chamber	g. Retina	k. Optic nerve head (optic disc)
c. Iris	h. Choroid	l. Fovea
d. Lens	i. Sclera	m. Optic nerve
e. Conjunctiva		

2. What bones make up the walls of the orbit?

The ethmoid, frontal, lacrimal, maxillary, palatine, sphenoid, and zygomatic bones make up the walls of the orbit.

3. What are the general categories of eye injuries?

Physical injuries, chemical injuries, thermal injuries, radiation injuries, and electrical injuries.

4. What type of physical injuries can occur?

- **Concussional injury**—a severe blow or impact from a blunt object or a high-pressure shock wave of air or water (e.g., an explosion)
- **Penetrating injury**—entry into a structure without traversing its entire substance
- **Perforating injury**—entering, traversing, and exiting a structure
- **Intraocular foreign body**—may be virtually anything, including skin, eyelashes, vegetable matter, glass, rock, plastic, or metal
- **Surgical injury**

5. A mechanic has splashed battery acid in his eyes. How should this injury be managed?

Chemical splashes to the eyes represent an emergency. The eyes should be flushed immediately and copiously with clean water even before the patient is examined. After thoroughly flushing out the eyes, the patient should be seen by a physician, who should check the pH of the eyes. If the pH is outside the normal range (7.0–7.5), irrigation using a liter of sterile saline should be resumed. Irrigation can be done in a variety of ways. One method is to use a commercially available plastic lens (such as the Morgan lens) that fits on the eye and connects to the saline flush via plastic tubing. Irrigation is continued until the pH normalizes. No attempt should be made to neutralize the eyes' pH by adding alkali for an acid exposure or vice versa. After topical anesthetic has been instilled, the eyes are examined closely and any particulate matter and debris is carefully removed with a cotton swab soaked with anesthetic. Topical antibiotics are applied, and the patient should be referred to an ophthalmologist for follow-up.

6. What are the clinical findings in ocular chemical injuries?

Mild injuries result in erosion of the corneal epithelium and little (if any) corneal haze. Moderate burns denude the corneal epithelium, causing corneal clouding that begins to blur the view into the eye and damaging blood flow to the sclera and conjunctiva. Severe burns result in significant tissue destruction, with necrosis of affected tissues. The cornea becomes cloudy, making the pupil difficult to see.

7. Which type of burn results in a more severe eye injury, acid or alkali?

Alkali saponifies fatty components of cell membranes, resulting in cell destruction and ongoing tissue penetration. Acid exposure, on the other hand, causes the formation of insoluble acid proteinates that then inhibit further penetration of the acid.

8. A dry cleaner experiences sharp pain, tearing, photophobia, and mildly blurred vision in the right eye after accidentally scraping that eye with the edge of a coat hanger. How should the patient be evaluated?

1. Observation of the eye for anything grossly wrong
2. Measurement of visual acuity (with glasses, if prescribed), preferably with a card or chart that can quantify (e.g., 20/20)
3. Pupillary reactions and shape
4. Ocular motility
5. Flashlight examination or slit lamp biomicroscopy of eyelids, conjunctiva, sclera, cornea, anterior chamber, iris, and lens
6. Fluorescein dye examination: after fluorescein (available in a dropper bottle or impregnated in paper strips that need to be moistened) is instilled into the eye, the cornea is examined with a cobalt blue light (most direct ophthalmoscopes and all slit lamps have such a setting). Areas of damaged or missing corneal epithelium will stain with fluorescein, appearing bright yellow under the blue light.

9. The examination of the right eye of the patient described in question 8 disclosed 20/50 vision, normal pupil reactions, mild conjunctival hyperemia, and an area of fluorescein staining on the cornea measuring 4 mm in diameter. What is the diagnosis and treatment?

The diagnosis is corneal abrasion. If large (> 5–10 mm) corneal abrasions are treated with an antibiotic ointment, such as erythromycin or bacitracin, and pressure-patched for 24 hours. After removing the patch, antibiotic ointment is used 3–4 times a day until the abrasion is completely healed (usually not more than 2–3 days). If the abrasion is small, patching may be omitted. **Note:** Patients should never be given or prescribed topical anesthetic for ongoing use because it may delay epithelial healing and lead to a corneal ulcer.

10. A construction worker sustained severe femur fractures after a crushing leg injury a few days ago and now complains of blurry vision. How may the fractures be causing blurry vision?

Severe long bone fractures, head trauma, and crushing chest or abdominal injuries may result in Purtscher's angiopathic retinopathy, with findings of retinal hemorrhages, exudates, and cotton-wool spots (infarctions of the nerve fiber layer of the retina). The pathophysiology is not well-understood, but the retinal changes are speculated to result from a combination of emboli (fat, fibrin/platelet, or air) in the retinal arterioles and increased pressure in the retinal venules from Valsalva-type maneuvers.

11. While operating a machine that punches holes in sheet metal, a worker experiences a sudden, burning sensation in one eye. The pain goes away shortly after, but vision in the eye has deteriorated. On arrival at the clinic, your examination of the affected eye finds hand motions vision, a nonreactive large pupil, a small area of subconjunctival hemorrhage, and a poor view to the retina and optic nerve. The eye appears otherwise normal. What is the likely diagnosis?

The most likely diagnosis is penetrating injury to the globe with an intraocular foreign body.

12. How should the case in question 11 be managed?

As in any injury assessment, the mechanism(s) of injury must be considered. In the present case involving a metal tool striking sheet metal with high impact, the production of small, high-velocity flying metal fragments may have resulted. Because of the impaired vision and poor view to the fundus, a penetrating or perforating injury should be suspected, despite the lack of pain or significant external hemorrhage. Manipulation of an eye suspected to be penetrated, perforated, or ruptured must be minimized. Intravenous antibiotics and a tetanus booster should be given, and a hard shield should be taped over the eye to guard the globe without touching it. The patient should be immediately referred to an ophthalmologist to assess the need for urgent surgery. In this particular case, careful slit lamp biomicroscopy discovered a subtle, 1.5 mm scleral wound under the focal subconjunctival hemorrhage. Fundus examination discovered a streak of vitreous hemorrhage leading to a metal fragment embedded in the retina. If a suspected intraocular foreign body is suspected but not found on clinical examination, computed tomography (CT) of the orbits should be performed. Scans of the orbit to rule out foreign bodies should be done in axial and coronal planes with fine cuts (1.5–3.0 mm thick), because routine 5 mm axial sections may miss small intraocular or intraorbital foreign bodies.

13. Does the composition of an intraocular foreign body influence the complications that may result from it?

Yes. Some intraocular foreign bodies may be relatively inert, such as glass and some plastics. Others, such as vegetable matter, cause immediate and serious inflammation or infection. The reactivity to a metallic foreign body depends on its constituents. Gold, silver, and platinum cause little reaction; their deleterious effects are related to mechanical damage during movement. Aluminum has intermediate reactivity, but copper, iron, and their alloys may have severe detrimental effects. Iron damages photoreceptors, detectable by an abnormal electroretinogram soon after injury. Iron also can diffuse throughout the eye and be taken up by the retina, ciliary body, lens, and cornea, eventually imbuing a brownish discoloration. Pure copper can cause a purulent reaction manifesting with hypopyon (a collection of white blood cells in the anterior chamber), vitreous abscess, and retinal detachment. Alloys with lower amounts of copper may elicit minimal inflammation, but the copper may diffuse throughout the eye and cause retinal degeneration, a greenish-blue ring in the peripheral cornea, and a sunflower-shaped cataract.

14. What is the most important and effective strategy for preventing eye injuries?

Use of appropriate eye protection with adequate impact strength and side shields is the best preventive measure. Although convenient, eye protection is frequently not worn. Consequently, the availability of eye protection must be accompanied by appropriate attitudes towards using the right eye safety equipment to prevent avoidable ocular injury.

15. Six hours after welding without a mask, a welder complains of severe pain, tearing, photophobia, and blurry vision in both eyes. Examination under a cobalt blue light after fluorescein dye instillation reveals diffuse staining of the cornea and conjunctiva. What happened?

The diagnosis is welder's flash, or photokeratoconjunctivitis. Exposure to the ultraviolet radiation generated by the welder's arc damages the corneal and conjunctival epithelium. After several hours, the injured epithelial cells slough, resulting in severe pain and a sensation of sand in the eyes. Welder's flash is treated by applying topical antibiotic ointment and pressure-patching the eyes. Daily follow-up examinations are important. Normally, the epithelium heals within a few days, restoring normal vision. Another concern in this patient is photic injury to the retinae; visual acuity testing and fundoscopy should be performed.

16. After being punched in the eye, a bartender experiences double vision and numbness in the cheek but has normal visual acuity. What is the most likely diagnosis?

The most likely diagnosis is an orbital wall fracture, also known as a blowout fracture. Blunt trauma is the usual cause of this type of fracture. The typical presentation may include pain on eye movements, diplopia due to limited ocular motility, enophthalmos (which may be masked by eyelid edema and ecchymosis), and epistaxis. Common findings on orbital CT include a fracture of the orbital floor and/or medial orbital wall, fluid in the maxillary or ethmoid paranasal sinuses, and, less commonly, entrapment of the inferior rectus muscle or orbital fat. Fractures of the lateral and superior orbital walls are rare because these bones are much thicker than the medial and inferior walls.

17. Why is the bartender's cheek numb?

Orbital floor fractures may be accompanied by injury to the infraorbital nerve (a branch of the maxillary division of the trigeminal nerve) as it traverses below the orbital floor or exits the infraorbital rim.

18. A hog farmer stepped on a rake head, which causes the handle to hit him in the eye and results in severe pain and poor vision. List the potential eye injuries and their clinical findings.

1. **Corneal abrasion:** sharp pain, foreign body sensation, fluorescein staining where the corneal epithelium is missing
2. **Hyphema:** blood layered inferiorly in the anterior chamber between the cornea and iris; blood will layer over the iris and pupil if the patient has been supine
3. **Traumatic iritis:** photophobia; mild anisocoria (unequal size pupils) with sluggish pupillary reaction; white blood cells in the anterior chamber
4. **Iris sphincter damage:** irregular pupil, often dilated
5. **Traumatic cataract:** opacification of a previously clear lens
6. **Lens dislocation/subluxation:** eccentric or apparently missing lens; the lens may be located in the vitreous
7. **Commotio retinae:** an area of retinal whitening; called Berlin's edema if the macula is involved
8. **Vitreous hemorrhage:** cloudy, reddish view to the fundus; a retinal tear or detachment may be associated
9. **Retinal detachment:** flashes, floaters, shadows; pigment clumps in the vitreous; elevated gray retina that moves with eye movements; often associated with vitreous hemorrhage
10. **Choroidal rupture:** white or yellow crescent-shaped streak concentric to the optic nerve head
11. **Ruptured globe:** pain; severe subconjunctival hemorrhage; hyphema; prolapse of black uveal tissue; usually associated with other significant ocular injury

19. While operating a "weed-eater" a landscaper experiences the sensation of something in one eye. When irritation and redness in the eye persist, the patient seeks medical attention. Examination with fluorescein reveals superior, vertically-oriented corneal abrasions but no obvious foreign body. What should the clinician's concern be?

Although not readily visible, the eye may contain a foreign body such as a rock chip or piece of organic material. Thus, the undersurface of the eyelid must be carefully examined. In this case, flipping the upper eyelid revealed a foreign body embedded in the conjunctival lining the eyelid (palpebral conjunctiva). With each blink, the foreign body scraped the cornea in a vertical fashion. Also, because infection (especially of the cornea) is a potential complication, the corneal abrasions should be examined for evidence of a white infiltrate. The presence of a corneal infection indicates the need for more aggressive treatment.

20. How should a laceration involving the margin of the eyelid be managed?

A person hit hard enough to sustain such a laceration should have a complete ocular evaluation to rule out concomitant injuries, including damage to the tear drainage apparatus or intraocular derangement. Lacerations of the eyelid margin should be repaired by an ophthalmologist or facial plastic surgeon. Exact apposition of the eyelid margins is essential to avoid a notched eyelid that incompletely closes and may result in corneal scarring or infection.

21. Several months ago, a young, previously healthy delivery truck driver was involved in a minor traffic accident while on the job, sustaining a right brow abrasion. The patient now complains of poor vision in the right eye and chronic neck pain. Examination of the right eye discloses a visual acuity capable only of counting fingers and a constricted visual field. No other abnormalities are detected in the right eye, including brisk pupillary reactions and no afferent pupillary defect. The left eye was entirely normal. What is the most likely explanation for the poor vision?

Functional visual loss, such as malingering, is likely. The thorough and creative examiner usually can find several pieces of objective evidence to prove that vision is actually better than claimed by the patient.

22. What is an afferent pupillary defect, and why is its absence relevant in the case described in question 21?

Normally, both pupils constrict equally when light shines into either eye. If an eye has optic nerve disease or severe retinal damage, the afferent pathway involved in this reflex will not function properly. Consequently, the pupil will constrict consensually with light in the other eye but fully or partially dilate, rather than stay constricted, when the light is shined directly into it. The absence of an afferent pupillary defect in the patient described in question 21 provides objective evidence for the absence of optic nerve damage, such as from traumatic optic neuropathy, or significant retinal damage.

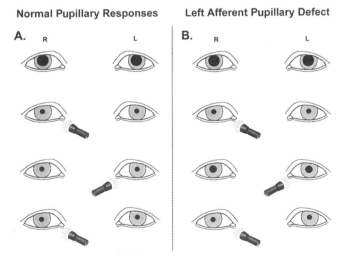

Normal pupillary responses to light compared to left afferent pupillary defect responses.

23. After examining tissue sections through a light microscope, a medical student experiences aching eye pain and blurry distance vision. Examination of the eye reveals no abnormality other than mild myopia (near-sightedness). What is the diagnosis?

Ciliary muscle spasm. Focusing at a near point for some period, as in light microscopy, can cause spasm of the ciliary muscle responsible for focusing, which results in ocular pain. The poor relaxation of the ciliary muscle renders the patient temporarily more myopic. This can be avoided by periodically looking up from the microscope and looking at a distant object, such as one outside a window, thereby relaxing the ciliary muscle.

24. A young rubber factory worker experiences a slowly progressive deterioration in vision. Examination of both eyes reveals identical abnormalities: 20/100 acuity; cecocentral scotomas (areas of decreased visual perception in the center of the visual field that incorporate the physiologic blind spots), and pale optic nerve heads. What is the probable diagnosis?

The patient most likely has toxic optic neuropathy, which may be caused by numerous substances. For example, carbon disulfide, a highly volatile liquid used in rayon, silk, and rubber factories, causes toxic optic neuropathy that may be accompanied by a peripheral sensory neuropathy with paresthesias and pain, especially in the lower extremities.

BIBLIOGRAPHY

1. Cullom DR Jr, Chang B: The Wills Eye Manual: Office and Emergency Room Diagnosis and Treatment of Eye Disease, 2nd ed. Philadelphia, J. B. Lippincott, 1994.
2. Eckenfelder DJ: Values-Driven Safety. Rockville, Government Institutes, 1996.
3. Goodner EK: Eye injuries. In LaDou J (eds): Occupational Medicine. Norwalk, Appleton & Lange, 1990, pp 80–93.
4. Grant WM, Schuman JS: Toxicology of the Eye, 4th ed. Springfield, IL, Charles C. Thomas, 1993.
5. Klintworth GK, Hitchcock ME: The Eye. In Craighead JE (ed): Pathology of Environmental and Occupational Disease. St. Louis, Mosby, 1995, pp 601–631.
6. MacCumber MW (ed): Management of Ocular Injuries and Emergencies. Philadelphia, Lippincott-Raven, 1998.
7. Morris DA: Ocular trauma. In Gardner A, Klintworth GK (eds): Pathobiology of Ocular Disease: A Dynamic Approach, 2nd ed. New York, Marcel Dekker, 1994, pp 387–432.
8. Palay DA, Krachmer JH (eds): Ophthalmology for the Primary Care Physician. St. Louis, Mosby-Year Book, 1997.
9. Spoor TC: An Atlas of Ophthalmic Trauma. London, Martin Dunitz, 1997.
10. Vaughan DG, Asbury T, Riordan-Eva P (eds): General Ophthalmology, 14th ed. Norwalk, Appleton & Lange, 1995.

47. LIVER TOXICOLOGY

Robert Harrison, M.D., M.P.H.

1. What are the common causes of occupational liver disease?

Epidemiologic studies have been performed among many groups of workers exposed to hepatotoxic agents, but relatively few workplace hepatotoxic agents have been studied in humans. Epidemiologic studies generally provide the best evidence of toxicity; however, they may be limited by inadequate study design and other factors that make conclusions difficult.

Cross-sectional studies that include biochemical liver tests have been conducted among many groups of workers exposed to hepatotoxic agents. Serum aminotransferase elevations have been found in workers exposed to polychlorinated and polybrominated biphenyls (PCBs, PBBs) and in painters exposed to various solvents. Hepatocellular liver enzyme abnormalities have been found among microelectronics equipment maintenance technicians and pharmaceutical industry workers exposed to mixed solvents. Increased levels of liver enzymes have been found among chemical plant operators exposed to carbon tetrachloride and workers exposed to methylene chloride, hydrazine, and tetrachlorodibenzo-p-dioxin. Using the noninvasive antipyrine clearance test, induction of the microsomal enzyme system has been demonstrated in workers exposed to various pesticides (chlordecone, phenoxy acids, dichlorodiphenyltrichloroethane [DDT], lindane), halothane, PCBs, and solvents. Functional abnormalities of liver metabolism—measured by antipyrine clearance or other noninvasive tests of liver function—are not accompanied by other clinical or laboratory signs of toxicity and so may provide a sensitive index of biologic change.

Cohort mortality studies have shown an increased mortality rate from liver cirrhosis among newspaper pressmen, spray painters, and oil refinery workers and from liver cancer among vinyl chloride, rubber, dye, and shoe factory workers. Case-control studies have shown a statistically significant association between primary liver cancer and exposure to organic solvents, particularly among laundry workers, dry cleaners, gasoline service attendants, asphalt workers, and bartenders.

2. What are the mechanisms of hepatotoxicity?

Inhalation is the most important route for hepatotoxic material, particularly volatile solvents. Several chemicals are lipophilic and may be absorbed through the skin in sufficient quantities to contribute to hepatotoxicity (e.g., trinitrotoluene, 4,4-diaminodiphenylmethane [MDA], tetrachloroethylene, PCBs, dimethylformamide). The liver is especially vulnerable to chemical injury by virtue of its role in the metabolism of foreign compounds (xenobiotics). Xenobiotic lipid-soluble compounds are well absorbed through membrane barriers and poorly excreted by the kidney as a result of protein binding and tubular reabsorption. Increasing polarity of nonpolar molecules by hepatic metabolism increases water solubility and urinary excretion. The mixed-function oxidase systems attached to the membrane layers of the smooth endoplasmic reticulum activate many hepatotoxic agents and hepatocarcinogens to a toxic or carcinogen metabolite. Examples include carbon tetrachloride, vinyl chloride, PCBs, bromobenzene, azo dyes, dimethylamine [DMA], and allyl compounds. Electrophilic intermediates react with enzymes and regulatory structural proteins and lead to cell death. Experimental studies show that many other factors also may affect the metabolism of xenobiotics: diet, age, cigarette smoking, endocrine status, genetic factors, diurnal variation, underlying liver disease, and stress. Inter- and intraindividual variation in xenobiotic metabolism is considerable, and the relative importance of these factors in the occupational setting is unknown.

3. What are the two major categories of hepatotoxic agents?

1. **Agents intrinsically toxic to the liver**—directly or indirectly—cause a high incidence of dose-dependent hepatic injury in exposed persons and similar lesions in experimental animals.

The interval between exposure and onset of disease is consistent and usually short. **Direct hepatotoxins** or their metabolic byproducts injure the hepatocyte and its organelles by a direct physicochemical effect, such as peroxidation of membrane lipids, denaturation of proteins, or other chemical changes that lead to destruction or distortion of cell membranes. Carbon tetrachloride, the prototype and best-studied example, causes centrolobular necrosis and steatosis in humans and experimental animals. Reactive metabolites of carbon tetrachloride bind to critical cellular molecules that interfere with cell function or cause lipid peroxidation of cell membranes. Chloroform, trichloroethylene, carbon tetrabromide, and tetrachloroethane also may cause direct dose-dependent hepatic damage. The hepatotoxic potential of the haloalkanes is inversely proportionate to chain length and bond energy and directly proportionate to the number of halogen atoms in the molecule and the atomic number of the halogen. **Indirect hepatotoxins** are antimetabolites and related compounds that produce hepatic damage by interference with metabolic pathways. Such compounds may result in cytotoxic damage (degeneration or necrosis of hepatocytes) by interfering with pathways necessary for the structural integrity of the hepatocyte (morphologically seen as steatosis or necrosis) or may cause cholestasis by interfering with the bile secretory process. The cytotoxic indirect hepatotoxins include chemicals of experimental interest (ethionine, galactosamine), drugs (tetracycline, asparaginase, methotrexate, mercaptopurine) and botanicals (aflatoxin, cycasin, mushroom alkaloids, tannic acid). MDA is the only industrial chemical categorized as a cholestatic indirect hepatotoxin.

2. A few agents may cause liver damage by virtue of **host idiosyncrasy**. Liver damage occurs sporadically and unpredictably, has low experimental reproducibility, and is not dose-dependent. The injury may be due to allergy (hypersensitivity) or production of hepatotoxic metabolites. A good example is halothane, which causes acute hepatitis in a small percentage of people with a hypersensitivity immune response.

4. What are the three basic disease patterns of hepatic injury?

Occupational exposure to xenobiotics may lead to acute, subacute, or chronic liver disease. Clinical syndromes may be associated with several types of morphologic changes as seen by light microscopy. Hepatic injury may be clinically overt or discovered only as a functional or histologic abnormality.

5. Discuss the symptoms and morphology of acute hepatic injury.

Acute hepatic injury results in degeneration or necrosis of hepatocytes (cytotoxic injury) or arrested bile flow (cholestatic injury). The latent period is relatively short (24–48 hours), and clinical symptoms are often of extrahepatic origin. Anorexia, nausea, vomiting, jaundice, and hepatomegaly are often present. Severely exposed people who have sustained massive necrosis may have coffee-ground emesis, abdominal pain, clinically detectable reduction in liver size, rapid development of ascites, edema, and hemorrhagic diathesis. Such symptoms often are followed within 24–48 hours by somnolence and coma. Morphologically, hepatic necrosis may be zonal, massive, or diffuse. Various degrees of fatty change or steatosis also may be seen.

6. What agents are associated with acute hepatic injury?

The classic example of acute hepatic injury is carbon tetrachloride, used commonly in the past as a liquid solvent, dry cleaning agent, and fire extinguisher. Tricloroethylene has been reported to cause acute hepatotoxicity when used as a dry cleaning agent and may cause centrilobular necrosis following recreational "solvent sniffing" of cleaning fluids. Trichloroethane has been reported to cause both fatal and acute, reversible hepatitis with fatty infiltration in several workers. A liver biopsy from one trichloroethane-exposed printer showed focal bridging fibrosis and nodule formation with evidence of parked portal tract fibrosis, a pattern suggestive of macronodular or early cirrhosis. Carbon tetrabromide has been reported to cause a syndrome in chemists similar to that of acute carbon tetrachloride hepatotoxicity. Several cases of acute fulminant hepatitis have been reported after exposure in confined spaces to 2-nitropropane, a nitroparaffin used as a solvent in epoxy resin paints and coatings. The solvent dimethylformamide may cause increased levels of liver enzymes. Liver biopsy shows focal hepatocellular necrosis with microvesicular steatosis. Fulminant hepatic failure also has been reported in a recreational solvent abuser exposed to a mixture of isopropyl alcohol, methyl amyl alcohol, and butylated hydroxytoluene and in workers exposed to dichlorohydrin during tank cleaning. Cholestatic jaundice has occurred among community residents (Epping jaundice) and workers exposed to MDA used as a hardener for epoxy resins.

7. Discuss the symptoms and morphology of subacute liver disease. How common is it?

Subacute hepatic necrosis is a smoldering illness, with delayed onset of jaundice after repeated exposure to relatively low doses of a hepatotoxin. Anorexia, nausea, and vomiting accompanied by hepatomegaly and jaundice may develop after several weeks to months of exposure leading to recovery or fulminant hepatic failure. A few patients are reported to have developed macronodular cirrhosis. Morphologic features include various degrees of necrosis, fibrosis, and regeneration. Postnecrotic scarring with subacute hepatic necrosis also has been observed. Subacute liver disease has been attributed to trinitrotoluene (TNT) but is fortunately rare today.

8. What agents are associated with hepatic cancer?

Many occupationally encountered chemical agents are known to cause hepatocellular carcinoma in experimental animals, but only a few are demonstrated human carcinogens. Vinyl chloride causes hepatic angiosarcoma, with pathology showing sequential progression from focal hepatocyte hyperplasia to sinusoidal dilatation, peliosis hepatis, and sarcomatous transformation of the lining of the cells of sinusoids and portal capillaries. Hepatic angiosarcoma also has developed in vintners with long exposure to inorganic arsenicals; in patients with psoriasis treated with inorganic potassium (Fowler's solution) in the 1940s and 1950s; and in patients injected with a colloidal suspension of thorium dioxide (Thorotrast), which was used for carotid angiography and liver-spleen scans from 1930–1955. Case-control studies have shown elevated odds ratios for the development of liver cancer in a variety of occupations, including clerical and hotel/motel workers, food service workers, distillery workers, transport equipment operators, and workers exposed to welding fumes. Known risk factors for liver cancer have generally not been associated with these occupations, and the significance of such findings is unknown.

9. Discuss the other forms of chronic liver disease and their common causes.

1. The histologic pattern of **progressive necrosis** accompanied by regenerating nodules, fibrosis, and architectural distortion of the liver (toxic cirrhosis) has been described after exposure to TNT, tetrachloroethane, PCBs, and chloronaphthalenes.

2. **Cirrhosis** has been reported after prolonged, repeated low-level exposure to carbon tetrachloride in dry cleaning plants and to inorganic arsenical insecticides among vintners. Micronodular cirrhosis was described in a worker with repeated exposure to a degreasing solvent containing a mixture of trichloroethylene and 1,1,1-trichloroethane. The anesthetic halothane has been reported to cause cirrhosis after acute exposure. Increased mortality due to cirrhosis has been observed among pressmen, shipyard workers, metal fabrication employees, marine inspectors, and anesthesiologists. However, the relationship to occupational exposures and the role of confounding factors such as ethanol or viral hepatitis remain to be determined.

3. **Chronic active hepatitis** also has been reported after acute exposure to halothane.

4. A few cases of **porphyria** cutanea tarda have been attributed to occupational exposure to the herbicide 2,4,5-triclorophenoxyacetic acid, probably caused by contamination with dioxin. Turkish peasants developed liver disease and hepatic porphyria after ingesting wheat contaminated with the fungicide hexachlorobenzene.

5. Beryllium and copper exposure may result in **granulomatous liver disease**, with hepatic granulomas located near or within the portal tracts.

6. **Steatosis** may result from acute occupational exposure to elemental phosphorus, TNT, arsenical pesticides, dimethylformamide, and certain chlorinated hydrocarbons (carbon tetrachloride,

methyl chloroform, and tetrachlorethane). Intracellular hepatic lipid formation results from xenobiotic effects on fat metabolism.

7. Minimal-to-moderate elevation in transaminase levels may be seen after acute occupational exposure, with resolution in several weeks after removal.

10. What is recommended for medical diagnosis and surveillance of occupational liver disease?

In an occupational setting, a screening test with a high sensitivity (to identify correctly all workers with disease) and specificity (to identify correctly all workers without disease) is needed. Clearance tests (e.g., antipyrine test, serum bile acids, urinary D-glucaric acid) have been successfully used in research settings but are not recommended for daily clinical or surveillance practice until further prospective studies are available. With current knowledge, the consequences of changes in microsomal enzyme activity cannot be accurately assessed.

Serum transaminases have a relatively high sensitivity for detection of liver disease, but their low specificity limits the practical utility of periodic measurements in a worker population exposed to potential hepatotoxins. Nevertheless, serum transaminases remain the test of choice for routine diagnosis and surveillance of such populations. Preplacement baseline measurement of serum transaminases may be helpful in establishing causality for purposes of workers' compensation when industrial liver disease is alleged. Routine medical surveillance involving measurement of serum transaminase levels should be conducted only when exposure assessment suggests potential for hepatic injury. When the prevalence of liver disease in the population is low, the poor predictive value of an abnormal serum transaminase level after routine screening may lead to many diagnostic evaluations for nonoccupational liver disease.

Patients with chronic elevations of serum transaminase levels may continue to work if exposure to potential hepatotoxins is minimized through appropriate workplace controls and exposure assessment.

11. Discuss the appropriate history and physical examination of patients with suspected occupational liver disease.

A **careful history** of occupational exposure to known human hepatotoxins should be obtained in every case of suspected occupational liver disease. Medical history of liver disease should be noted. The review of symptoms should include symptoms of acute central nervous system toxicity, such as headache, dizziness and lightheadedness, which may indicate excessive solvent exposure. Nonoccupational risk factors for liver disease—such as steroid use, glue-sniffing, travel to areas with endemic parasitic or viral diseases, hobbies with hepatotoxic exposures, previous blood transfusion, percutaneous exposures, and intravenous drug use—should be evaluated carefully. Use of protective work practices (such as respiratory protection, gloves, and work clothes) should be elicited and may help to indicate the extent of pulmonary and skin absorption. Material safety data sheets and airborne contaminant monitoring data should be requested and reviewed. The employer should be asked about other employees with possible liver disease.

Physical examination for suspected acute liver disease should include palpation of the right upper quadrant for tenderness or hepatosplenomegaly, and inspection for jaundice. Chronic liver disease may result in stigmata such as spider angiomata, palmar erythema, testicular atrophy, ascites, or gynecomastia.

12. What other measures are appropriate for the management of occupational liver disease?

1. Other causes of liver disease should be ruled out, particularly infectious and alcohol- and drug-induced hepatitis. The most common cause of elevated serum transaminase is ingestion of ethanol. If a history of excessive ethanol ingestion is elicited, the serum transaminase should be repeated after 3–4 weeks of abstinence. If serum transaminase levels are normal on follow-up, ethanol should be suspected as the probable cause. Persistent transaminase elevation may represent chronic alcoholic hepatitis or continued occupational exposure.

2. If an occupational cause of liver disease is suspected, the patient should be immediately removed from exposure for 3–4 weeks. The serum transaminase measurement should then be repeated; with few exceptions, serum transaminase concentrations normalize after removal from exposure. A persistently elevated serum transaminase concentration suggests a nonoccupational cause of liver disease or, rarely, chronic occupational liver disease.

3. Although little evidence indicates that patients with nonoccupational liver disease are more susceptible to further liver damage due to occupational exposure, it is prudent to monitor them carefully for evidence of worsening liver damage. Appropriate engineering controls and personal protective equipment should be made available to reduce potential hepatotoxic exposure. If there is evidence of worsening liver disease or if exposure cannot be satisfactorily reduced, the worker should be reassigned. Persistent abnormalities in liver function tests after removal from exposure have rarely been reported, and a thorough search for other causes should be conducted. Occasionally, chronic liver disease may follow acute chemical hepatitis or years of low-dose exposure.

BIBLIOGRAPHY

1. Chen JD, Wang JD, Tsai SY, Chao WI: Effects of occupational and nonoccupational factors on liver function tests in workers exposed to solvent mixtures. Arch Environ Health 52:270–274, 1997.
2. Cohen C, Frank AL: Liver disease following occupational exposure to 1,1,1-trichloroethane: A case report. Am J Indust Med 26:237–241, 1994.
3. Lynge E, Anttila A, Hemminki K: Organic solvents and cancer. Cancer Causes Control 8:406–419, 1997.
4. Neghab M, Qu S, Bai CL, et al: Raised concentration of serum bile acids following occupational exposure to halogenated solvents, 1,1,2-trichloro-1,2,2-trifluoroethane and trichloroethylene. Int Arch Occup Environ Health 70(3):187–194, 1997.
5. Swanson GM, Burns PB: Cancer incidence among women in the workplace: A study of the association between occupation and industry and 11 cancer sites. J Occup Environ Med 37:282–287, 1995.
6. Wu MT, Kelsey KT, Mao IF, et al: Elevated serum liver enzymes in coke oven and by-product workers. J Occup Environ Med 39:527–533, 1997.
7. Zimmerman HJ: Hepatotoxicity. Dis Month 39:675, 1993.

48. MULTIPLE CHEMICAL SENSITIVITY

Iris R. Bell, M.D., Ph.D., and Carol M. Baldwin, R.N., Ph.D.

1. What is multiple chemical sensitivity (MCS)?

MCS is a chronic, polysymptomatic condition in which patients report severe illness in multiple systems from exposures to low levels of environmental chemicals that most people find neutral. It is a highly controversial diagnosis within mainstream medicine.

2. Give Cullen's criteria for a diagnosis of MCS.

MCS is an acquired disorder characterized by recurrent symptoms, referable to multiple organ systems, in response to demonstrable exposure to many chemically unrelated compounds at doses far below those established as biologically harmful in the general population. Re-exposures trigger acute flares of illness, and removal from the exposures leads to remission of symptoms. No single widely accepted test of physiologic function can be shown to correlate with symptoms. The Cullen criteria require the identification of a specific chemical exposure that initiated the deterioration in health. This last criterion is under debate because of findings by several different investigators that a subset of patients otherwise meet MCS criteria but report gradual onset of illness rather than an identifiable initiating exposure.

3. Name the most frequent symptoms reported by patients with MCS.

Patients typically give a large number of nonspecific symptoms, such as feeling unreal or "spacy," memory problems, dizziness or lightheadedness, difficulty with focusing eyes, muscle ache, and irritability. Other commonly reported symptoms include headache, shortness of breath or chest discomfort, depression, joint pains, digestive problems, and numbness or tingling in fingers and toes. Comorbid medical conditions may include rhinitis and sinusitis, irritable bowel, migraine headache, menstrual disturbances, and ovarian cysts.

4. Does MCS affect more men or women?

Most studies have found that many more women than men have MCS (up to 70–80% of the patient populations studied).

5. At what age do patients with MCS commonly present to the clinician?

Patients typically present with MCS in their 30s to 40s.

6. Do patients with conditions other than MCS also report illness from low levels of environmental chemicals?

Patients with other controversial diagnoses, such as chronic fatigue syndrome, fibromyalgia, Persian Gulf Syndrome, and solvent encephalopathy, report chemical odor intolerance at increased rates. Unlike patients with these conditions, however, patients with MCS give universal reports of marked chemical odor intolerance.

7. Does MCS count as a disability in some arenas?

The Americans with Disability Act and the U.S. Department of Housing and Urban Development recognize MCS as a disability. Most persons diagnosed with MCS report some degree of occupational or social disability. Occupational medicine physicians often see a skewed sample of patients with MCS, such as those applying for disability or pursuing litigation against a building owner or chemical company. The overall clinical issues of such patients should be considered related to but not a necessary part of MCS.

8. List the psychiatric disorders and problems found in many patients with MCS.

Structured interviews of patients with MCS suggest that many, but not all, also have increased rates of past or current diagnoses of major depression, panic disorder, and somatization disorder in comparison with controls. Other observers have suggested that MCS is an atypical or subclinical form of posttraumatic stress disorder (PTSD), especially in view of increased rates of early sexual or other abuse histories in affected patients. Studies have found increased rates of abuse histories but not of PTSD. Patients with MCS who have an identifiable initiating chemical exposure history have lower rates of psychiatric morbidity than patients with gradual onset. Although psychiatric patients in general have increased rates of comorbid alcohol and drug abuse, patients with MCS, including those with psychiatric comorbidity, generally report abstention because of alcohol and drug intolerances.

9. What factors have been implicated in initiating MCS?

Patients clinically implicate certain types of chemicals, such as pesticides and solvents. Other patients may report major life stress, surgery, or other traumas as initiating events. A substantial subset of patients with an MCS-like syndrome cannot identify any particular initiating chemical or event.

10. What factors have been implicated in triggering established MCS?

Patients with MCS tend to report that symptoms are triggered by substances that used to be benign, such as perfumes and other scented products, natural gas, gasoline and car exhaust, fresh newspapers, new carpet odors, rubber and soft plastics, drying paints, cleaning agents, bleach, and chlorinated water. Specialists in MCS refer to this finding as a "spreading phenomenon," in which chemical sensitivity or intolerance involves increasing numbers of agents over time. Eliciting chemicals do not necessarily share structural or chemical properties with each other or with the initiating agent.

11. Are there any diagnostic tests for MCS?

No routine laboratory tests help in the diagnosis of MCS. Research tests that eventually may provide adjunctive evidence of central nervous system problems include single-photon emission computerized tomography (SPECT), positron emission tomography (PET), and functional magnetic resonance brain scans for patchy areas of dysfunction in specific regions, especially during cognitive task performance; quantitative electroencephalography (EEG) for increased resting alpha-band activity; or altered auditory- and visual-evoked potentials. Most standard neuropsychological test batteries have not shown definitive objective support for the cognitive symptoms, but some specialized tests of visual memory performance and/or divided attention may differentiate a subset of patients with MCS from non-MCS patients. Some clinicians have reported that certain markers of autoimmunity, such as specific autoantibodies and immune complexes, are elevated; helper-to-suppressor T-cell ratios are altered; and other immune system parameters are disturbed. Controlled studies, however, have not replicated these claims. Others believe that patients with MCS have an atypical form of porphyria and use specialized blood or urine tests for the diagnosis of porphyria to support their claims.

12. Describe the epidemiologic tools available for assessment of MCS.

Validated questionnaires include a 122-chemical item comprehensive survey asking for one of four possible responses for each agent: current symptoms; no symptoms; formerly symptomatic, now avoid; and no known exposure/do not know. A score of 23 or more out of 122 has sufficient sensitivity and specificity to distinguish patients with MCS from other types of patients or normal controls. A separate, validated 5-item screening index asks for ratings of frequency of illness from the odor of pesticide, paint, perfume, car exhaust, and new carpet on a 5-point Likert scale (from almost never to almost always, yielding a possible range of 5–25). Patients with MCS score an average of 22 on the 5-item index. Another commonly used brief scale asks patients to indicate on a true/false basis whether they have made four different types of lifestyle changes (e.g., in diet, clothing, home furnishings, restaurant or shopping habits) because of chemical sensitivity. A lifestyle change score of at least 2–4 out of 4 distinguishes patients with MCS from controls and correlates with level of reported disability. Approximately 30% of patients answer positively the general clinical screening question, "Do you consider yourself to be especially sensitive to certain chemicals?"

13. Do patients with MCS report intolerances to environmental factors other than chemicals?

Almost all patients with MCS report multiple food intolerances, often to commonly eaten foods such as milk, wheat, yeast, corn, egg, beef, potato, and sugar. The types of implicated foods tend to differ in patients with documented immunologically mediated food allergies (e.g., shellfish). Most patients with MCS also give a history of multiple drug and/or anesthesia intolerances. Most report that they can no longer ingest even small amounts of alcohol without experiencing severe adverse acute effects and persistent hangovers.

14. What are possible similarities and differences between MCS and sick building syndrome (SBS)?

Both MCS and SBS may involve complaints of fatigue, difficulty in concentrating, mucous membrane irritation, headache, and gastrointestinal problems. In some cases, the conditions may overlap; some patients with MCS report that their health problems began with SBS. However, patients with MCS report illness from multiple chemicals in any setting in which they believe that they encounter these agents. Patients with MCS also report food and drug intolerances. In contrast, patients with SBS usually report feeling ill only in a particular building or part of a building; their symptoms resolve away from the building and do not occur in other locations.

15. What is the time course of an adverse reaction to an environmental substance in a patient with MCS?

Patients usually report onset within seconds to minutes after a chemical inhalant exposure, but some adverse reactions, especially to foods, may be delayed for up to 24 hours. Typical duration of symptom flares, once triggered, varies from a few minutes to several days.

16. Is MCS an allergic condition?

Historically, an allergist named Theron Randolph first described MCS. He and others suggested that MCS is an allergy in the original sense of the word, i.e., "altered reactivity" to the environment. However, both proponents and critics of MCS as a valid condition acknowledge that immunoglobulin E, the antibody of atopy, does not mediate MCS. Studies have shown some overlap in conditions between patients with hay fever, asthma, eczema, and urticaria diagnoses and patients with MCS, but presently it is not known if atopic allergy and MCS share common mechanisms.

17. What is the distinction between chemical intolerance and MCS?

MCS is a chronic illness of unknown etiology, involving multiple symptoms in multiple different systems. Chemical intolerance (CI) is one symptom that all patients with MCS report. CI involves the experience of a negative hedonic reaction and some degree of illness (e.g., headache, nausea, dizziness) from the odor of low levels of environmental chemicals. CI is synonymous with chemical sensitivity or cacosmia but does not imply any specific mechanism or any specific chemical. Non-MCS patients may experience CI without disability and without fulfilling criteria for a diagnosis of MCS.

18. How common is mild CI in the general population?

CI is surprisingly common in the general population. Various studies suggest that 15–30% may experience some degree of CI, often with concomitant polysymptomatic syndromes similar to but less severe than MCS. It is not known whether they are vulnerable individuals who will develop MCS in the natural course of the condition or whether they remain stable or improve over time. Studies suggest that nondisabled persons with mild CI may exhibit disturbed polysomnographic sleep, elevations and lability in plasma beta endorphin after meals, poorer performance on visual divided attention tests, and sensitization (progressive increases in power or magnitude) of certain EEG frequency bands and/or cardiovascular variables over multiple sessions compared with controls.

19. Do family histories indicate familial or genetic vulnerabilities in patients with MCS or in non-MCS populations with mild CI?

Some research suggests that the family histories of patients with MCS may have a higher prevalence of rhinitis and diabetes mellitus. Non-MCS patients with mild CI also report increased family histories of respiratory problems such as rhinitis, hay fever, and asthma; heart disease; and diabetes mellitus. Of note, despite their own intolerance of alcohol and drugs, preliminary findings indicate more reports of alcohol and/or drug problems in the families of patients with mild CI or MCS than in the family histories of normal controls.

20. Do any patients with MCS recover fully?

Few longitudinal studies are available to document the natural course of MCS. Clinically, a subset of patients remain occupationally and socially disabled for years to decades. Most improve, to varying degrees, and resume a modified active lifestyle over the years. A few report complete remission of problems. The probably multiple factors that contribute to different clinical outcomes need further study.

21. What are the generally accepted treatments for MCS?

Because of the continuing debate about the existence and nature of MCS, medical authorities have not agreed on guidelines for treatment of MCS. Doctors who specialize in the care of patients with MCS, often termed "clinical ecologists" in the past, use an array of controversial medically oriented interventions:

1. Strict avoidance of chemical exposure by relocation of home to a remote area and modification of home furnishings to eliminate carpet, natural gas, cleaning agents, pesticides, and other suspected eliciting agents

2. Dietary changes, including elimination of identified offending foods and rotation diet for currently tolerated items (no food is eaten more often than once in 4 days to avoid activating intolerances)

3. Saunas to remove presumptive toxicants stored in fat

4. Neutralization therapy with sublingual drops or intradermal injections, relying on certain doses of diluted chemicals and foods to turn off or prevent symptom flares on reexposures

5. Nutritional therapies to boost metabolic and/or immune functions

6. Other complementary or alternative therapies

Many proponents and skeptics agree that diagnosis of a comorbid psychiatric condition may indicate a need for psychotropic medications and/or psychotherapy (e.g., supportive psychotherapy for adjustment problems, behavioral desensitization for phobic avoidance, cognitive-behavioral therapy for some cases of panic disorder or depression). Experimental treatments may include use of anticonvulsants such as gabapentin to treat a presumptively sensitized but subconvulsive disturbance in the limbic nervous system. However, because most patients with MCS report poor tolerance for medications, including antidepressants, conventional care is difficult. Patients also resist psychiatric referrals, believing that they imply a purely psychogenic rather than medical etiology for their health problems and indicate rejection or abandonment by the provider. Some patients report that the controversial therapies outlined above provide satisfactory treatment for their psychological distress.

22. What types of specialist referrals may be helpful in determining the problems of a patient with MCS?

As in any presenting problem, some patients' needs may include referrals to specialists: occupational medicine specialists, allergists, rheumatologists, pulmonologists, gastroenterologists, psychiatrists, neuropsychologists, or neurologists. At times industrial hygienists are needed to determine chemical exposure levels at home or work.

23. List the major theories about possible mechanisms for MCS.

Although proponents of different models often emphasize only their own perspective, it is possible and perhaps likely that multiple mechanisms contribute to and interact in MCS. Hypothesized mechanisms include the following:

1. Irritant effects—nonspecific activation of somatic dysfunction (e.g., vasomotor rhinitis), including, but not limited to, trigeminal nerve-mediated irritation.

2. Immune dysregulation—non-IgE-mediated disturbances that produce somatic and CNS symptoms.

3. Atypical porphyria—a disturbance of heme metabolism with prominent central nervous system and gastrointestinal manifestations.

4. Psychogenic effects—psychological factors, including suggestion and expectation, trigger symptoms without direct biologic effects of chemicals.

5. Misattribution of psychiatric symptoms—symptoms of depression, panic disorder, or somatization disorder overlap those of MCS, thereby underlying the clinical picture, but patients mistake chemicals as the cause of their symptoms.

6. Classical conditioning—the learned association from repeated pairing of an initially neutral stimulus without biologic effects, such as a low-level odor (conditioned stimulus [CS]), to a biologically active stimulus, such as a toxic chemical (unconditioned stimulus [US]) so that the CS eventually elicits effects without the presence of the US. This theory requires an initiating toxic chemical exposure as US, and symptoms should fade (i.e., extinguish) on their own over time without re-pairing of the CS with the US.

7. Neurogenic inflammation—a nonimmunologically mediated form of inflammation involving C-fiber pain nerves, at which irritant chemicals activate release of a cascade of endogenous mediators, including substance P. This theory accounts for many of the somatic symptoms of MCS.

8. Neural sensitization—a nonimmunologically mediated form of amplification of responses in behavioral, neurochemical, autonomic, hormonal, or immune pathways by repeated intermittent exposures to a stimulus. Drugs, chemicals, and stress may initiate and elicit heightened reactivity and cross-sensitize with each other. This theory accounts for the recurrent and worsening long-term nature of MCS in addition to various psychiatric disorders, including substance abuse, PTSD, depression, panic disorder, eating disorders, and somatization disorder. A special form of sensitization, limbic kindling, is an animal model for temporal lobe epilepsy (TLE); MCS involves some TLE-like symptoms.

24. Discuss the controversies surrounding MCS.

MCS has engendered intense debate and disagreement among professionals as to its nature, course, and treatment. Critics charge that doctors specializing in MCS offer unproven therapies that put patients at risk for negative outcomes, ranging from disappointment and financial loss to iatrogenic social isolation and occupational disability. Some skeptics report remission of MCS symptoms in selected patients treated with conventional behavioral approaches. Proponents insist that patients worsen without aggressive chemical avoidance and detoxification programs. Methodologic problems make it extremely difficult to perform properly designed double-blind, placebo-controlled challenge studies in MCS. One issue is blinding odorants at suprathreshold concentrations. Masking odors used as placebo may or may not be neutral on first or later reexposures. In addition, MCS advocates suggest that cross-reacting chronic exposures leave many patients in a habituated state, unable to respond acutely to test exposures without full avoidance in a special, environmentally controlled hospital unit for 4–7 days. Research units for this purpose are not available. Many patients pursue workers' compensation claims and/or litigation against employers and building owners, forcing much of the discussion into the adversarial legal rather than scientific area. Previous research on MCS is often flawed by the recruitment biases of patient samples chosen from clinical settings in which disability applications are under evaluation. In addition, the debate within medicine has taken a dualistic direction, pitting psychogenic models against toxogenic models of illness. Ironically, the fields of psychiatry and psychosomatic medicine actively pursue a far more multivariate, integrative view of psychiatric and psychophysiologic illnesses, involving biologic, psychological, and social factors, than occurs in the MCS debate. Research is further hampered by lack of a generally accepted case definition, in contrast with other controversial illnesses such as chronic fatigue syndrome or fibromyalgia. Nevertheless, researchers are slowly delineating the characteristics of MCS and beginning to find evidence for clinically different subtypes. Regardless of diagnostic labeling, the mechanisms by which patients with MCS develop illness are likely to be far more complex than current understanding allows. More rigorous research and rational discussion outside the courtroom will help advance the field in coming years.

BIBLIOGRAPHY

1. Ashford NA, Miller CS: Chemical Exposures: Low Levels and High Stakes, 2nd ed. New York, Van Nostrand Reinhold, 1998.
2. Bell IR, Baldwin CM, Schwartz GE: Illness from low levels of environmental chemicals: Relevance to chronic fatigue syndrome and fibromyalgia. Am J Med 105(Suppl):745–825, 1998.
3. Bell IR, Peterson JM, Schwartz GE: Medical histories and psychological profiles of middle-aged women with and without self-reported illness from environmental chemicals. J Clin Psychiatry 56:151–160, 1995.
4. Cullen MR: The worker with multiple chemical sensitivities: An overview. Occup Med State Art Rev 2(4):655–662, 1987.
5. Fiedler N, Kipen H: Chemical sensitivity: The scientific literature. Environ Health Perspect 105(Suppl 2):409–415, 1997.
6. Fiedler N, Kipen HM, DeLuca J, et al: A controlled comparison of multiple chemical sensitivities and chronic fatigue syndrome. Psychosom Med 58:38–49, 1996.
7. Kipen HM, Hallman W, Kelly-McNeil K, Fiedler N: Measuring chemical sensitivity prevalence: A questionnaire for population studies. Am J Public Health 85:574–577, 1995.
8. Kreutzer R, Neutra RR, Lashuay N: The prevalence of people reporting sensitivities to chemicals in a population based survey. Am J Epidemiol, in press, 1998.
9. Miller CS: Toxicant-induced loss of tolerance—An emerging theory of disease? Environ Health Perspect 105(Suppl 2):445–453, 1997.
10. Miller CS, Mitzel HC: Chemical sensitivity attributed to pesticide exposure versus remodeling. Arch Environ Health 50:119–129, 1995.
11. Ross GH: History and clinical presentation of the chemically sensitive patient. Toxicol Industr Health 8:21–28, 1992.
12. Simon GE, Katon WJ, Sparks PJ: Allergic to life: Psychological factors in environmental illness. Am J Psychiatry 147:901–906, 1990.
13. Sparks PJ, Daniell W, Black DW, et al: Multiple chemical sensitivity syndrome: A clinical perspective. I: Case definition, theories of pathogenesis, and research needs. J Occup Med 36:718–730, 1994.
14. Sparks PJ, Daniell W, Black DW, et al: Multiple chemical sensitivity syndrome: A clinical perspective. II: Evaluation, diagnostic testing, treatment, and social considerations. J Occup Med 36:731–737, 1994.
15. Sullivan J, Bell IR, Meggs W: Multiple chemical sensitivity and low level chemical intolerance. In Sullivan JB, Krieger GR (eds): Clinical Principles of Environmental Health, 2nd ed. Baltimore, Williams & Wilkins, 1998.
16. Szarek MJ, Bell IR, Schwartz GE: Validation of a brief screening measure of environmental chemical sensitivity: The chemical odor intolerance index. J Environ Psychol 17:345–351, 1997.

V. Practice of Occupational Medicine

49. PULMONARY FUNCTION TESTS

Russell P. Bowler, M.D.

1. What are pulmonary function tests?

Pulmonary function tests (PFTs) aid in understanding the mechanisms of ventilation and respiration. Spirometry, lung volumes, diffusing capacity, airway mechanics, and airway reactivity are the most common PFTs. Spirometry is the cheapest, easiest, and most frequently used (yet still clinically underutilized) measurement.

2. How are spirometry measurements made?

Spirometry measures the volume and flow rate of air at the mouth over time. The patient is coached to expire maximally, to make a good seal on the mouthpiece, and then to attempt maximal inspiration followed by maximal expiration. At least three measurements are made, and the best effort is recorded. Measurements can be displayed as either volume vs. time or flow rate vs. volume. Lack of coaching, poor patient effort, incorrect technique, and equipment malfunction contribute to unreliable measurements. Many spirometry devices are inexpensive and portable; however, spirometric measurements are most reliable when performed by a trained technician in a pulmonary function laboratory. The American Thoracic Society (ATS) has published additional guidelines to ensure reproducibility.

3. What data are obtained from spirometry?

The most useful data obtained from spirometry are forced expiratory volume at one second (FEV_1), forced vital capacity (FVC), and the FEV_1/FVC ratio. Spirometry also is used to measure peak expiratory flow rates, forced expiratory flow from 25–75% of FVC, abnormal inspiratory flow loops, and response to inhaled drugs or antigens. Spirometry may be diagnostic of abnormal airway resistance (obstructive lung disease). Although spirometry may suggest restrictive lung disease, it is insufficient to make the diagnosis. Formal lung volume measurements are necessary to diagnose restrictive lung disease.

4. What are flow-volume loops?

Flow-volume loops plot volumes on the horizontal axis and flows on the vertical axis (see figure, top of next page).

5. How are lung volumes measured?

Total lung capacity (TLC) represents the volume of air in the lungs after maximal inspiration. Residual volume (RV) is the volume left in the lungs after maximal expiration. TLC and RV cannot be measured with spirometry but can be calculated by several techniques. Helium dilution relies on an inert gas (helium) to measure lung volumes. Nitrogen washout also uses dilution to measure volumes. After 7 minutes of 100% inspired oxygen, expired gas is collected and the concentration of nitrogen is measured. Lung volumes from both methods are calculated by extrapolation of the dilution of the measured gases. A much different technique, plethysmography, uses Boyle's law (pressure times volume of a gas yields a constant at fixed temperature) to measure volumes. Plethysmography is the most accurate measurement of lung volumes, because dilution techniques measure only the volume that freely communicates with the larger airways. Dilution

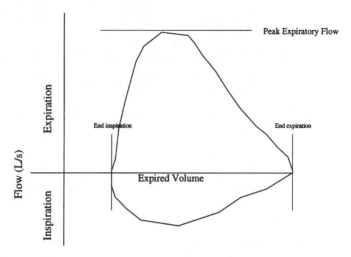

Normal flow-volume loop.

techniques may underestimate true lung volumes in patients with noncommunicating lung segments (e.g., bullae).

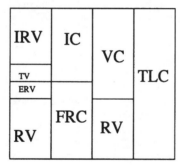

Lung volumes. Total lung capacity (TLC), vital capacity (VC), residual volume (RV), inspiratory capacity (IC), tidal volume (TV), inspiratory reserve volume (IRV), expiratory reserve volume (ERV), and functional residual capacity (FRC).

6. What is the forced oscillation technique?

The forced oscillation technique (FOT) measures induced flow oscillations from sinusoidal pressure variations applied by an external generator at the mouth. It measures resistive, elastic, and inertial properties of the respiratory system. The role of FOT in detecting early respiratory impairment in pneumoconiosis is under study.

7. What is DL_{CO}?

DL_{CO} is the diffusing capacity for carbon monoxide (CO) in the lung. In Europe it is called the transfer factor. The DL_{CO} measures the volume of CO gas that diffuses across the alveolar capillary membrane. It is a good measure of the cross-sectional area of the alveolar capillary membrane in the lung. Any disease that impairs alveolar capillary beds decreases the DL_{CO}. Nonpulmonary factors may change DL_{CO} measurement. Smokers have elevated levels of CO in the blood, which tends to lower CO uptake during the test. Patients with anemia have less hemoglobin to bind CO and therefore have lower DL_{CO}. Finally, patients at high altitude have lower oxygen saturations and therefore high DL_{CO}. Decreased DL_{CO} can be found in interstitial lung diseases (e.g., pneumoconioses), emphysema, and pulmonary vascular disease.

8. What are normal values for PFTs?

The wide range of normal values depends on the patient's demographic group. Age, height, race, and sex are all-important predictors of spirometry and lung volumes. For instance, African-Americans have a 10–14% decrease in FEV_1 and FVC compared with non-Hispanic Caucasians. Without the appropriate reference group or regression formula, PFTs cannot be determined to be normal or abnormal.

9. How much change is considered significant in spirometry measurements?

On repeated testing FEV_1 and FVC may vary up to 5% per day, 12% per week, and 15% per year in normal people. In patients with obstructive lung disease the variation may be twice as high. A rise of at least 200 ml and 12% in FVC or FEV_1 after bronchodilator is considered a significant response. Lack of a significant bronchodilator response does not preclude the use of a bronchodilator if clinically indicated.

10. What is obstructive lung disease?

Obstructive lung disease results from an impediment to airflow on expiration. A reduction of airflow without a reduction in FEV_1 does not currently define an obstructive defect. Obstructive lung disease is therefore diagnosed with spirometry. A decrease in FEV_1 of more than 20% of normal is considered abnormal. FVC may be normal or decreased. The FEV_1/FVC ratio is decreased. When measuring lung volumes one often finds an elevated RV and TLC. Occupational asthma is the most common occupational obstructive lung disease. Airflow obstruction may be reversible; therefore, one cannot exclude the diagnosis of obstructive lung disease when spirometry is normal. A typical flow loop from a patient suffering from acute airflow obstruction during an occupational asthma attack is shown in the figure below.

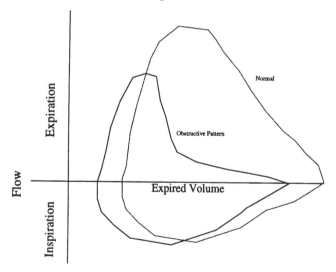

Flow loop from a patient with obstructive lung disease with a marked decrease in expiratory flow rates at lower lung volumes.

11. What role do PFTs play in diagnosing occupational asthma?

An isolated PFT is often not helpful in making the diagnosis of occupational asthma. Serial spirometry performed before and after a period of work is most helpful in establishing an association between asthma and the workplace. The worker can obtain peak expiratory flow rates (PEFR) every 2 hours at the workplace to identify the interval between exposure and airway obstruction. Patient compliance with self-testing is often a problem. Serial bronchial challenge tests and specific bronchial challenge tests also may be useful in correlating asthma with the workplace.

12. What is the difference between PEFR and spirometry?

Portable flow meters (e.g., the Wright peak-flow meter) are invaluable in allowing patients to self-monitor changes in airflow (e.g., to assist in the diagnosis of occupational asthma). PEFR is the highest flow rate in the expiratory cycle and is typically reported in liters/minute. Flows also can be obtained from spirometry measurements but are reported in liters/second. One can obtain PEFR from spirometry by measuring the top of the flow loop and multiplying by 60 to obtain PEFR in liters/minute. Spirometry requires more training than PEFR; however, it measures the more clinically useful FEV_1 and FVC. Neither PEFR nor spirometry is useful without proper technique and full patient effort.

13. What is an inhaled bronchial challenge?

Normally asthma is characterized by reversible small airway obstruction, airway inflammation, and airway hyperresponsiveness. When the clinical history suggests asthma in patients with normal spirometry and no response to bronchodilators, measurement of airway hyperresponsiveness is a useful laboratory test. Inhaled bronchial challenge testing uses various aerosolized agents to provoke airway hyperresponsiveness. The most common agents are methacholine and histamine, which nonspecifically induce airway hyperresponsiveness. Specific agents suggested by the occupational history, such as toluene diisocyanate, also can be tested. Before testing the patient is asked to withhold all medicines that may affect airway caliber (e.g., bronchodilators). The patient is then placed in an enclosed space and exposed to increasing concentrations of the aerosolized agent. A positive test occurs when the inhaled methacholine level is < 8 mg/ml and there is either a 40% fall in airway conductance (Sgaw) or a 20% and at least 200 ml fall in FEV_1. Bronchoconstriction may occur early (within 30 minutes), late (4–8 hours), or both early and late. Patients with obstructive lung disease and airway hyperresponsiveness may have a worse prognosis. The sensitivity of methacholine challenge is 90–95% in asthmatic patients, but its specificity is low.

14. What are restrictive lung diseases?

Restrictive lung diseases are characterized by reduced compliance or stiffening of the lung that leads to decreased lung volumes. On spirometry FVC and FEV_1 are reduced, but the FEV_1/FVC ratio may be normal or elevated. Measurement of lung volumes usually reveals diminished RV and TLC. A pattern of restrictive lung disease on PFTs may be seen with hypersensitivity pneumonitis, inhalational fevers, hard metal disease, beryllium disease, chronic silicosis, and asbestosis.

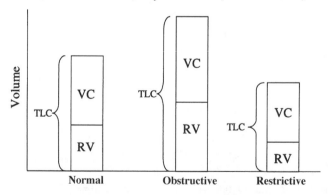

Lung volumes in normal controls and patients with obstructive or restrictive lung disease.

15. When is the pressure-volume curve useful?

Pressure-volume (PV) curves measure the compliance of the lung at different lung volumes. An esophageal balloon is placed to allow measurement of transpulmonary pressure. Compliance is calculated by measuring the change in volume divided by the change in transpulmonary pressure.

The PV curve is used mainly for the diagnosis of interstitial lung disease (low compliance) and emphysema (high compliance). The PV curve also helps to distinguish obesity (chest wall) from parenchymal lung disease.

16. How does one evaluate occupational disability secondary to respiratory disorders?

The FEV_1, FVC, FEV_1/FVC ratio, and DL_{CO} are the primary tests recommended for the determination of respiratory impairment. In 1986 the ATS adopted arbitrary percentages of mean predicted values to indicate different levels of impairment. Because the respiratory system has substantial reserve, usually only moderate-to-severe impairment becomes limiting in the workplace. A patient who has no or mild impairment but continues to exhibit occupationally related respiratory symptoms should be considered a candidate for further testing such as inhaled bronchial challenge or clinical exercise testing. Attributing impairment to occupational exposures requires clinical judgment.

Rating of Pulmonary Impairment

IMPAIRMENT	FVC (%)	FEV_1 (%)	FEV_1/FVC (%)	DL_{CO} (%)
Normal	> 80	> 80	> 75	> 80
Mild	60–79	60–79	60–74	60–79
Moderate	51–59	41–59	41–59	41–59
Severe	< 51	< 41	< 41	< 41

17. When should cardiopulmonary exercise testing be ordered in the occupational medicine setting?

Cardiopulmonary exercise testing (CPET) measures gas exchange, oxygen uptake, ventilation, and cardiovascular function during symptom-limited maximal exercise. It is useful in determining the origin of dyspnea for suspected cardiac or pulmonary disease as well as assessing the functional exercise capabilities of the patient for occupational limitations or compensation. CPET is useful in documenting progressive exercise impairment in patients with restrictive lung disease. Oxygen uptake (V_{O_2}) has been estimated for various activities, but the results should be applied to specific occupational tasks in an individual worker with caution. CPET does not distinguish occupational asthma from nonoccupational asthma.

Oxygen Uptake during Various Activities

ACTIVITY	V_{O_2}
Office work	5–7 ml/kg/min
Moderate labor	15 ml/kg/min
Strenuous heavy labor	20–30 ml/kg/min

BIBLIOGRAPHY

1. American Thoracic Society: Evaluation of impairment/disability secondary to respiratory disorders. Am Rev Respir Dis 133:1205–1209, 1986.
2. American Thoracic Society: Standardization of spirometry—1987 update. Am Rev Respir Dis 136:1285–1298, 1987.
3. American Thoracic Society: Lung function testing: Selection of reference values and interpretative strategies. Am Rev Respir Dis 144:1202–1218, 1991.
4. Chan-Yeung M: Assessment of asthma in the workplace. American College of Chest Physicians Consensus Statement. Chest 108:1084–1117, 1995.
5. Clausen JL, Coates AL, Quanjer PH: Measurement of lung volumes in humans: Review and recommendations from an ATS/ERS workshop [editorial comment]. Eur Respir J 10:1205–1206, 1997.
6. Glindmeyer HW, Lefante JJ, JOnes RN, et al: Exposure-related declines in the lung function of cotton textile workers. Relationship to current workplace standards. Am Rev Respir Dis 144:675–683, 1991.

7. Harving H, Dahl R, Molhave L: Lung function and bronchial reactivity in asthmatics during exposure to volatile organic compounds. Am Rev Respir Dis 143:751–754, 1991.

8. Mannix ET, Dresser KS, Aukley D, et al: Cardiopulmonary exercise testing in the evaluation of patients with occupational asthma and reactive airways dysfunction syndrome. J Investig Med 46:236–242, 1998.

9. Pham QT, Bourgkard E, Chau N, et al: Forced oscillation technique (FOT): A new tool for epidemiology of occupational lung diseases? Eur Respir J 8:1307–1313, 1995.

10. Rijcken B, Shouten JP, Weiss ST, Ware JH: ERS/ATS workshop on longitudinal analysis of pulmonary function data, Barcelona, September 1995. Eur Respir J 10:758–763, 1997 [published erratum appears in Eur Respir J 10:1197, 1997].

11. Stocks J, Quanjer PH: Reference values for residual volume, functional residual capacity, and total lung capacity. ATS Workshop on Lung Volume Measurements. Official Statement of the European Respiratory Society. Eur Respir J 8:492–506, 1995.

12. Sue DY: Exercise testing in the evaluation of impairment and disability. Clin Chest Med 15:369–387, 1994.

50. WORKPLACE SMOKING AND DRUG AND ALCOHOL USE

Marilyn Thatcher, Ph.D.

1. What are the divisions between social substance use, abuse, and dependence?

Use: I like
Abuse: I want
Dependence: I need

The physician often makes the initial diagnosis of substance-related problems. Interviews can determine patients' substance use. Quantity is not a valid criteria. "One glass of wine a day" may be one large tumbler in the patient's translation. The crucial question is whether substance use has affected at least one area of daily living (e.g., legal issues, job, finances, family life, emotional health, socialization, or physical health).

2. Why is early identification of substance abuse important in the workplace?

Alcohol and other substances affect cortical functioning over time. If early assistance is not provided, the patient may not have the residual brain capacity to maintain sobriety. For example, frontal lobe functions are a common site of damage from heavy use of alcohol, cocaine, or methamphetamines. The brain's ability to determine cause and effect, to apply higher-order reasoning, and to inhibit ongoing behavior may well be impaired. In addition, impairment of work performance may increase the risk of on-the-job injuries. Use of heavy machinery, driving work vehicles, and executive tasks requiring higher-order reasoning may be impaired. Alcohol particularly disturbs global processing, response time, and capacity for divided attention.

3. Why not refer the patient directly to a psychiatrist?

Psychiatric intervention may be appropriate for prescription of medication and addressing concomitant psychological issues. It is a general principle that substance abusers should not receive insight-oriented therapy for at least 1 year. Too rapid a reduction of defense mechanisms may increase substance use. The exception may be cognitive-behavioral therapy which attempts to change belief systems.

4. How important is an extended family medical history?

Genetic research shows a 50% chance of alcoholism if one parent is an alcoholic. The risk increases to almost 90% if both parents are alcoholics. Research suggests that 60% of substance abuse cases are hereditary and 40% environmental.

5. What if the patient firmly denies any problem with substances?

Denial plays a large part in the presentation of substance abuse. Observe the patient's manner of denial. Excessive protestations with emotional charge and escalating statements of denial are a red flag. The clinicians should deal with denial in the following ways:

1. Name it.
2. Confront the patient as an ally with a nonjudgmental stance.
3. Offer hope.

6. What important questions should be asked during a patient visit?

Formal interview schedules such as the Michigan Alcohol Screening Test (MAST) are available. Briefer formats include the **CAGE** and **FOY** questionnaires:

CAGE
- Have you ever felt the need to   **cut** down on your drinking?
- Have you ever felt   **annoyed** by criticism of your drinking?
- Have you ever felt   **guilty** about your drinking?
- Have you ever taken a morning   **eye-opener**?

FOY
- Has your   **family** ever objected to your drinking?
- Have   **others** ever said that you drank too much for your own good?
- Did   **you** ever think that you drank too much in general?

Ask patients specifically to **qualify** and **quantify** their substance use. For example, what is the longest period without substance use? Ask patients to describe the role of alcohol in their life. For example, does it facilitate social interactions? Reduce stress? Help with sleep? Look for a preoccupation with substances. How much of the patient's day revolves around alcohol? Be aware of faulty self-reporting and overelaborate responses to persuade you that alcohol use is within normal limits. Ask about the patient's behavior when he or she is drinking.

7. What physical symptoms are expected in alcoholic patients?

Difficulty with sleep, frequent accidents by falls and in vehicles, complaints of heartburn, increased heart rate when drinking, and weight loss.

8. What laboratory tests are related to a diagnosis of alcoholism?

Results may not be positive in early phase but are useful to help break the patient's denial.

Blood Alcohol

- Alcohol abuse (National Council on Alcoholism criteria):
  - \> 100 mg/dl at the time of routine medical exam
  - \> 150 mg/dl without gross evidence of intoxication
  - \> 300 mg/dl at any time
- Elevated mean corpuscular volume
- Elevated aspartate aminotransferase, alanine aminotransferase, lactate dehydrogenase
- Elevated gamma-glutamyl transpeptidase (particularly sensitive)
- Decreased albumin, vitamin B_{12}, folic acid
- Increased uric acid, elevated amylase

---

9. What if the patient reports numerous stressors and describes substance use as temporary?

Faulty attribution is common among substance abusers. Until denial is resolved, substance use is often attributed to external causes. Overuse of the word "stress" should be noted.

10. How is the patient's family relevant to the physician?

Determine whether the patient has lost close relationships in the past year and, if so, why. It is often necessary to obtain collateral information from family members about substance use.

11. Is adequate or superior job performance a contraindication to a substance problem?

Many users function well in their daily job but use alcohol or other substances excessively in the evening. The ability to maintain performance at work is not a valid criterion.

12. Does substance abuse occur only as a result of faulty internal psychological dynamics?

Substance use may occur in isolation without psychological concomitants. Many users are highly intelligent, successful people with a well-integrated psychological make-up.

13. Is age a significant factor in substance-abusing patients?

Be aware of the older population and alcohol use. Many older people grew up in a time when social drinking was a natural transition from day to evening ("the cocktail hour"). Issues of loneliness, isolation, loss of family, and altered job role may move the older social drinker into abuse. A secondary issue is the combining of alcohol with prescribed medication and the patient's lack of sophistication about the dangers involved.

14. How does alcoholism fit with the model of disease?
Alcoholism is a chronic, progressive illness with an insidious onset. It affects all areas of the person's life. Prolonged alcohol use typically results in diverse organ system damage, affecting the liver, heart, endorphin system, gastrointestinal tract, and nervous system, as well as increasing rate of infections. It has been estimated that over 93% of alcoholics presenting for treatment have serious medical problems. Alcoholics are likely to die 15 years earlier than the general population.

15. How does alcohol differ neurochemically from other substances?
Alcohol does not have a specific receptor site in the body.

16. Where is the site of action for addiction in the brain?
The mesolimbic system, in which instinctual drives and ability to experience emotions and pleasure reside, is believed to be the site of addiction. Specifically, the medial forebrain bundle (MFB) is considered the pleasure pathway. Impaired control of drug use is theorized to be related to a person's perception that the drug is necessary for existence, much like breathing, hunger, thirst, and sex.

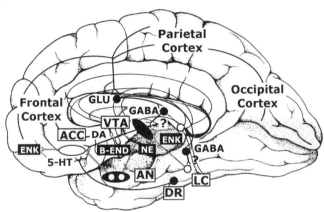

Mesolimbic system as it is involved in addiction to drugs. ACC, nucleus accumbens; VTA, ventral tegmental area; AN, arcuate nucleus; LC, locus ceruleus; DR, dorsal raphé; GLU, glutamate; GABA, gamma-aminobutyric acid; ENK, enkephalin; NE, norepinephrine; DA, dopamine; β-END, beta endorphin; 5-HT, 5-hydroxytryptamine (serotonin). (Modified from Crossman AR, Neary D: Neuroanatomy: An Illustrated Colour Text. New York, Churchill Livingstone, 1995, p 97.)

17. What brain chemicals have a dominant role in addiction?
Scientific theory suggests that addiction results from neurochemical dysfunction with a chemical deficiency in one or more parts of the MFB. Specific chemicals include the following:

1. Dopamine   3. Endorphin
2. Serotonin   4. Gamma-aminobutyric acid (GABA)

Drug dependence (addiction) is a disease over which the patient has minimal control. New treatments with neuropharmacology may soon be available. Drug abuse (misuse) is a behavioral problem that responds to education and environmental changes.

18. Why is cocaine the most addictive drug?
Cocaine produces intense and prolonged cravings. Stimulants produce almost the same effects as normal actions of the sympathetic nervous system and have a molecular structure similarity to that of neurotransmitters. The primary mechanism of action is the blockade of the reuptake of

dopamine. After an initial "rush," intense craving probably results from depletion of dopamine and serotonin. Laws of learning predict that elimination of an aversive state (craving), coupled with feelings of euphoria, creates a behavior likely to be repeated.

19. Where does nicotine fit in the pattern of addiction?

Nicotine is a prototype for addiction: ingestion occurs despite known dangers; smokers believe that they can quit any time but do not; the rate of relapse is high; genetic factors play a role in use; cessation attempts usually involve titration of dose; and the user denies smoking-related problems that are obvious to others.

20. What treatment approaches are effective for smoking cessation?

A combination approach should be used, including relief of withdrawal symptoms, education, and behavioral therapies. Hypnosis is successful in a small percentage of cases. Maintaining a high motivational state for cessation appears to be a key factor.

21. Do some psychiatric disorders have a high concomitant rate of substance use?

Patients with bipolar disorder (manic depression) are more likely to abuse substances because of the urge for excessive behaviors. Attention deficit-hyperactive disorder has a 40% comorbid risk for substance abuse in adolescents and adults.

22. What is the next step if substance abuse appears to be a diagnostic issue?

Approach the patient directly in a nonjudgmental manner about your concerns for his or her physical health. Have a list of available resources at hand, including employee assistance programs, Alcoholics Anonymous, and short- and long-term rehabilitation facilities. Have cards available with the appropriate phone numbers. Schedule a follow-up visit to verify follow-through.

23. What important caveats should be kept in mind with substance-abusing patients?

1. Be aware of your own opinions and judgments about substance users: hopeless cases? Character defect in will power?

2. Do not collude with the patient's denial.

3. Tell the truth about your concerns.

4. Do not use an early intervention of psychotropic medications that may mask and/or delay treating a substance-related problem.

5. Discuss issues of confidentiality, particularly in relation to job security.

6. Assure patients that help is available. People who are already in the workforce have a much higher success rate for attaining sobriety.

BIBLIOGRAPHY

1. Berman SM, Soyenobu B, Zaidel E: Multiple callosal channels: Evidence from alcohol and event-related potentials. Presented at the Twenty-sixth Annual International Neuropsychology Society Meeting, February, 1998.
2. Brick J, Erickson CK: Drugs, the Brain and Behavior. The Pharmacology of Abuse and Dependence. New York, Hawthorne Medical Press, 1998, pp 159–165.
3. Deckel AW, Bauer L, Hesselbrock V: Anterior brain dysfunctioning as a risk factor in alcoholic behaviors. Addiction 90:1323–1334, 1995.
4. Knight RG, Longmore BE: Clinical Neuropsychology of Alcoholism. East Sussex (UK), Lawrence Erlbaum Associates, 1994, pp 31–50.
5. Lavine R: Personal correspondence, March, 1998.
6. Parsons OA, Butters N, Nathan PE (eds): Neuropsychology of Alcoholism: Implications for Diagnosis and Treatment. New York, Guilford Press, 1987, pp 153–173.
7. Schuckit MA: Drug and Alcohol Abuse: A Clinical Guide to Diagnosis and Treatment. New York, Plenum Press, 1995.
8. Tarter RE, Van Thiel DH, Edwards KL (eds): Medical Neuropsychology. The Impact of Disease on Behavior. New York, Plenum Press, 1988, pp 84–89.
9. White WL: Slaying the Dragon. The History of Addiction Treatment and Recovery in America. Illinois, Chestnut Health Systems/Lighthouse Institute, 1998.

51. WORKFORCE VIOLENCE

Robert Harrison, M.D., M.P.H.

1. What is workplace violence?

The scope of workplace violence ranges from offensive language to homicide and includes actions that make one person uncomfortable in the workplace; threats and harassment; and bodily injury inflicted by one person on another.

The National Institute for Occupational Safety and Health (NIOSH) defines workplace violence as "violent acts, including physical assaults and threats of assault, directed towards persons at work or on duty." These acts may include beating, obscene telephone calls, rape, suicide, attempted suicide, intimidation, shooting, stabbing, harassment, threat, following someone, or swearing or shouting at someone. A workplace is any location, either permanent or temporary, where an employee performs any job-related duty. It may include buildings, surrounding premises, parking lots, field locations, clients' homes, and vehicles used to travel to and from work assignments.

The U.S. Bureau of Labor Statistics classifies workplace homicide according to the type of circumstance, such as business disputes (including actions of a coworker or former coworker), customer or client disputes, disputes involving a relative of the victim (such as spouse or ex-spouse, boyfriend or ex-boyfriend), incidents involving police or security guards in the line of duty, and incidents in which death occurred during a robbery or crime.

The California Division of Occupational Safety and Health has defined three types of workplace violence. Type 1 involves assailants with no legitimate relationship to the workplace (generally in the course of a robbery or other criminal act). Type II involves customers of a service provided by an establishment or clients, patients, passengers, criminal suspects, or prisoners. Type III involves current or former employees, supervisors, managers, and other persons with employment-related involvement with an establishment, such as an employee's spouse, boyfriend, friend, relative, or a person who has a dispute with an employee.

2. Why is workplace violence an important occupational health problem?

Workplace violence is a major contributor to occupational injury. Homicide at work is the second leading cause of occupation-related death after motor vehicle-related deaths. According to estimates from the National Crime Victimization Survey of the U.S. Department of Justice, approximately 1 million persons per year are assaulted while at work or on duty. Workplace violence represents about 15% of all acts of violence experienced by U.S. residents aged 12 or older. Furthermore, the epidemiology of workplace violence suggests that prevention strategies may be different from strategies to prevent violent injuries in general.

For example, the circumstances of occupational homicides are different from the circumstances of homicides in general. Robbery is a factor in about 75% of occupational homicides, whereas robbery is involved in only about 9% of all homicides. Although almost one-half of all murder victims in the general population were related to or knew their assailants, most occupational homicides involve persons not known to one another. Workplace violence also disproportionately affects certain occupations. More than one-half of workplace homicides and more than three-quarters of all nonfatal workplace assaults occur in retail trade and service industries. Therefore, the risk of workplace violence is associated with specific factors that largely involve dealing with the public (e.g., clients, patients, inmates, or customers).

3. What are the major causes of workplace homicides?

NIOSH reports that over the past 10–15 years homicides have surpassed machine-related deaths as the second leading cause of fatal occupational injuries. Work-related homicides are primarily an urban problem; eight of the largest U.S. metropolitan areas account for almost one-half of the total number of incidents. The average workplace homicide rate for 1980–1992 was 0.70/100,000 workers. The majority (80%) of workplace homicides occur among men, although homicides are the leading cause (42%) of occupational fatalities among women. The risk of homicide among men is more than three times the risk among women. Most homicides among men occur in retail, service, public administration, or transportation industries; most homicides among women occur in the retail and service industries. The largest number of workplace homicides occurs in the 25–34-year-old group, but the highest rate occurs in workers aged 65 or older. Most homicide victims are Caucasian, although African-American workers have rates 2–3 times higher than Caucasian workers.

Firearms account for an increasing percentage of all workplace homicides and are now involved in over three-quarters of all fatal injuries at work. The largest number of deaths occur in grocery stores, eating and drinking places, taxicab services, and justice/public order establishments. Taxicab services also have the highest rate of work-related homicide, followed by liquor stores, detective/protective services, gas service stations, and jewelry stores. For occupational groups, the highest rates occur among taxicab drivers/chauffeurs, sheriffs/bailiffs, police and detectives, gas station/garage workers, and security guards. The U.S. Bureau of Labor Statistics (BLS) reports that robbery was involved in over three-quarters of all workplace homicides; a business dispute or conflict with a coworker or associate, customer, or client accounts for less than one in five deaths on the job.

4. What are the major causes of nonfatal violent injuries?

More limited data are available about the major causes of nonfatal violent injuries. The BLS estimates that most nonfatal assaults occur in the service and retail trades. Among service employees more than 50% occur in nursing homes, social services, or hospitals. The source of injury in most cases was a patient. Most injuries involve hitting, kicking, or beating. A survey completed by a major life insurance company estimated that 2.2 million workplace assaults occurred between July 1992 and July 1993. A household survey by the U.S. Department of Justice from 1987–1992 indicated that each year about 1 million persons were assaulted at work or on duty. Workplace assaults represented 15% of all acts of violence experienced by Americans during that period. Women workers were more likely to be attacked by someone they knew. Government workers accounted for disproportionately more work-related violence, suggesting a great risk in dealing with the public or delivering services to clients.

Workers' compensation data have recently been used to describe the major causes of nonfatal workplace injury. Data from California indicate that the greatest risk of nonfatal workplace assaults is among police, correctional employees, bus drivers, hospital workers, and security guards. The overall rate of nonfatal occupational assaults was 72.9 per 100,000, approximately 50 times the rate of fatal occupational injury. When police reports of workplace assault were included for eight cities, the combined annual rate of workplace assault was 184.7 per 100,000 workers, almost twice the rate found by either source individually. Almost two-thirds of all nonfatal workplace injuries are type II—involving a customer or client. Minnesota workers' compensation claims data show that women have an assault rate twice that of men. The greatest number of assaults occurred among nursing aides, orderlies, and attendants. Social service workers had the highest rate of injury (169 per 100,000 workers). Most assailants were people with whom the workers were in contact as part of their jobs (e.g., patients, clients, inmates, or customers). An analysis of 600 nonfatal workplace violence claims at a large workers' compensation insurance carrier found that over one-half of cases were caused by a criminal act (e.g., type I), whereas 38.5% of cases were caused by a patient, client, customer, or student (type II). The highest percentage of nonfatal workplace violence claims were filed by school and health care employees.

5. What are the risk factors for workplace assault?

NIOSH has identified many factors that increase the risk of workplace assault:
• Contact with the public

- Exchange of money
- Delivery of passengers, goods, or services
- Mobile workplace, such as a taxicab or police cruiser
- Working with unstable or volatile persons in health care, social service, or criminal justice settings
- Working alone or in small numbers
- Working late at night or during early morning hours
- Working high-crime areas
- Guarding valuable property or possessions
- Working in community-based settings

6. How can the risk factors for workplace violence be reduced?

The risk factors for workplace violence can be reduced by attention to environmental design, administrative controls, and behavioral strategies. For example, the use of drop safes, carrying small amounts of cash, and posting of signs that limited cash is available may help to reduce assaults in retail establishments. Bullet-resistant barriers or enclosures may be used in gas stations or convenience stores, hospital emergency departments, and social service agencies. Other issues such as visibility, lighting, access/egress, and use of security devices also should be considered. Increasing the number of staff on duty may help to reduce the risk of assault in retail establishments or may reduce frustration among patients, customers, or clients in public service settings. Employee training in hazard recognition, nonviolent response, and conflict resolution is essential.

7. What should be the components of a workplace violence prevention program?

Specific guidelines have been published by federal and state agencies for effective workplace violence prevention programs for health care and social service providers and retail stores. An effective violence prevention program should include the following components:

- Management commitment and employee involvement
- Workplace security analysis
- Hazard prevention and control measures
- Incident reporting and follow-up procedures
- Employee and supervisor training
- Recordkeeping
- Evaluation

One of the first steps in developing a workplace violence prevention program is to establish a system for documenting violent incidents. A written policy should specify zero tolerance of violence at work and establish a threat assessment team to which all incidents should be reported. An existing labor-management committee or a joint committee responsible for workplace violence prevention should develop written policies and procedures. The workplace security analysis includes a step-by-step inspection of all areas in and near the workplace to identify potential hazards as well as review of records documenting past incidents. The engineering, administrative, or work practice control measures are selected based specifically on the results of the security analysis. Prevention programs should include posttrauma counseling services for employees and supervisors.

CONTROVERSY

8. Do perpetrator profiles help to identify people who may commit a violent act?

Violent behavior is often difficult to predict. Nevertheless, a history of violence and certain other psychosocial factors often indicate that a person may become violent at work. Indicators of higher risk may include a history of drug or alcohol abuse, serious stress or multiple life stressors, depression, vocational dissonance, poor interpersonal relationships, romantic obsessions, domestic disputes or sexual harassment, severe personality disorders, impaired neurologic functioning, behavioral disintegration, and psychotic and/or paranoid behavior. Many experts suggest that a profile of a typical perpetrator can help to identify the future assailant. However, perpetrators vary widely in age, gender, and background, and it is important to avoid illegal discrimination in developing intervention and prevention measures.

BIBLIOGRAPHY

1. Askari E: Violence on the Job: A Guidebook for Labor and Management. Berkeley, CA, Labor Occupational Health Program, 1997.
2. Baron SA: Organizational factors in workplace violence: Developing effective programs to reduce workplace violence. Occup Med 11:335–348, 1996.
3. Hashemi L, Webster BS: Non-fatal workplace violence workers' compensation claims (1993–1996). J Occup Environ Med 40:561–567, 1998.
4. Howard J: State and regulatory approaches to preventing workplace violence. Occup Med 11:293–302, 1996.
5. Kraus JF, McArthur DL: Epidemiology of violent injury in the workplace. Occup Med 11:201–218, 1996.
6. Lamar WJ, Gerberich SG, Lohman WH, Zaidman B: Work-related physical assault. J Occup Environ Med 40:317–324, 1998.
7. National Institute for Occupational Safety and Health: Violence in the Workplace, Risk Factors and Prevention Strategies [Current Intelligence Bulletin 57.DHHS (NIOSH) 96-100]. Washington, DC, National Institute of Occupational Safety and Health, 1996.
8. Peek-Asa C, Schaffer KB, Kraus JF, Howard J: Surveillance of non-fatal workplace assault injuries, using police and employers' report. J Occup Environ Med 40:707–713, 1998.
9. State of California: Guidelines for Security and Safety of Health Care and Community Service Workers. Sacramento, CA, Division of Occupational Safety and Health, Department of Industrial Relations, 1993.
10. U.S. Department of Labor, Occupational Safety and Health Administration: OSHA Guidelines for Preventing Workplace Violence Among Health Care and Social Service Workers. Washington, DC, Occupational Safety and Health Administration, 1996.
11. U.S. Department of Labor, Occupational Safety and Health Administration: OSHA Guidelines for Workplace Violence Prevention Programs for Night Retail Establishments. Washington, DC, Occupational Safety and Health Administration, 1996.

52. DISABILITY EVALUATION

Stephen L. Demeter, M.D., M.P.H.

1. What are the definitions of impairment, disability, and handicap?

An **impairment** is the inability to complete successfully a specific task based on insufficient intellectual, creative, adaptive, social, or physical skills. A **disability**, on the other hand, is a medical impairment that prevents remunerative employment, desired social or recreational activities, or other personal activities. According to the American Medical Association's guidelines, "An impaired individual is **handicapped** if there are obstacles to accomplishing life's basic activities that can be overcome only by compensating in some way for the effects of the impairment. Such compensation or accommodation often entails the use of assisted devices."

An example serves well. A person who has had an amputation of the fifth digit on the right hand has a medical impairment. Loss of function results from the anatomic deficit. If the person is a physician, this medical impairment may translate into no disability. On the other hand, if the person is a concert pianist, the same medical impairment may create total disability. Thus, disability is task-specific, whereas impairment merely reflects an alteration from normal body functions.

2. What is an impairment evaluation?

An impairment evaluation is a medical evaluation. Its purpose is to define, describe, and measure the differences in a particular individual compared with either the average person (e.g., an IQ of 86 compared with the normal expected average of 100) or the individual's prior capabilities (e.g., a preinjury IQ measured at 134 compared with the current level of 100). Such differences may take the form of anatomic deviations (e.g., amputations), physical abnormalities (e.g., decreased motion of a joint, decreased strength surrounding that joint, or abnormal neurologic input), physiologic abnormalities (e.g., diminished ability to breathe or electrical conduction disturbances in the heart), or psychological (e.g., diminished ability to think and reason or to remember).

3. Who performs an impairment evaluation?

Impairment evaluation should be performed only by professionals with a background in medical practice. Doctors of medicine and osteopathy are the logical choices. However, other professionals also possess such training and background and often perform impairment evaluations. Examples include doctors of chiropractic, dentists, optometrists, psychologists, and physical therapists.

4. How does an impairment evaluation differ from a normal history and physical examination?

The goal of an impairment evaluation is to define deviations from normalcy. Having or arriving at a specific diagnosis/diagnoses is often useful and helpful. However, a specific diagnosis is not the end result in an impairment evaluation as it is in the standard history and physical examination. Both evaluations require appropriate educational background, skill, thoroughness, and dedication. The results of the standard history and physical belong to the patient. The results of an impairment evaluation often do not; they usually are given to attorneys, insurance companies, or governmental agencies (e.g., workers' compensation boards or the Social Security Department). This point often raises an interesting legal concept. Physicians are not allowed to disclose medical information to anyone but the patient. To whom does such confidentiality apply in an impairment evaluation? Usually it exists between the physician and the referring agency or party as opposed to the person evaluated.

Another basic distinction is that the impairment evaluation report centers on the questions that were asked by the referring party. For example, if the physician is asked to evaluate a person for a specific injury, such as arm amputation or dysfunction, the entire process centers on the arm. The end result is a report that describes the injury, differences in the function level of the arm from a normal person's, and a prognosis for future recovery. This information is then used by other parties to determine appropriate compensation. Other diagnoses discovered during the evaluation may be irrelevant.

5. How does a disability evaluation differ from an impairment evaluation?

A disability evaluation is a comprehensive evaluation based on various factors. One of these factors is medical impairment. Other factors may include a person's age, educational background, educational capabilities, and other social factors. Such elements are used by the system to which the worker has applied for relief. For example, a person whose right arm has been amputated may be capable of entering the work force in some other capacity. If the person is young enough, smart enough, and sufficiently motivated, he or she may be capable of performing remunerative activities in some other job market. The referring agency uses such factors when determining whether a person is totally or partially disabled and which benefits are applicable.

6. What is workers' compensation?

According to Elisburg, "Workers' compensation is a disability program to provide medical economic support to workers who have been injured or made ill from an incident arising out of and in the course of employment. It is a complex $70 billion a year program in the United States that involves nearly sixty different systems." This program originated as a social experiment by Bismarck in Germany in the 1880s. It is a "no-fault" compensation system designed to replace the traditional tort system, under which a worker had to sue his employer to get benefits. Unfortunately, the deck was stacked against the employee for various reasons. To rectify this problem, many states developed workers' compensation systems. The last state to do so was Mississippi in 1949. The federal government has similar systems. These systems often are industry-specific and have variable rules regarding impairment, disability, and compensation.

7. What is Social Security Disability (SSD)?

According to the Social Security Administration, SSD is defined as "the inability to engage in any substantial gainful activity by reason of any medically determinable physical or mental impairment(s) which can be expected to result in death or which has lasted or can be expected to last for a continuous period of not less than 12 months." In addition, for a person under the age of 18, disability can exist "if he or she has a medically determinable impairment(s) that is of comparable severity" to impairment in an adult. To comply with these definitions, a person may have a single medical impairment or multiple impairments that, when combined, are of such severity that the person can no longer perform his or her previous occupation or sustain any remunerative activity after age, education, and prior work experience are considered.

Two groups of people are eligible for SSD. Under Title II, Social Security Disability Insurance (SSDI) provides cash benefits for disabled workers and their dependents who have contributed to the Social Security Trust Fund through taxes. Title XVI (Supplemental Security Income [SSI]) provides a minimal income level for the needy, aged, blind, and disabled. People qualify for SSI because of financial need. Under SSI, financial need is said to exist when a person's income and resources are equal to or below an amount specified by law.

8. What is the cost of disability?

This question is difficult to answer. For example, if a worker is injured on the job, what defines the cost of disability? Is it the cost of time off work? Is it the medical expenses (e.g., physician's fees, operative costs, prescription costs, physical therapy, rehabilitation costs)? Is it the cost of paying the worker while he or she is out of work? Is it offset by the fact that the worker's spouse had to return to work? Is it the money to fund the social programs and human resource departments needed to fill out the forms and provide the benefits? Ultimately, of course, all of these factors must be considered.

The aggregate cost of disability in the United States in 1980 was $177 billion or approximately 6.5% of the gross domestic product. Medical expenditures in 1987 totaled $336 billion. Approximately 51% of disability costs are for medical care and other goods and services provided to the disabled. Approximately 39% of the overall cost comes from lost earnings and approximately 10% from the labor market losses of household members or persons with disabilities.

9. Who wrote the "rules" for impairment evaluation?

Disability is a big business in the United States and other countries. Various institutions pay the costs, such as state governments (workers' compensation), the federal government (e.g., veterans or longshoremen), insurance companies, or self-insured employers. Many systems that pay for disability have their own rules and regulations, including rules about the performance and rating of the impairment evaluation. The most commonly used system is a formal set of rules developed by the American Medical Association, which is constantly updated. Another major source of guidelines is the Social Security System. The rules and regulations found in these sources are vastly different. For example, the Social Security Administration recognizes only total impairment. The AMA *Guides* fractionates impairment from 1% to 100%. Highly specific rules are applied to these impairments in each set of guidelines. The impairment evaluator must be thoroughly familiar with the system that he or she is required to use.

10. Define the concept "whole person impairment."

In the AMA *Guides*, whole person impairment reflects the amount of impairment in a given individual. A person who is totally impaired has 100% whole person impairment. A person whose right arm was amputated at the shoulder has a 60% impairment of the whole person. A person with coronary disease may have whole person impairment ranging from 0% to 100%. It depends on the degree of deviation from normal.

11. What is maximum medical improvement (MMI)?

This concept, which is used in impairment evaluation, states that a person has achieved MMI if no more substantial improvement is anticipated with time and/or further treatment. Treatment may include medications, surgery, physical therapy, or other types of rehabilitation. Most impairment systems demand that the person achieve MMI before a final impairment rating can be given. This rating is then used as a basis for the final disability settlement.

12. What is apportionment?

A few states use a concept called apportionment. For example, if a male worker applies for disability benefits because of a toxic gas inhalation, some states take into consideration the fact that he was a two pack per day smoker for the past 20 years. The fact that he was a smoker may have contributed to loss of lung function. The physician evaluating the worker for impairment can quantitate only the current amount of loss of lung function. This loss may have occurred because of the toxic inhalation, the smoking, or a combination of both. When a state or system uses apportionment, it requires the physician to estimate the amount of impairment created by a specific injury or factor as opposed to all other factors that contribute to the total impairment value. Some states ignore this concept and recognize that for any impairment that may have been caused by occupational injury, the occupational injury must be considered the sole cause. California, on the other hand, requires apportionment; the physician in the above case is required to state, for example, that 60% of the impairment was caused by toxic inhalation and 40% by cigarette smoking. Clearly, apportionment requires a great deal of skill and educational background.

13. How does one perform an impairment evaluation?

One starts with the questions that are asked by the referring party. For example, if the examinee's right arm has been amputated, one centers on the amputation. One does not do a complete history and physical examination if it is not requested, called for, or appropriate. On the other hand, the body part that was injured and/or specified in the referral is evaluated thoroughly. This evaluation may take the form of a history, physical examination, specialized physical examination techniques, radiographs and other types of body imaging studies, physiologic testing, and other types of examinations. The evaluation must answer specific questions not only in respect to specific body parts but also in respect to the evaluating system. For example, some evaluating systems require certain tests to be performed and ignore the results from other types of testing. The impairment evaluator must understand thoroughly the system so that the appropriate diagnostic examinations can be performed.

14. What is a functional capacity assessment?

This concept, derived from ergonomists and physical therapists, has been extended to involve other body systems and other types of tests. A functional capacity assessment basically refers to how much a person is capable of doing. In other words, we can measure a person's flexibility in a given joint, the neurologic input to the muscle surrounding that joint, and the strength of the muscles. Then we can determine the physical capability of that joint. This capability may be measured in terms of how much weight can be lifted, how many times it can be lifted, or for how long the person can perform the same activity. These results, called functional capacity assessment, are linked to the specifications of a job. For example, if a man is capable of lifting, on a sustained basis, only 20 pounds (although on a rare basis he is capable of lifting as much as 50 pounds) and the job entails lifting, on an infrequent basis, 60–80 pounds, we might determine that the man is not fit or qualified for the job.

15. What is the Americans with Disabilities Act?

In 1990 Congress passed the Americans with Disabilities Act (ADA). This law protects people with disabilities from discrimination and mandates accommodations for disabled employees, customers, clients, patients, and others. It prohibits discrimination in public or private employment, governmental services, public accommodations, public transportation, and telecommunication. The ADA defines a person with a disability in three ways: "(1) any person who has a physical or mental impairment that substantially limits one or more of the individual's major life activities, (2) any person who has a 'record of' a substantially limiting impairment, and (3) any person who is 'regarded as' having a substantially-limiting impairment, regardless of whether the person is in fact disabled."

According to the ADA, before an offer for a job, an employer may not inquire about an applicant's impairment or medical history. In addition, inquiries about past injuries and/or workers' compensation claims are expressly prohibited. An employer, however, may conditionally offer a position based on completion of a medical examination or medical inquiry—but only if such examinations or inquiries are made of all applicants for the same job category and the results are kept confidential. A postoffer medical evaluation may be more comprehensive. A job offer may be withdrawn only if the findings of the medical examination show that a person is unable to perform the essential functions of a job, even with reasonable accommodation, or if the person poses a direct threat to his or her own health or safety or to the health and safety of others, even with reasonable accommodation. Obviously, it is important to have the list of the essential functions of a job for comparison.

16. How do I fill out back-to-work forms?

Functional capacity assessment(s) often comes into play. Some of the basic principles from the ADA are also applicable. One starts with a description of the job—primarily its essential functions, although peripheral functions that, on occasion, may arise also may be included. For assembly-line workers, the job description may include where they have to stand, how many times they have to bend over, whether they have to pick up a part, how heavy the part is, how often they do this activity, and various other ergonomic issues. Ideally, one then matches the person's capability with the requirements of the job. For example, if we can measure how long examinees can stand, how often they can bend, how much bending they are capable of doing, and what strength they have, we should be able to say whether they are capable of returning to their job or whether they need to be assigned to modified and/or restricted duties.

In most circumstances, we do not achieve this perfect state of knowledge and blending of worker with job. When faced with this decision, we have two choices: we can either refer the person for appropriate testing, or we can make an "educated guess," based on experience, knowledge, and background. The more educated the examiner and the better his or her understanding of the job requirements, the more valid his or her determination will be.

17. How do I fill out the forms from the Social Security Department?

Social Security forms frequently cross a physician's desk. They are often multipaged evaluation questions and can be daunting. They are intended to provide background information to the impairment and disability evaluator in the Social Security System. An independent impairment examination also may be performed on such patients. Your report is used to provide background information so that a more accurate and appropriate evaluation can be made. As the patient's treating physician, often you have insights and background that otherwise would not be available to the medical or disability evaluator. You are *not* performing an impairment evaluation when you fill out such forms; that is someone else's job.

EXAMPLES

18. A man with a job-related rotator cuff injury has achieved MMI. Your evaluation discloses that he is capable of abduction of the right shoulder to 60°, adduction of 20°, flexion of 40°, extension of 20°, internal rotation of 60°, and external rotation of 60°. Strength and neurologic sensation around the shoulder joint are normal. Does the man have an impairment? If so, how much? Does he have a disability? If so, for what jobs?

Certainly the man has an impairment. Restricted range of motion is an anatomic and physical impairment and/or deviation from normalcy. Using the AMA *Guides*, the man has a 13% impairment of the whole person. Under the Social Security System, he does not have a disability, which is defined as a permanent condition preventing a person from performing any remunerative activity.

The injury may or may not pose a disabling condition; it depends on his job. Once the essential activities of the job are known, one can determine whether the man has a disability.

19. During the course of her job, a woman performs repetitive motion activities. She now has numbness and tingling in the first three fingers of both hands. What is your diagnosis? Does she have an impairment? If so, how much?

The woman has bilateral carpal tunnel syndromes, as documented by her history. The physical examination is expected to be abnormal, consisting of diminished sensation in the affected fingers, a positive Phalen's sign, a positive Tinel's sign, and normal strength except in severe and prolonged cases, in which diminished strength and even muscle atrophy may be seen. The diagnosis is further verified by abnormalities on a nerve conduction study.

To determine impairment, one must ask whether the woman has achieved MMI. She has had no form of treatment, which may include rest, medications, braces, and, possibly, surgery. Only after she has achieved MMI can an impairment percentage be given. The impairment percentage often depends on the symptoms (amount and frequency), as well as nerve conduction study abnormalities. The AMA *Guides* divides cases into mild, moderate, and severe impairment and provides a percentage for each (6, 12, and 24% whole person impairment, respectively).

20. During his work, a man slips on ice while delivering packages. He has sudden onset of pain and discomfort in his lower back. The pain radiates down the right leg. In addition, numbness and tingling also radiate down the right leg after rest and pain relievers. He is given physical therapy, with some relief. Unfortunately, 2 years later, he has a similar injury. An MRI discloses a herniated disc at the L4–L5 interspace. He has surgery because of persistent and disabling symptoms. He has a successful outcome and has now returned to the work force. He is basically asymptomatic except for mild discomfort in the lower back with prolonged sitting and standing. Does the man have an impairment? If so, how much?

Certainly the man has an impairment because of anatomic deviation from normalcy. Using the AMA *Guides*, he has 10% impairment of the whole person because of the herniated disc and neurologic abnormalities, despite the fact that he has had a successful operation and is relatively asymptomatic.

21. The same man returns to work and slips and falls again. His symptoms are severe. He has pain with minimal activity. He can no longer do sports activities, which he enjoyed in the past. Sexual intercourse is uncomfortable. Does he have an impairment? If so, how much?

The man continues to have impairment caused by the first and second injuries and exacerbated by the third. However, no further impairment is awarded. The 10% impairment that he received originally (although he was essentially asymptomatic) was given because of the known risk for further problems as time passes. Thus, there is no increase in the impairment rating.

22. After exposure to toxic fumes, a man is hospitalized with severe shortness of breath. Corticosteroids and bronchodilators are administered. One year later he continues to have shortness of breath with wheezing, cough, and sputum production. His symptoms may be triggered by exposure to cold air, fumes, dust, or cigarette smoke and by exertion. Spirometry is performed before and after bronchodilator treatment. Before treatment, forced vital capacity (FVC) is 60% of predicted and forced expiratory volume in one second (FEV$_1$) is 40% of predicted. After treatment, FVC is 70% and FEV$_1$ 60% of predicted. Does the man have an impairment? If so, how much? Does it make a difference whether he is currently on medication? Does it make a difference whether he was a two pack per day smoker for 30 years before the toxic inhalation?

The man certainly has an impairment, as measured by physiologic testing (spirometry). He has a 10–25% impairment of the whole person. Using the AMA *Guides*, it is immaterial whether he is currently on medication or whether he continues to smoke although some would argue that he cannot, by definition, achieve MMI if he continues to smoke and does not take medication. This concept is addressed poorly in the present edition of the *Guides*. In addition to its effect on MMI, smoking also may raise the question of apportionment, as described above.

23. A 43-year-old man is diagnosed with cardiomyopathy after a viral illness. One year later he is taking digoxin, diuretics, and other medications. He continues to have poor exertional capabilities and is capable of walking only one-half flight of stairs without stopping because of severe shortness of breath. His ejection fraction, as measured echocardiographically, is 19%. Does the man have an impairment? If so, how much?

Certainly the man has an impairment in terms of heart performance. Using the AMA *Guides*, he has an 80% impairment of the whole person. He is considered to be at MMI because 1 full year has elapsed from the time of the initial diagnosis and he appears to be stable. He may well qualify for Social Security Disability. One may argue that he could perform a sedentary job that represents "sustained remunerative activity," but the Social Security Department often does not apply a strict 100% rule. Otherwise almost no one would qualify. For example, a quadriplegic could possibly do telemarketing, which represents "sustained remunerative activity." Thus, he would not be disabled from a strict definitional standpoint.

24. A man has had an amputation of the lower part of his left extremity 3 inches below the knee because of a work accident. Does he have an impairment? If so, how much? One year after the initial injury he presents with a well-healed, below-the-knee amputation of the left leg but complains of phantom limb pain, which at times is excruciating and interferes with activities of daily life. Does this bestow additional impairment? If so, how much?

According to the AMA *Guides*, below-the-knee amputation constitutes 28% impairment of the whole person. However, the phantom pain needs to be assessed separately. In most circumstances, the AMA *Guides* take into account pain and suffering when an impairment percentage is given for an alteration in function, especially orthopedic. However, because phantom limb pain involves pain beyond that associated solely with the amputation, the AMA *Guides* includes rules used only in special and/or rare circumstances. The impairment percentage is left to the discretion of the evaluator. Discretionary judgment is frequently debated by both defense and plaintiff attorneys in determining the eventual award.

25. An employee at a fast-food restaurant witnessed the killing of five people and the wounding of several others by a man with an automatic rifle. Although the employee was not injured in any way, he has become totally dysfunctional. He is afraid of leaving his home. He breaks into a cold sweat and hyperventilates whenever he is asked to attend a social function. For this reason he is no longer able to find a job, and his social contacts are greatly limited. He spends most of his day in the house watching television. Is he impaired? If so, how much?

Certainly this man is impaired. He has a deviation from normalcy and from his prior level of activity. The diagnosis is posttraumatic stress disorder. Impairment should be assessed by using the psychiatric section of the system under which he is evaluated. In earlier editions of the AMA *Guides*, impairment percentages for psychiatric illnesses were based on certain criteria. At present, however, no impairment percentages are given. Thus, assessment relies on the discretion and expertise of the evaluator. Of course, the effects of medications, the amount of medications, and the patient's response to medications and/or other forms of therapy are taken into account when impairment is rated. MMI also needs to be applied in this and other circumstances.

BIBLIOGRAPHY

1. American Medical Association: Guides to the Evaluation of Permanent Impairment, 4th ed. Chicago, American Medical Association, 1993.
2. Barth PS: Economic costs of disability. In Demeter SL, Andersson GBJ, Smith GM (eds): Disability Evaluation. St. Louis, Mosby, 1996, pp 13–19.
3. Bell C: Overview of the Americans with Disabilities Act and the Family and Medical Leave Act. In Demeter SL, Andersson GBJ, Smith GM (eds): Disability Evaluation. St. Louis, Mosby, 1996, pp 582–591.
4. Demeter SL: Appendix A. In Demeter SL, Andersson GBJ, Smith GM (eds): Disability Evaluation. St. Louis, Mosby, 1996, pp 606–607.
5. Demeter SL: Contrasting the standard medical examination and the disability examination. In Demeter SL, Andersson GBJ, Smith GM (eds): Disability Evaluation. St. Louis, Mosby, 1996, pp 68–72.
6. Demeter SL, Smith GM, Andersson GBJ: Approach to disability evaluation. In Demeter SL, Andersson GBJ, Smith GM (eds): Disability Evaluation. St. Louis, Mosby, 1996, pp 2–4.
7. Elisburg D: Workers' compensation. In Demeter SL, Andersson GBJ, Smith GM (eds): Disability Evaluation. St. Louis, Mosby, 1996, pp 36–44.
8. Greenwood JG, History of disability as a legal construct evaluation. In Demeter SL, Andersson GBJ, Smith GM (eds): Disability Evaluation. St. Louis, Mosby, 1996, pp 5–12.
9. Mather JH: Social Security disability systems. In Demeter SL, Andersson GBJ, Smith GM (eds): Disability Evaluation. St. Louis, Mosby, 1996, pp 45–51.
10. Matheson LN: Functional capacity evaluation. In Demeter SL, Andersson GBJ, Smith GM (eds): Disability Evaluation. St. Louis, Mosby, 1996, pp 168–188.
11. Smith GM, Demeter SL, Washington RJ: The disability-oriented medical evaluation and report. In Demeter SL, Andersson GBJ, Smith GM (eds): Disability Evaluation. St. Louis, Mosby, 1996, pp 68–72.
12. Social Security Administration, U.S. Department of Health and Human Services: Disability Evaluation under Social Security. Social Security Administration Publication No. 64-039/ICN 468600, Washington, DC, 1994.

53. OCCUPATIONAL MEDICINE AND THE LAW

Elaine A. Lisko, J.D.

BACKGROUND

1. What is occupational medicine?

Occupational medicine is a form of preventive medicine that attempts to evaluate the health-related hazards of the workplace, to maintain the health of workers, and to return workers who have been injured or exposed to hazards at work to good health. In addition, occupational medicine physicians are asked to conduct job fitness evaluations and drug tests on workers. Many of these medical functions have legal implications of which the occupational medicine physician needs to be aware.

2. Name the different types of occupational health care delivery mechanisms.

Occupational health services are delivered through two basic types of mechanisms:

1. On-site or in-plant services provided by occupational health care practitioners employed by the organization

2. Off-site or community-based services by occupational health care practitioners who may be employed by the organization or serve as independent contractors.

3. Describe the primary issues that occupational medicine physicians face in their practices.

- Health and safety of workers
- Understanding of occupational setting
- Understanding of unique occupational health laws
- Confidentiality of workers' medical information
- Employers' right to know certain information
- Potential conflict of interest between rights of workers and employers

Concern for these issues is reflected in the Code of Ethical Conduct adopted by the American College of Occupational and Environmental Medicine. The code provides that physicians should do the following:

1. Accord the highest priority to the health and safety of individuals in both the workplace and the environment

2. Practice on a scientific basis with integrity and strive to acquire and maintain adequate knowledge and expertise upon which to render professional service

3. Relate honestly and ethically in all professional relationships

4. Strive to expand and disseminate medical knowledge and participate in ethical research efforts as appropriate

5. Keep confidential all individual medical information, releasing such information only when required by law or overriding public health considerations or to other physicians according to accepted medical practice or to others at the request of the individual

6. Recognize that employers may be entitled to counsel about an individual's medical work fitness but not to diagnoses or specific details, except in compliance with laws and regulations

7. Communicate to individuals and/or groups any significant observations and recommendations concerning their health or safety

8. Recognize medical impairments in oneself and others, including chemical dependency and abusive personal practices, that interfere with one's ability to follow the above principles and take appropriate measures

PHYSICIAN-PATIENT RELATIONSHIP

4. Who are the players in the occupational health setting?
- Physician
- Patient
- Employer
- Union
- Regulatory agency
- Workers' compensation carrier

As a result, the occupational medicine physician may be required to interact with many more individuals or entities than the general medicine physician, who is concerned primarily with the patient and secondarily with the patient's insurance carrier or third-party payor.

5. When does the physician-patient relationship arise in general medicine?

In general medicine, the physician-patient relationship arises when an individual chooses a physician and the physician agrees to provide or provides medical services. The relationship is contractual in nature.

6. When does the physician-patient relationship arise in the occupational health setting?

In the occupational health setting, the employer, not the worker, retains the physician. As a result, a physician-patient relationship may not arise automatically between the worker and the physician. When a distinction is drawn between an individually chosen physician and an employer-provided physician, courts consider the following factors in determining whether a physician-patient relationship has been formed:

1. Whether the physician is treating or merely examining the worker
2. For whose benefit the physician is performing the service

When the object of the medical examination is to determine fitness for employment or when the physician performs the service for the benefit of the employer, courts generally have not found a physician-patient relationship to exist. However, if the physician renders treatment to the worker or if the physician performs the service for the benefit of the worker, a physician-patient relationship may be found to exist.

7. What other factors may be considered in determining whether a physician-patient relationship exists?

In addition to treatment and benefit considerations, the following factors may influence whether a physician-patient relationship is found to exist:

1. The period over which the physician sees the worker
   - An isolated examination suggests no relationship
   - An ongoing series of examinations suggests a relationship
2. The reasonable expectations of the physician and the worker about the nature of the relationship
   - Such expectations may be based on expressed or implied statements or conduct
   - If the physician does not intend to form a physician-patient relationship with the worker, the physician should make this clear to the worker and act in a manner consistent with that intent
3. The nature of the worker's consent to the medical examination
   - Consent to a limited examination suggests no relationship
   - Consent to a complete examination, including diagnosis and treatment, suggests a relationship

8. What conflicts of interest are peculiar to occupational medicine physicians?

Because the worker and the employer may have competing interests, unavoidable conflicts may result, as outlined in the table (top of next page).

Potential Conflicts of Interest

NATURE OF CONFLICT	WORKER'S INTEREST	EMPLOYER'S INTEREST
Confidentiality	Expects physician to hold all medical information in strict confidence.	Expects physician to disclose any medical information that may relate to work fitness.
Disability	Worker who wants reasonable accommodations for disability expects physician to document disability. Worker who does not want employer to know of disability expects physician not to report.	Expects physician to report any disability as soon as physician becomes aware of it.
Work status	Worker who wants to avoid returning to work expects physician to state that he or she is not fit due to work-related injury or illness.	Expects physician to state that worker is fit to return to work as soon as possible after any work-related injury or illness.
Medical surveillance	Expects physician to disclose any potential long-term health hazards and offer treatment.	Expects physician to monitor potential long-term hazards without disclosing hazards to worker.

PHYSICIAN'S DUTIES AND POTENTIAL LIABILITY

9. Assuming that a physician-patient relationship exists, what is the applicable standard of care?

When a physician-patient relationship exists, the physician is required to use the degree of care, skill, and knowledge of the average practitioner engaged in the field under the same or similar circumstances. Members of a medical specialty are held to a higher standard of care—namely, that of the average practitioner of the medical specialty of which the physician is a member.[1] The appropriateness of the physician's conduct is based on the state of medical knowledge at the time that medical services are performed.[2]

10. Assuming that a relationship exists, what duties does the occupational medicine physician owe to the patient?

When a patient-physician relationship exists, the occupational medicine physician has the following duties in conducting a medical examination:

1. The duty to inform the patient of the patient's medical condition and of all medical facts that the patient reasonably should know
2. The duty to notify the patient of the results of any tests and of the physician's diagnosis, including impairment and work-related issues
3. The duty to inform the patient of the need for treatment
4. The duty to give the patient proper instructions for self-care
5. The duty to advise the patient of any conditions that may aggravate the illness
6. The duty to preserve the confidentiality of the patient's medical information
7. The duty to refer the patient to a specialist, if appropriate

The mnemonic **MANIACS** summarizes the occupational medicine physician's seven major duties to the patient:

M = **M**edical condition
A = **A**ny test results
N = **N**eed for treatment
I = **I**nstructions for self-care
A = **A**ggravating conditions
C = **C**onfidentiality
S = **S**pecialist

When no physician-patient relationship exists, the occupational medicine physician should owe no greater duty than to avoid injuring the worker during the course of the examination and, in some circumstances, to use reasonable care in giving medical advice.

11. Is an employer-retained occupational medicine physician subject to liability?

In most instances, no. As discussed in question 2, an occupational medicine physician is an employee of or an independent contractor for the employer. As a result, the physician is immune from employee lawsuits generally. This immunity is founded on two principles:

1. A legal duty to act with reasonable care will not be imposed in the absence of a physician-patient relationship.

2. Workers' compensation laws preclude an employee from suing a coemployee, including a coemployee physician, for work-related injuries.

12. What are the exceptions to immunity from liability?

1. When a physician-patient relationship is found to exist and the physician has failed to exercise reasonable care in examining, testing, diagnosing, advising, or treating the patient.

2. When no physician-patient relationship is found to exist but the physician has caused injury to the worker during the course of the examination.

3. When the physician is an independent contractor and makes a negligent medical assessment that results in an improper job placement.

OCCUPATIONAL HEALTH AND FEDERAL LAW

Americans with Disabilities Act (ADA)

13. What is the ADA?

The ADA is the first comprehensive federal law to prohibit discrimination based on actual or perceived physical or mental disabilities. Two sections of the ADA receive frequent attention. Title I prohibits employment discrimination and applies to all private employers with 15 or more employees. Title III prohibits discrimination in public accommodations, which include health care services and housing.[3]

14. What constitutes a disability under the ADA?

1. A physical or mental impairment that substantially limits one or more major life activities:
   - Caring for one's self
   - Performing manual tasks
   - Walking
   - Seeing
   - Hearing
   - Speaking
   - Breathing
   - Learning
   - Working
   - Being able to reproduce and bear children[4]
2. A record of such an impairment
3. Being perceived or regarded as having such an impairment[5]

15. How does the ADA affect the practice of occupational medicine?

Occupational medicine physicians conduct medical examinations of job applicants and employees to assess their health status and job fitness. They also may be asked to assist in determining reasonable accommodations to be provided to a person with a disability so that the person can perform the job. The ADA regulates the permissible scope of job-related medical examinations.[6] The scope depends in part on whether an offer has been made.

The ADA and Employment-related Medical Examinations

EMPLOYMENT STAGE	PROHIBITED INQUIRIES	PERMITTED INQUIRIES
Preemployment (before offer has been extended)	All medical examinations and inquiries prohibited	Prospective employer may inquire into applicant's ability to perform job-related functions (e.g., if job requires driver's license, applicant may be asked to provide proof of current license; if job requires lifting of 100-lb boxes, applicant may be asked to demonstrate ability to lift 100-lb weight)
Preplacement (after conditional offer of employment)		Medical examination permitted, provided: 1. All entering employees are subjected to such an examination regardless of any disability 2. Any information obtained about applicant's medical condition or history is collected and maintained on separate form and in separate file and treated as confidential medical record (with certain limited exceptions) 3. Examination results are used only in accordance with ADA (i.e., not to discriminate against applicant on basis of disability)
Employed	Any inquiries designed to elicit: 1. Whether applicant has disability 2. Nature or severity of any disability *unless* the inquiry is shown to be job-related and consistent with business necessity	Medical examination permitted, provided: 1. It is voluntary and part of employee health program available to employees at work site, or 2. Inquiry relates to employee's ability to perform job-related functions

16. What can an occupational medicine physician do to ensure compliance with the ADA, especially at the preplacement stage?

To be safe, an occupational medicine physician may want to limit medical examinations conducted after an offer has been made but before employment has begun to assess medical conditions that bear directly on the person's ability to perform the offered job. Examples include:

1. Carefully tailoring the medical examination to specific job requirements (e.g, checking ability to reach or lift weights when reaching or lifting weights is an integral part of the job);

2. Using medical screening procedures with a high positive predictive value (e.g., precluding the use of low-back x-ray studies for screening out asymptomatic people); and

3. Designing the medical examination to correspond with the demands of the job (e.g., the less physically demanding the job, the less detailed and comprehensive the examination).

The occupational medicine physician also may want to consider advising the applicant that the medical examination, by its very nature, is limited. It is not intended to substitute for a comprehensive examination by the applicant's personal physician and is not intended to establish a physician-patient relationship.

Occupational Safety and Health Act (OSH Act)

17. What is the OSH Act?

The OSH Act (1970) was enacted by Congress to ensure a healthy workplace environment by eliminating dangerous conditions and instituting needed safeguards.[7] The OSH Act charges the United States Department of Labor (DOL) with a number of responsibilities aimed at regulating and improving workplace safety. DOL discharges its duties under the OSH Act through the Occupational Safety and Health Administration (OSHA).

18. What is NIOSH?

The OSH Act charges the United States Department of Health and Human Services (DHHS) with a number of responsibilities aimed at monitoring workplace health and safety issues. DHHS discharges its duties under the OSH Act through the National Institute for Occupational Safety and Health (NIOSH), which is part of the Centers for Disease Control and Prevention.

19. Describe the difference between OSHA and NIOSH.

OSHA	NIOSH
Arm of DOL	Arm of DHHS
Regulatory agency	Research agency

20. How does OSHA affect the practice of occupational medicine?

Occupational medicine physicians may be asked to conduct OSHA-mandated medical examinations of employees. Such examinations are required to be performed on employees with exposure to specifically enumerated toxic substances. When an examination is required:

1. The physician must provide the employer with a statement of the employee's suitability for employment in the regulated area;

2. The employer must offer the employee periodic medical examinations (typically on an annual basis); and

3. The employer must provide the employee with a medical examination upon termination of employment.[9]

21. How does NIOSH affect the practice of occupational medicine?

In conducting research activities, NIOSH may require occupational medicine physicians as agents of the employer to allow access to confidential employee medical and exposure records. Government access to such records is subject to certain restrictions:

1. Unless written consent is obtained from the employee or access is sought in consultation with the employer's physician on an occupational health or safety issue, the government representative's request to examine or copy personally identifiable employee medical information must be made pursuant to a written access order, the issuance of which requires the following:

• The medical information must be relevant to a statutory purpose.
• A need must exist to gain access to the information.
• The information must be limited only to that needed to accomplish the purpose for access.
• The authorized personnel examining the information must be limited to those who have a need for access and appropriate professional qualifications.

2. The written access order must be posted at the employment site without specifically identifying the employee for whom the information is sought.

3. Any medical information taken from the employment site with direct personal identifiers must be coded to protect the employee's identity and ensure its confidentiality.[10]

In conducting its regulatory and investigative activities, OSHA also may require disclosure of medical and exposure records. The same restrictions that apply to NIOSH's access apply to OSHA's access. Employers are not required to prepare employee medical and exposure records. However, once prepared, employers are required to maintain exposure records for 30 years and medical records for the duration of employment plus 30 years with few exceptions.[11] Occupational medicine physicians need to clarify with the employer in advance their obligation to maintain such records.

OCCUPATIONAL HEALTH AND OTHER LAWS

22. What other laws regulate occupational medicine?

Occupational medicine is also regulated by workers' compensation law and general common law. Historically, common law was the unwritten law, as distinct from statutory or written law. Today common law is reflected in written court decisions (e.g., the application of *Daubert* requirements to expert testimony).[12]

Workers' Compensation

23. What is workers' compensation?

Workers' compensation is a system of state and federal laws that provide for income replacement, medical expenses, and rehabilitation services for people suffering from work-related injuries or illnesses. In general, it relieves the employee from having to prove fault on the part of the employer and limits the amount that the employee can recover from the employer. The law of the state in which the occupational medicine physician practices should be consulted to determine precise eligibility requirements and procedures. However, certain features are common:

- The employee must notify the employer of the claim.
- The employee must file a claim with the state workers' compensation board within a specified period after becoming aware of the injury or illness.
- The employee must wait a specified period after filing the claim before becoming eligible for benefits.
- Contested claims are presented to an administrative agency for adjudication.

Federal law also provides for compensation for work-related injuries for certain classes of employees, including federal civilian employees, longshoring and harbor workers, sailors, railroad workers, and coal miners.

24. How does workers' compensation law affect the practice of occupational medicine?

To qualify for workers' compensation benefits, an employee must obtain medical documentation that (1) the employee is suffering from an injury or illness and (2) the injury or illness is work-related. The occupational medicine physician may be asked to make this two-part determination.

In addition, the occupational medicine physician may be asked to determine the disability status of the employee, including (1) a rating of the employee's physical impairment, (2) a decision about the employee's ability to return to work at all, and (3) whether the employee can return to work and the type of work that the employee can perform. Because the work environment may influence greatly the employee's ability to return to work, the occupational medicine physician, especially one who practices off site, must have a good understanding of job tasks and exposure potential. This information should be gathered as part of the medical history.

25. Name the disability classifications applicable to workers' compensation law.

1. **Temporary partial:** employee is unable to perform regular job but is able to perform other gainful employment.
2. **Temporary total:** employee is unable to work at all for a limited period.
3. **Permanent partial:** employee experiences residual impairment or loss of physical function to body part for remainder of life.
4. **Permanent total:** employee is unable to return to work at all.

JOB-RELATED DRUG TESTING

26. Is drug testing legal?

The legality of drug testing depends on a number of factors:

- Whether the tested employees are in the public or private sector
- Whether the drug testing is government-mandated
- Whether the employees have union representation
- Whether the state in which the employer is located has enacted a drug-testing law
- Whether the testing is directed at employees in safety-sensitive jobs

The law generally gives private employers broad discretion in drug testing

27. What are the occupational medicine physician's special concerns about drug testing?

Legal counsel should be obtained when any question about the legality of drug testing arises. Factors that the occupational medicine physician is well advised to keep in mind include the following:

1. The ADA does not consider drug testing to be a medical examination; therefore, testing may be performed at any time, although some commentators suggest that it should not be done until an offer has been extended.

2. The results of any drug tests must be treated as confidential information.

3. Drug screening tests should be confirmed using the latest technology (e.g., gas chromatography/mass spectrometry).

4. Employees will more than likely challenge observed urination as an invasion of privacy.

5. Courts tend to disfavor random testing, except when a clear public safety concern is demonstrated.

ACKNOWLEDGMENT

The author thanks Mark A. Rothstein, Director of the Health Law and Policy Institute, University of Houston Law Center, Hugh Roy and Lillie Cranz Cullen Distinguished Professor of Law, and a leading authority on occupational health law, for his generous guidance and permission to use portions of his chapter on *The Americans with Disabilities Act, Workers' Compensation, and Related Issues of Occupational Medicine Practice* in the preparation of this chapter.

CITATIONS OF LAWS, CODES, AND REGULATIONS

1. See, e.g., *Mitchell v. United States*, 141 F.3d 8, 13 (1st Cir. 1998) (setting forth standard of care applicable when physician-patient relationship exists); see also *Zarow-Smith v. New Jersey Transit Rail Operations*, 953 F. Supp. 581, 590 (D.N.J. 1997) (involving occupational disease claim against employer based, in part, on company doctor's alleged failure to take lateral x-ray and setting forth standard of care applicable in occupational disease case).
2. See, e.g., *Hall v. Arthur*, 141 F.3d 844, 850 (8th Cir. 1998) (noting physician's conduct is judged based on state of medical technology at time of treatment).
3. 42 U.S.C. § 12101 et seq. (1990). Title I of the ADA is found in 42 U.S.C. §§ 12101–12117 (§ 12102(2) defines "disability" and § 12112(d) outlines permissible scope of employment-related medical examinations and inquiries). Title III of the ADA is found in 42 U.S.C. §§ 12181–12188. Title II applies to state and local governments.
4. 29 C.F.R. § 1630.2(I) (1997) (listing major life activities for ADA purposes); see also *Bragdon v. Abbott*, 118 S.Ct. 2196 (1998) (recently recognizing reproduction as major life activity).
5. 42 U.S.C. § 12102(2).
6. 42 U.S.C. § 12112 (d).
7. 29 U.S.C. § 651 et seq. (1970) (§ 655(b)(7) discusses OSHA-mandated medical examinations).
8. 29 U.S.C. § 655(b)(7). Because one or more of the specified toxic substances must be present for an examination to be required, the occupational medicine physician may never be asked to conduct this type of medical examination.
9. 29 C.F.R. § 1910.120(f)(3) (1997) (outlining requirements related to OSHA-mandated medical examinations).
10. 29 C.F.R. § 1913.10 (1997) (setting forth restrictions applicable to government requests for access to employee medical and exposure records).
11. 29 C.F.R. § 1910.1020(d) (1997) (specifying maintenance requirements for employee medical and exposure records).
12. See *Daubert v. Merrell Dow Pharmaceuticals, Inc.*, 509 U.S. 579 (1993) (setting forth requirements for introduction of expert testimony).

BIBLIOGRAPHY

1. American College of Occupational and Environmental Medicine Code of Ethical Conduct (adopted 10/25/93) [found at <http://www.acoem.org/code/code.htm>].
2. Guidotti TL, Cowell JWF, Jamieson GG: Occupational Health Services: A Practical Approach. Chicago, American Medical Association, 1989.
3. Jacobstein JM, Mersky RM, Dunn DJ: Fundamentals of Legal Research. Westbury, NY, Foundation Press, 1994.
4. Richards EP, Rathbun KC: Law and the Physician: A Practical Guide. Boston, Little, Brown, 1996 [found at <http://plague.law.umkc.edu/default.htm>].
5. Rothstein MA: The Americans with Disabilities Act, Workers' Compensation, and Related Issues of Occupational Medical Practice. In Rosenstock L, Cullen MR (eds): Textbook of Clinical Occupational and Environmental Medicine. Philadelphia, W.B. Saunders, 1994, pp 77–83.
6. Rothstein MA: Medical Screening of Workers. Washington, DC, Bureau of National Affairs, 1984.
7. Sandler HM: Legal aspects of occupational medicine. In Rom WN (ed): Environmental and Occupational Medicine. Boston, Little, Brown, 1992, pp 1347–1350.
8. Squillante NJ: Expanding the potential tort liability of physicians: A legal portrait of "nontraditional patients" and proposals for change. UCLA Law Rev 40:1617–1689, 1993.

INDEX

Page numbers in **boldface type** indicate complete chapters.